DEMENTIA:
Molecules, Methods and Measures

DEMENTIA:
Molecules, Methods and Measures

Edited by

I. Hindmarch
Human Psychopharmacology Research Unit,
University of Surrey, UK

H. Hippius
Psychiatric Department, University of Munich, Germany

and

G. K. Wilcock
Department of Care of the Elderly,
University of Bristol, Frenchay Hospital, Bristol, UK

JOHN WILEY & SONS
Chichester · New York · Brisbane · Toronto · Singapore

Other Wiley Editorial Offices

John Wiley & Sons, Inc., 605 Third Avenue,
New York, NY 10158-0012, USA

Jacaranda Wiley Ltd, G.P.O. Box 859, Brisbane,
Queensland 4001, Australia

John Wiley & Sons (Canada) Ltd, 5353 Dundas Road West, Fourth Floor,
Etobicoke, Ontario M9B 6H8, Canada

John Wiley & Sons (SEA) Pte Ltd, 37 Jalan Pemimpin   05-04,
Block B, Union Industrial Building, Singapore 2057

Library of Congress Cataloging-in-Publication Data

Dementia : molecules, methods, and measures / edited by I. Hindmarch,
  H. Hippius, and G. Wilcock.
       p.   cm.
    Includes bibliographical references and index.
    ISBN 0 471 92874 7
    1. Senile dementia—Chemotherapy. 2. Senile dementia—Molecular
aspects. I. Hindmarch, I. (Ian), 1944–   II. Hippius, Hanns.
III. Wilcock, G. K. (Gordon K.)
    [DNLM: 1. Dementia.   WM 220 D376376]
RC524.D46 1991
616.89′83061—dc20
DNLM/DLC
for Library of Congress   91-21552
                                                                 CIP

British Library Cataloguing in Publication Data

A catalogue record for this book is
available from the British Library

ISBN 0 471 92874 7

Typeset by Dobbie Typesetting Limited, Tavistock, Devon
Printed in Great Britain by Courier International, East Kilbride

Contents

Contributors   vii

Preface   xi

Foreword (*P. Stonier*)   xiii

1 Molecules for Modelling Cognitive Impairment
   J. M. Rusted and D. M. Warburton   1

2 A Comparison of the Animal Pharmacology of Nootropics and
   Metabolically Active Compounds
   C. D. Nicholson   19

3 New Anti-dementia Molecules
   B. Costall and R. J. Naylor   33

4 Some Considerations on the Methodology of Clinical Trials with
   Potential Anti-dementia Compounds in Patients with Alzheimer's
   Disease
   K. R. Siegfried   47

5 Scientific Basis for Therapeutic Developments in Alzheimer's Disease
   G. K. Wilcock   61

6 The Predictive Value of Volunteer Studies with Anti-dementia Drugs
   R. Spiegel   67

7 European Approaches to the Design of Drug Trials in Dementia
   R. R. Engel, H. Hippius and W. Satzger   79

Contents

8   International Development of Anti-dementia Drugs
    B. Musch and J. L. Robin   89

9   The Development of the SKT Project
    H. Erzigkeit   101

10 Appropriate Psychometric Testing of Cognitive Enhancers in
    Human Pharmacological Studies with Healthy Volunteers
    H. Ott   109

11 Clinical Assessment Instruments and Neuropsychological Tests
    L. Israel, DJ. Kozarevic and J. M. Orgogozo   127

12 EEG Brain Mapping in Dementia and Gerontopsychopharmacology
    B. Saletu   151

13 Age-related Memory Impairment: A Longitudinal and Cross-
    sectional Comparison
    S. G. Kilminster   161

14 Critical Flicker Fusion in Gerontological Research: Clinical
    Implications for Alzheimer's Disease
    S. Curran   169

15 The Assessment of Quality of Life in Nootropic Drug Research:
    Some Questions
    W. Deberdt and A. Brems   177

16 Intrusion Errors in Dementia: A New Look at an Old Measure
    T. Lorscheid and S. Thompson   185

17 Molecules, Measures and Methods: Issues and Comments
    C. Shillingford   197

Index   201

Contributors

A. BREMS
Pasteelsblokweg 3, B-3010 Kessel-Lo, Belgium

B. COSTALL
Postgraduate Studies in Pharmacology, The School of Pharmacy, University of Bradford, Bradford, BD7 1DP, UK

S. CURRAN
Department of Psychology, The University, Leeds, LS2 9JT, UK

W. DEBERDT
UCB – Pharmaceutical Sector, Chemin de Foriest, B-1420 Braine L'Alleud, Belgium

R. R. ENGEL
Psychiatric Department, University of Munich, Nussbaumstrasse 7, D-8000 Munich 2, Germany

H. ERZIGKEIT
Psychiatric Department, University of Erlangen-Nuremberg, Schwabachanlage 6, D-8520 Erlangen, Germany

H. HIPPIUS
Director, Psychiatric Department, University of Munich, Nussbaumstrasse 7, D-8000 Munich 2, Germany

L. ISRAEL
Internal Medicine and Gerontology Department, Grenoble University Hospital, Unit Elisse Chatin, 38043 Grenoble Cedex, France

S. G. KILMINSTER
Head of Psychometrics, Interphase UK, Pond Court, Loxwood, Billingshurst, West Sussex, RH14 0SA, UK

DJ. KOZAREVIC
Chief, Research Department, Pasterova 2, University Clinical Centre, Belgrade, Yugoslavia

T. LORSCHEID
Clinical Research Department, F. Hoffmann-La Roche AG, Grenzacherstrasse 124, CH-4002, Basel, Switzerland

B. MUSCH
The Upjohn Company, 10 Rue de Geneve, 1040 Brussels, Belgium

R. J. NAYLOR
Postgraduate Studies in Pharmacology, The School of Pharmacy, University of Bradford, Bradford, BD7 1DP, UK

C. D. NICHOLSON
Department of Pharmacology, Organon Laboratories Ltd, New Edinburgh Road, Newhouse, Lanarkshire, ML1 5SH, UK

J. M. ORGOGOZO
Neurology Department, Raymond Pellegrin Hospital, Bordeaux Cedex 33076, France

H. OTT
Department of Pharmacopsychology, Schering AG, Postfach 650311, D-1000 Berlin 65, Germany

J.-L. ROBIN
Rhone-Poulenc Rorer, Research and Development, 20 Avenue Raymond Aron, 92165 Antony Cedex, France

J. M. RUSTED
Laboratory of Experimental Psychology, University of Sussex, Brighton, Sussex, BN1 9QG, UK

B. SALETU
Department of Psychiatry, School of Medicine, University of Vienna, Wahringer Gürtel 18-20, A-1090 Vienna, Austria

W. SATZGER
Psychiatric Department, University of Munich, Nussbaumstrasse 7, D-8000 Munich 2, Germany

C. SHILLINGFORD
Director, Clinical Research, Interphase House, 1 London Road, Hindhead, Surrey, GU26 8AB, UK

K. R. SIEGFRIED

Clinical Research/Neuroscience, Hoechst AG, Postfach 80 03 20, D-6230 Frankfurt 80, Germany

R. SPIEGEL

Clinical Research, CNS Department, SANDOZ Pharma Ltd, CH-4002, Basel, Switzerland

S. THOMPSON

Clinical Research Department, F. Hoffmann-La Roche, AG, Grenzacherstrasse 124, CH-4002, Basel, Switzerland

D. M. WARBURTON

Department of Psychology, University of Reading, Building 3, Earley Gate, Whiteknights, Reading, Berkshire, RG6 1HR, UK

G. K. WILCOCK

Department of Care of the Elderly, University of Bristol, Frenchay Hospital, Bristol, BS16 1LE, UK

Preface

There is an increasing public and medical concern over the devastating effects of Alzheimer's Disease, not only as regards the clinical management of the sufferer, but also as regards the quality of life and well-being of the carer—particularly when the dementia patient is cared for at home. The response of professionals concerned with Alzheimer's disease and related disorders has been three-fold.

There has been an increase in the number of molecules developed as putative anti-dementia agents. Psychometricians have questioned the methodological and theoretical basis of the systems for assessing dementia and of recording, objectively, the impact of psychopharmacology on clinical and psychological manifestations of Alzheimer's disease. Furthermore, there has been a renewed interest in the appropriate ways and methods for assessing the severity of the disease and the impact of therapy.

It is clear that modern strategies for the clinical management of the dementia patient must take account of the molecules and the ways of quantifying the effects of the drug, as well as placing more reliance on appropriately designed rating scales and techniques for assessing the impact of therapy on the demented patient.

This book brings together the contributions of an international panel of speakers who were present at a symposium on dementia organized under the aegis of the Human Psychopharmacology Unit, Robens Institute, University of Surrey, by Interphase (UK) Ltd. The intention in drawing together leading researchers in pharmacology, psychology, psychiatry, geriatric medicine, gerontology, psychopharmacology, psychometrics and neurology was to explore the ways in which the various disciplines could interact to provide the modus operandi by which new molecules could be measured and assessed within an appropriate theoretical and methodological framework. This book has no sponsorship which causes it to toe a particular party line. It is a collection of opinions of recognized experts and in its entirety can be regarded as a source of information and practice for those companies, groups or individuals who seek to conduct valid and reliable work to alleviate the tragic impact of Alzheimer's disease and related disorders within a contemporary context.

Preface

Foreword

In ageing Western societies, the causes and treatment of degenerative diseases including those of the central nervous system, notably dementia, represent a significant challenge to medical research.

As a major participant and sponsor of such research efforts the international pharmaceutical industry is investing heavily in projects to discover, develop and register new medicines to treat dementia, which represents to many people a truly frightening prospect of premature or accelerated intellectual decline.

The oft-quoted prevalence figure for dementia is that 10% of people aged over 65 years have some degree of cognitive impairment, which means that by the year 2000 the European community will have in its midst some 6 million people afflicted with dementia and perhaps up to 25 million family members and carers with some degree of responsibility and personal involvement with the sufferers.

Whilst it could be said, generously, that some progress has been made in the diagnosis and clinical management of dementia, in establishing its place in community and institutional care and in the recognition of its social and political impact, little progress has been made in the therapeutic treatment of the condition. It is not surprising that the pharmaceutical industry sees the potential of satisfying the medical need in this sphere by providing new medicines, and justifies the investment in research projects on new molecules, which in turn will stimulate further competition in academic research with the promise of real progress in the quest to discover the cause of the disease and provide measures to reduce or eradicate the problem.

Nevertheless, several important questions need still to be answered before much confidence can be placed in a successful outcome to this research effort. It is regrettable that, at this stage, just as many of these questions need to be addressed to clinicians as to pharmacologists. To list the challenges facing dementia research is beyond this preface and even the book, but suffice it to say that considerably more assumptions must be made about the medical model for this condition as a basis for molecular research than about many other diseases which have succumbed to pharmaceutical breakthrough.

Whilst the condition may be recognized in the clinic in aberrations of cognitive and physical behaviour, and clinical progress can be charted over an inexorable downward path, little else is certain or agreed. Apart from continuing difficulties over diagnostic nomenclature, there is also little known or agreed on the genetic background, the presence or absence of environmental triggers, the social or cultural influences on clinical presentation, the mechanism or extent of compensatory psychological processes, the heterogeneity of the condition and, most importantly for pharmaceutical research, the pathology, pathophysiology and neurochemistry of the central nervous pathways involved in the aetiology and clinical manifestations of the disease. This uncertainty is reflected in weak diagnostic criteria, including difficulties differentiating dementia from depression and other mental conditions. There is an absence of robust measures of the degree of intellectual impairment or of the change in cognitive function over time, with or without the intervention of therapeutic agents.

The implications of this for the selection of suitable clinical trial subjects for multicentre (possible multinational) clinical trials is all too apparent. The difficulties faced in devising appropriate protocols and agreeing batteries of tests of cognitive and clinical variables is already clear to many working in the field. Hospitalized patients are usually too advanced to be suitable as trial subjects for agents expected to slow down or improve the disease process at an earlier stage. The introduction of the concept of 'age-related mental impairment' in an attempt to define a potentially drug-sensitive population within the community is no real answer to this problem. As a means of circumventing difficulties obtaining patients from the clinic it blurs the boundaries between healthy volunteer and patient requiring treatment, and also has a dubious relationship with the disease process itself.

Moreover there is little to be gained in comparing the performance of 65-year-olds with 25-year-olds. Only through longitudinal studies using individuals and groups as their own controls can reliable and robust methodology be developed from which to gather data on the efficacy and safety of new medicines.

From the pharmacological standpoint, the evidence that the condition is due to a defect in one neurotransmitter system comes from several sources but remains speculative. Even more speculative is the idea that the development of products influencing one neurotransmitter system, for example the cholinergic system, will ameliorate the global clinical condition. Such products may produce palliation and behavioural change in some individuals, but are unlikely to become widely available medicines.

Laboratory models to simulate memory impairment, such as the scopolamine test, are so far little other than sophisticated pharmacological tools to tinker at the periphery of the problem. Indeed, despite earlier hopes, the idea of single systems being solely responsible for any condition for which psychopharmacological agents have been developed has proved short-sighted. Depression, anxiety and other mental disorders have proved to have multifactorial causation, but at least some of these have clearcut pathognomonic features and improvement outcome measures, which are still a distant hope in dementia research. It must be remembered, however, that in this difficult area such research efforts and product developments are, however, the state of the art today, and hopes for future breakthrough are based on these principles.

In the meantime, such considerations also raise broader issues about the aim of treatment. The obvious medical model is an interventive one with the aim of improving or slowing down a demonstrable process presenting in the clinical setting. However, much of the thinking in dementia research rests on the hope that patients can be found early enough to prevent the disease from either starting at all or at least from reaching an advanced, untreatable stage. Thus the thinking leaps from intervention to prophylaxis, but prevention involves the development of totally different methodologies for screening, measuring change and assessing the risk-benefit of any treatment – a very far cry indeed from the aim of symptomatic intervention seen in today's research.

Even these fairly tough challenges to research progress in dementia are, however, overshadowed by the pressing need to define the whole research milieu, for in this condition it is insufficient to investigate molecules in isolation. Without a sociocultural model for treatment and care in the community for the millions of dementia sufferers, and without due consideration for the quality of life of the patients and their relatives, no true assessment of the cost-benefit of new treatments can be made. Without this, one wonders whether governments will be keen to sanction widespread prescription of new products for degenerative diseases in an elderly population for whom resources are already stretched.

The aims of research must be clearly defined before the large sums which will inevitably be required can be invested confidently in clinical development programmes. It may be that, as in the past, the beneficence of serendipity will come to the rescue of researchers already engaged on the problems, and this would be welcomed. Nevertheless, serendipity cannot be a factor built into the rational and strategic planning of complex research projects.

What follows in this book is a reasoned argument for the development of potential molecules, methods and measures for a therapeutic approach to dementia, made in the awareness of the uncertainties and debates about the condition and the aims of treatment both in the clinic and in the community. It is a timely contribution prepared in the confidence that where there are patients, of whatever age, in need of treatment, a concentration of knowledge, expertise and resources will ultimately, however gradually, bring about an improvement in their, and our, lot.

PETER D. STONIER

1

Molecules for Modelling Cognitive Impairment

*Jennifer M. Rusted and †David M. Warburton

*Laboratory of Experimental Psychology, University of Sussex, Brighton, UK and †Department of Psychology, University of Reading, UK

Introduction

Senile dementia of the Alzheimer type (SDAT) is associated with disruption of function in a large number of brain neurotransmitter systems, but the single transmitter system which has received the most attention is the cholinergic system. The cholinergic system has long been considered to have a modulatory role in information processing, attention and memory, and the emphasis on impaired cognitive functioning as an early and progressive symptom of SDAT appeared to support the significance of the relationship between the two (Sahakian et al., 1989). The clinical severity of SDAT correlates both with cognitive decline (Cutler and Narang, 1986) and decline in the activity of markers of cortical cholinergic activity (Perry et al., 1978) and also with chronic loss of subcortical cholinergic cell bodies in the basal forebrain (Whitehouse et al., 1981, 1982).

Psychopharmacological treatment strategies for the cognitive dysfunction in SDAT have, in consequence, examined the potential of direct enhancement of cholinergic function to counteract the loss of cholinergic neurons in the basal forebrain.

Early studies involving treatment with precursors of acetylcholine, such as choline or lecithin, were generally unsuccessful in producing significant improvements in cognitive performance (see review by Bartus et al., 1982). The results with cholinesterase inhibitors, such as physostigmine and tacrine hydrochloride (THA), which inhibit the breakdown of acetylcholine released into the synaptic cleft, have been marginally more positive. Kopelman (1986) provides a succinct review of experimental studies; small benefits have been reported in the better-designed studies, but the effects are far from dramatic, and the potential of the compounds in clinical practice is limited by the narrow therapeutic window for effective doses, and the adverse side effects associated with chronic administration.

Dementia: Molecules, Methods and Measures. Edited by I. Hindmarch, H. Hippius and G. K. Wilcock
© 1991 John Wiley & Sons Ltd

Finally attempts to drive the cholinergic pathway by administration of postsynaptic muscarinic agonists, such as arecoline, bethanecol and RS 86 have failed to produce reliable improvement in objective tests of cognitive performance (Palacios and Spiegel, 1986), although there are some claims that the compounds improve global functioning (Harbaugh *et al.*, 1984) and affect (Tariot *et al.*, 1988).

The limited success of these strategies has naturally led to a certain degree of scepticism about the cholinergic hypothesis of cognitive dysfunction. Kopelman (1987) and others have argued, for example, that while there is strong evidence for an association between decline in cognitive abilities and markers of cortical cholinergic activity, it is possible that the correlation may be due to some other factor, and that we should be more concerned with the involvement of multiple neurotransmitter systems.

Nevertheless, there is a strong association between the decline in cognitive abilities and markers of cholinergic activity, while the correlation is not at all convincing for other transmitter systems. Furthermore, our understanding of the cholinergic system and the mechanisms of action within this system has suggested alternative reasons for the failure of the current cholinomimetic strategies. For example, cholinesterase inhibitors only maintain the acetylcholine in the synaptic cleft but do not increase the total amounts of available acetylcholine (Stern *et al.*, 1987). Thus, the released acetylcholine, even if effectively maintained by cholinesterase inhibition, may still be too little to exert continued cholinergic stimulation (Sarter *et al.*, 1990).

The existence of subpopulations of muscarinic receptors with presynaptic autoreceptor function (Mash *et al.*, 1985) may counteract the effects of postsynaptic muscarinic agonists by down-regulating the release of naturally occurring acetylcholine. More significantly, there is substantial evidence for widely unchanged density and function of muscarinic receptors in SDAT. Coupled with the apparent ineffectiveness of muscarinic agonists, this would suggest that treatment strategies other than transmitter replacement or postsynaptic stimulation may be required to counteract the cognitive impairments associated with cholinergic denervation. For example, Warburton (1981), Sahakian *et al.* (1989) and Sarter *et al.* (1990) have suggested different alternative pharmacological strategies which focus on the amplification of presynaptic activity rather than direct influence on the normal patterning of cholinergic transmission. More detailed knowledge of the functional activity and pharmacological properties of the remaining cholinergic neurons is clearly needed if we are to effectively implement such strategies.

In this chapter, we will argue that cognitive psychopharmacology offers a valuable tool for a more in-depth exploration of the modulatory capacity of the cholinergic system in information processing and the extent to which and the route by which appropriate pharmacological intervention can enhance activity within that system and hence the cognitive functions which that activity maintains.

In order to make a strong contribution to psychopharmacology, information processing theory must provide a detailed framework for examining the effects of drugs. Such a framework must serve both an integrating and a predictive function. That is, it must indicate how drug-dependent phenomena are related, by providing a theoretical framework within which they can be drawn together, and, presented with new paradigms, it must predict which will show drug effects and which will not. Thus, the contribution of human information processing theory to psychopharmacology will be to enable us to organize and predict the complex pattern of cognitive functioning affected by drugs.

Structural and Processing Descriptions in Information Processing Theory

Human information processing theory provides two types of descriptions; structural and processing. Structural descriptions refer to the nature of the data stored in the memory and the functional components in which they reside. Processing descriptions are concerned with the states which the data may enter and the transitions between data representations and the stores in which they are held. Any account of drugs and information processing must consider both structures and processes.

Structural Descriptions

Short-term memory storage. Traditionally, short-term memory was conceived as a passive, temporary, limited capacity store, whose function was to maintain information long enough to allow more durable traces to be established in long-term memory. More recently, a more active conceptualization has emerged, in which short-term memory is viewed as active and multimodal with both storage and processing functions. In an influential model, Baddeley (1986) fractionates short-term working memory into an articulatory loop, a visuospatial scratch-pad, and the central executive mechanism (Baddeley and Hitch, 1974; Baddeley and Lieberman, 1980; Vallar and Baddeley, 1984a, 1984b; Baddeley, 1986).

The executive component of this system is the controller of the working memory, harnessing the other components as 'slave' systems for the processing of specific types of information. The articulatory loop is used for the passive recycling of auditory and phonological information, while the visuospatial scratch-pad is involved in the maintenance and manipulation of spatial representations and mental images. Both of these subsystems have been shown to be independent components of working memory, and to have limited capacities, such that simultaneous processing of two tasks which make use of the same system will result in deficits in performance in at least one of the tasks. Hence, paced repetition of a number sequence will impair digit span, a task which involves the maintenance of a series of digits in the articulatory loop, but would not be expected to disrupt a mental imaging task, which uses the visuospatial scratch-pad. Similarly, a spatial tapping task would be expected to impair performance on a mental rotation task, since they both make use of the visuospatial scratch-pad, but would not impair digit span, a task which involves the articulatory loop.

It is assumed that the central executive can itself store information, as well as control the processing of information held in other systems. Central resources are minimally involved in subcapacity slave system tasks, but may be allocated when capacity is exceeded or when the task becomes more difficult. However, the central executive has a limited capacity, and priority is given to controlling the flow of information and maintaining ongoing processing of information.

Thus, the central executive is regarded primarily as a resource rather than a storage location. Various processes compete for resources, and processes compete with storage requirements. The analogy with the resource limitations of attentional processing are clear, and we have argued elsewhere that they may represent two aspects of the same system (Warburton and Rusted, 1991).

Long-term memory storage. Recent theories of long-term memory have been influenced by computer models of associative memory structures (McClelland and Rumelhart, 1986).

These 'neural net' models adopt an approach in which the long-term representation of a given concept is distributed throughout the associative structure, in response to the short-term activation which characterizes working memory. No one node or structure corresponds to a particular mental entity, but instead its representation is constituted by the interneural weights within the entire net. As these change with exposure to new information, the mnemonic representation of that concept is constantly changing and being updated in response to new experiences.

Data structures. Several binary contrasts between data structures are considered in current descriptions of the data processed for storage.

(i) Semantic vs episodic. The distinction between semantic and episodic knowledge was originally suggested by Tulving (1972), in response to what he saw as a major change in the nature of the experimental work on memory. He distinguished between autobiographical (episodic) knowledge about the occurrence of events in a particular context, and general factual (semantic) knowledge which comprises our mental representation of the world. Experimental studies suggest qualitative differences between these two types of information, for example, in terms of their retention parameters, and the degree of affective overlay associated with each (Tulving, 1983).

(ii) Procedural vs declarative. The distinction between procedural and declarative knowledge has been described as the difference 'knowing how' and 'knowing that'. In theory, procedural knowledge underlies people's ability to perform certain acts or procedures, e.g. reading a word (perceptual), typing (motor) or solving equations (cognitive). Declarative knowledge concerns facts, not acts. The term declarative reflects the idea that such knowledge should be readily expressed in words. Despite some vague aspects of this distinction, it does seem to capture the fact that we can perform many acts, especially skilled ones, but cannot describe how we do them. The distinction is also reflected in the differential susceptibility of the two forms of information to disruption (i.e. the relative unsusceptibility of procedural memory) following head injury or organic amnesias (Cohen, 1984) or in progressive degenerative disorders such as SDAT (Weingartner *et al.*, 1983).

Processing Descriptions

Any description of information processing must include assumptions not only about the data structures but also about the processes that operate on the data.

Encoding processes. Encoding refers to the concomitant rehearsal and learning processes which occur in the course of an experience of an event.

(i) Elaborative processes. An important distinction between encoding strategies has been made within the 'levels of processing' framework, which postulates that the more meaningfully and distinctively an event is encoded, the better it will be remembered (Craik and Lockhart, 1972). This enhancement of subsequent recall by elaboration of an experience, for example by association formation or by imagery, may involve retrieving concepts and past experiences that are related to the current event. These are used to interpret and expand the new experience, and thus influence its representation in memory. Persuasive demonstrations have been made by a number of research groups to the effect that simple maintenance rehearsal (essentially Baddeley's articulatory process) does not enhance subsequent recall, although it can maintain the items and extend their availability for immediate memory tasks (e.g. Glenberg *et al.*, 1977).

(ii) Automatic vs controlled processes. A second important distinction is made between automatic and attentional processing (Hasher and Zacks, 1979). Specifically, it assumes that there are certain processes that lay down accessible traces in long-term memory without demanding attention. Such automatic encoding results in 'effortless', incidental learning of information.

Interestingly, Naveh-Benjamin and Jonides (1984) provided evidence that rote repetition is quickly automated (i.e. to the point where it does not produce dual-task interference), but that automation in this instance coincides with the point at which further repetition produces no further change in memory performance. In contrast, the practices grouped under 'elaborative' rehearsal do not become automatic; they consistently demand attention and pay off in retention. They involve meaningful inter-action with the material with the intention of placing the new information in a context which will be most effective in promoting its subsequent recall.

Retrieval processes. Remembering is a general term for the retroactive process of accessing information from previous events. Retrieval includes making the context of retrieval into an effective probe for the memory store, searching through the network of associations, decision-making about the editing of information found in the search, and generating a response.

The process of retrieval will essentially depend on the nature of the knowledge being retrieved. For example, episodic retrieval requires access to contextual information that specifies the episode of interest, whereas retrieval of semantic information is context-free by definition. Retrieval of declarative and procedural data also differs. Declarative data are accessed in the form of some explicit statement about the contents of memory ('I know these particular facts'). Procedural data may be retrieved by reenactment, perhaps without conscious awareness of remembering (Graf *et al.*, 1982). The attentional demands of these retrieval procedures are likely to differ considerably (but see Baddeley *et al.*, 1984).

Selective Deficit of Memory Subprocesses

A distinction has been made between encoding and retrieval processes in memory. Further distinctions are made among types of encoding processes, particularly elaborative, attentional and automatic encoding processes, and among the subprocesses of retrieval. There is accumulating evidence that ageing affects these subprocesses selectively, in particular elaborative encoding (or 'deep' processing) and the search subprocess of retrieval, which are demanding of system capacity.

Craik (1989) has argued that age-related differences in memory performance should be characterized in terms of the interaction between processing skills and 'environmental support', rather than notions of deficits in structural modules of memory. He suggests that the elderly rely more heavily on environmental cues or context to guide encoding and retrieval processes. Thus, their difficulties are not related to specific types of memory tasks, but rather to the application of appropriate strategies in a specific situation.

This view is consistent with the results from experimental studies which indicate that age-related changes reflect some type of suboptimal resource allocation. Memory tasks which show the clearest impairments in the elderly are those which are most likely to make heavy demands on resources. For example, Inglis and Caird (1963) reported age-related deficits in a dichotic listening task which requires concurrent storage, selection and output. Digit span shows no significant decline with age, suggesting unimpaired operations in the more passive component of working memory.

While Craik (1989) suggests that age-related deficits may relate to the inflexibility of central executive processes, Baddeley (1986) has argued for age-related deficits in total processing capacity. Both authors are in general agreement that ageing effects become more salient the greater the demands of the task under study. In other words, it could be argued that it is impaired functioning of the central executive control mechanism which places important constraints on information processing in the elderly.

In a series of studies, Morris (1984, 1986) presented experimental evidence to suggest a similar locus of impairment in patients with SDAT. Despite the fact that most patients with this disease demonstrate severe impairments on traditional measures of short-term memory, such as digit span, Morris found no evidence of impaired functioning of the articulatory loop itself. His patients showed no deficits in the word-length effect, their articulation rate was unimpaired, and the effects of concurrent articulation on memory span were of the same order as observed in the control group. Since the articulatory loop was still functional, Morris concluded that impairments on tasks of short-term memory must therefore reflect difficulties in accessing the articulatory loop as a consequence of dysfunction of the controlling central executive mechanism.

Summary

Theoretical models emerging from cognitive psychology are moving away from the structural approach to memory, emphasizing instead the significance of effective and efficient processing strategies in both the encoding and retrieval of information. Within this context, a crucial role is played by the supervisory control mechanism which coordinates the necessary operations, and dysfunction of this mechanism has been implicated in the information processing deficits associated with both normal and abnormal ageing.

In the next section we will present evidence from volunteer studies for the modulatory role of the cholinergic system in central executive function.

Cholinergic Drugs and Information Processing

Cholinergic drugs have long been associated with memory processes, and drug studies involving cholinergic blockade in healthy volunteers have generally produced a highly consistent pattern of deficits.

Cholinergic Blockade and Working Memory

Tasks associated with the output of items from immediate, short-term memory have generally been shown to be unaffected by cholinergic blockade. Digit span is not impaired by scopolamine (Ostfeld and Aruguete, 1962; Drachman and Leavitt, 1974; Rusted, 1988; Kopelman and Corn, 1988), even at the higher dose levels (Drachman and Leavitt, 1974 – 1.0 mg subcutaneously; Kopelman and Corn, 1988 – 0.4 mg intravenously). Word span is similarly unaffected (Mohs and Davis, 1985), and in tasks involving free recall of supraspan word lists, the recall of items from the last few positions (the recency component) is unimpaired (Crow and Grove-White, 1973; Mewaldt and Ghonheim, 1979; Frith *et al.*, 1984; Rusted and Warburton, 1989).

This difference has traditionally been interpreted in terms of the two-store memory model developed by Atkinson and Shiffrin (1968); subjects maintain the information in the short-term store and selected information is transferred to the more permanent, long-term store. In terms of this model, the cholinergic system was implicated in the process of establishing durable storage of information in longer term memory, but not in processes associated with the maintenance of information in short-term memory.

This simple dichotomy was brought into question by studies demonstrating impairments on certain types of short-term memory tasks. Caine *et al.* (1981) reported that scopolamine impaired performance on the Brown–Peterson memory task. In this task subjects are required to remember trigram letter sequences over varying delays, while rehearsal is prevented by a backwards counting task. The task provides a measure of the decay of information in short-term memory over time, under conditions in which concurrent processing of the distractor task prevents rehearsal of the to-be-remembered trigrams.

Kopelman and Corn (1988) reported similar effects. Subjects were required to complete the Brown–Peterson task with different distractor tasks which varied in level of difficulty from an easy task (repeating the word 'the' throughout the intervening interval) to more difficult tasks (counting backwards in twos or in sevens throughout the intervening interval). Differences between placebo and scopolamine-treated groups only emerged in the more difficult distractor conditions.

We have also found scopolamine-induced memory deficits on short-term memory tasks involving a heavier processing load (Rusted and Warburton, 1988). Following 0.6 mg of subcutaneously administered scopolamine, volunteers were tested on a non-verbal battery of tasks adapted from the CANTAB computerized test battery (Morris *et al.*, 1987). Performance on a simple task of recognition memory for a set of 12 abstract visual patterns was not impaired by the drug treatment. However, subjects were significantly impaired on a problem-solving task (involving sentence verification), memory for spatial location of a sequence of five boxes, and memory for location of visual shapes hidden inside a series of eight boxes.

This pattern of differential effects across a range of short-term memory tasks is not consistent with the two-store structural model of memory, which would anticipate an all-or-none disruption of short-term memory tasks. However, it is not incompatible with the characterization of working memory, and its role as a workspace for the different types of rapid and transitory mental processes which comprise a significant proportion of the everyday requirements of a memory system. All four of the tasks described above provide measures of short-term memory; although they differed in the type of processing involved, they all had processing requirements which were not contained within the articulatory loop or visuospatial subsystems, and hence involved processing resources under the direction of the central executive mechanism.

A study completed in our laboratory examined directly the interaction between scopolamine-induced deficits and working memory (Rusted, 1988). The question of interest was whether the scopolamine-induced impairments on short-term memory tasks with heavier processing requirements might be due to the selective effects of scopolamine on a single component of working memory, namely the central executive mechanism.

The effects of 1.2 mg scopolamine (oral administration) were examined on tasks associated with each of the three subcomponents of working memory (the articulatory loop, the visuospatial scratch-pad and the central executive mechanism). In order to demonstrate the sensitivity of each of those tasks to disruption, we incorporated secondary distractor tasks intended to make use of the articulatory loop (articulatory suppression task) and the visuospatial scratch-pad (spatial tapping task). Digit span was selectively impaired by the articulatory suppression task but was not impaired by scopolamine. Mental rotation was selectively impaired by concurrent spatial tapping, but was not impaired by scopolamine. In contrast, a supraspan free recall task, requiring central executive resources for encoding and organizing items for subsequent recall, was significantly impaired by drug treatment.

Immediate free recall was also disrupted by the requirement to complete a concurrent secondary task, but there was no differential effect of articulatory versus spatial processing. The occurrence of non-selective disruption is consistent with the idea that when the primary task demands central executive resources, the threshold for interference from other tasks, which themselves have only minimal recourse to central executive resources, is lowered.

Significantly, the requirement to complete a secondary task did not affect the size of the drug-induced deficit in performance. This again argues for a functional distinction between the components of working memory, with the drug affecting different components from those affected by the secondary tasks. The absence of interaction between secondary task and drug effects also argues against a complexity explanation of the scopolamine effects in working memory. If it were the case that the drug effects occurred only when the test situation exceeded some level of difficulty, then one would anticipate increased sensitivity to scopolamine when the free recall task is paired with another task, i.e. an interaction between drug effects and dual processing.

Consequently, we interpreted these effects as evidence for the specificity of the action of scopolamine in working memory, with cholinergic blockade reducing either the absolute level of resources or the effective allocation of resources in the working memory.

Cholinergic Blockade and Long-term Memory

Cholinergic blockade by scopolamine produces significant impairment on tasks involving the recall of information from long-term memory. Petersen (1977) reported a reduction in the number of words learned under scopolamine, with the acquisition rate apparently unaffected. Drachman and Leavitt (1974), Crow (1979) and Ghonheim and Mewaldt (1975) have reported impaired free recall of word lists with both visual and auditory presentation. This impairment is restricted to items presented early in the list and recalled from long-term memory, with recall of items in the recency portion of the list unaffected. All of these findings have been interpreted as evidence that the scopolamine-induced disruption of memory occurs primarily at the encoding stage, affecting the formation of durable memory traces or the transfer of information from short- to long-term storage (Drachman, 1977; Ghonheim and Mewaldt, 1977).

The effects of scopolamine at input have encouraged the examination of the effects of cholinergic blockade on the recall of different types of words. Frith *et al.* (1984) examined the possibility of differential effects of scopolamine on the recall of abstract versus concrete word lists. Abstract words are generally found to be harder to learn than concrete words, and Hasher and Zacks (1979) have suggested that both encoding and retrieval of low imagery words requires more effortful processing than high imagery words. Frith *et al.* (1984) found that scopolamine impaired performance on both types of list, with no differential effect on the superiority of concrete over abstract words. They also included lists of phonologically and semantically related words with the intention of examining the effects of scopolamine on homogeneous lists of items. Scopolamine had significant effects on measures of ordered recall with both types of lists.

However, if the recall was scored in terms of the number of correct items, irrespective of order, the authors noted that the deficit produced by scopolamine was significantly reduced. They suggested that while scopolamine does not differentially disrupt encoding operations for any specific type of word, the negative effects of scopolamine are attenuated for lists having intrinsic cues for list membership, providing the temporal order information is not important. Caine *et al.* (1981) have also noted an adverse effect of scopolamine on the ability to recall items in their correct sequence. However, they reported no differential effects of level of processing (semantic versus acoustic) on recall performance under scopolamine, suggesting that deeper processing *per se* could not compensate for the scopolamine-induced impairments.

These scopolamine-induced effects in long-term memory can be interpreted in terms of the resource model of working memory. It can be argued that scopolamine reduces the resources available for processing information for durable storage. While intrinsic cues such as homogeneous word sets may alleviate the problem (by providing ready-made organizational sets), they are not powerful enough to compensate entirely. Resource limitations may also be implicated in the failure to encode temporal order information for list items. What seems to be critical in determining the impact of scopolamine in these studies is the extent to which the task requirements involve storage of more than one aspect of the stimulus materials. Hence, little advantage can be gained by inducing semantic rather than acoustic processing, but differential effects of scopolamine are observed when both word stimuli and their temporal order within the list are required.

However, it should be noted that the scopolamine-induced recall deficits are not exclusively a function of acquisition failure. Caine *et al.* (1981) found that while free recall performance was impaired by the drug, cued recall performance was not affected. Dunne and Hartley (1985) reported no effect of drug treatment on recognition of items presented in a dichotic listening task, in which significant effects of scopolamine had been found for free recall. Finally, Rusted and Warburton (1989) reported that recognition memory following scopolamine was equivalent to recognition memory under placebo, despite the fact that volunteers in the scopolamine condition consistently failed to recall the recognized items over a sequence of eight acquisition trials. These retrieval deficits observed for unrelated word lists may be a consequence of inadequate organization of material which is processed sufficiently for durable storage. This, of course, could be interpreted as another manifestation of capacity overload.

Summary. The effects on human memory of cholinergic blockade, which have traditionally been interpreted within the structural two-store models, seem to be more easily accommodated in a capacity model of memory. According to this view, capacity limitations are exacerbated by cholinergic blockade as a consequence of drug-induced disruption of resource allocation. Our studies suggest that the source of these difficulties may be the central executive mechanism. This system determines processing strategies in immediate memory, is implicated in the organization of material for long-term storage, and is selectively impaired by cholinergic blockade.

Cholinergic mediation of this central executive mechanism is also consistent with the pathological degeneration of the cholinergic system associated with SDAT. As we pointed out earlier, Morris (1984, 1986) reported that on more sophisticated measures of performance, there was evidence that the functioning of the articulatory loop remained intact in a group of mild-to-moderate SDAT patients, and that digit span performance was impaired as a consequence of chronic disruption of central executive function, required in the normal course of events to access the articulatory slave system.

The less severe loss of cholinergic neurons in a healthy elderly population (Ball, 1977) would also be consistent with the idea of cholinergic modulation of central executive function. As we indicated earlier, healthy elderly individuals demonstrate memory deficits which reflect reduced capacity for elaborative processing and effective organization of material, and reduced flexibility of processing resources. The evidence of unimpaired digit span in this group, and, indeed, in studies of scopolamine-induced cholinergic blockade in healthy adults, indicate the quantitative differences in severity of functional loss between normal and abnormal ageing.

Cholinergic Drugs and Attention

The finding of selective effects of scopolamine on central executive function raises an interesting issue regarding the parallels between the capacity models of memory and the capacity models of attention. To what extent might the central executive mechanism be considered to subsume attentional functions, and how distinct would such functions be from the attentional components discussed in capacity models of attention? In working memory, the central executive mechanism determines the allocation of processing resources to the task in hand, a role required of the resource allocation mechanism of attention, and a function which has been repeatedly demonstrated to be susceptible to disruption by cholinergic blockade. Does this association with cholinergic modulation extend to other aspects of attention?

It has frequently been pointed out that attention cannot be thought of as a unitary concept. Posner and Boies (1971) suggested that we must consider alertness, selectivity and processing capacity as separate components of attention. Kinchla (1980) suggested three classes of experiment which were relevant to the issue of selectivity in information processing: namely, sustained attention tasks, attentional switching tasks and selective attention tasks.

Sustained attention. One classical type of sustained attention test is the vigilance task. In vigilance tasks, attention is directed to one or more sources of input for long periods of time and the subject is required to detect and respond to brief, infrequent changes in input. During a typical vigilance session, the detection rate decreases, a change called the vigilance decrement. We have used the Mackworth Clock task (Mackworth, 1950) as a task which produces a reliable vigilance decrement. In this task, the volunteer has to detect brief pauses in the movement of the minute hand of the clock. Oral doses of 0.6 mg and 1.2 mg scopolamine decreased the number of detections in this vigilance task to below that found in the placebo condition (Wesnes and Warburton, 1983).

In addition, we have used a completely different sustained visual attention task in which a series of digits is presented sequentially on a computer screen at a rapid rate (100 digits/min). Volunteers are required to detect three digit sequences of odd or even numbers as they occur. Measures of both speed and accuracy of detection are taken. Oral doses of 1.2 mg scopolamine administered prior to this rapid visual information processing task produce very clear deficits in performance relative to baseline. In contrast, the effects of methylscopolamine at the same dose of 1.2 mg were not different from placebo (Wesnes and Warburton, 1984). Scopolamine impaired both speed and accuracy, which is important because it shows that this was not a consequence of speed-accuracy trade-off in performance, but that there was an overall impairment in attentional processing efficiency.

Attentional switching. In an attentional switching task, volunteers must attend to more than one source of information and process material from both sources. One study which investigated the effects of scopolamine on this type of processing was reported by Drachman and his colleagues (Drachman *et al.*, 1980). In their dichotic listening task, items were presented simultaneously to both ears and the volunteers had to perceive, store and recall both sets of items. Undrugged volunteers could only process about 35% of the total amount of information presented, while scopolamine reduced performance to only 19% of the total of both sets of items.

Selective attention. A task which demonstrates selective attention and perceptual intrusions from unattended material is the Stroop task (Stroop, 1935). This is a complex information processing task in which volunteers are required to process information under conditions of distraction. The Stroop effect is the name given to the distracting effect of the to-be-ignored distractor stimuli on the processing of the attended material. Typically, a list of colour words may be presented, with the words written in different coloured inks. The ink colours are incongruent with the written words, for example, the word YELLOW may be written in red ink, and the word RED in green ink. The task is to move down the word list naming the colour of the ink in which each word is written, ignoring the actual printed word. Ink colour naming of incongruently printed colour words takes much longer than ink colour naming of non-colour words written in different inks. The difference in time required for these conditions provides a measure of the volunteer's capacity to selectively attend to the relevant dimension (the ink colour) while ignoring the irrelevant one (the printed word). Studies in our laboratory with scopolamine (Wesnes and Revell, 1984b) and elsewhere with atropine (Callaway and Band, 1958) have shown that both these cholinergic antagonists impair performance on this task.

Summary. Baddeley (1986) refers to working memory as corresponding approximately to the set of things we are attending to at any given moment. In his view, the function of the central executive mechanism is likely to be related to the control of attention, and he has associated the central executive with the supervisory attentional system developed by Norman and Shallice (1986).

According to Norman and Shallice (1986), the supervisory attentional system is used when tasks involve planning or decision making. It would be needed where new or poorly learned behavioural sequences are performed. The system would also be involved where some strong habitual response is competing with the appropriate response, or when an automatic process appears to be running into problems. The common thread running through these situations is the need for conscious control, or attention.

It should be noted that this type of supervisor is common to a number of information processing models in the form of the operating system (Johnson-Laird, 1983) or the executive system (Logan and Cowan, 1984). The supervisory attentional system proposed by Norman and Shallice (1986) is also assumed to have limited capacity, and in this sense, has conceptual similarities with the central processor in the Posner and Boies (1971) model of attention.

Experimental studies demonstrate that cholinergic blockade has marked adverse effects on sustained and selective attention and on attentional switching. We have already reviewed the evidence for its adverse effects on resource allocation in working memory. The most parsimonious explanation of these commonalities would be that the cholinergic modulation is acting on a single information processing mechanism responsible for resource allocation at all levels of on-going cognitive processing.

Enhancement of Function

An interesting new focus in cholinergic research which is relevant to the present discussion is the role of the nicotinic receptor within the cholinergic system.

Norman (1986) has suggested that the conscious control mechanism may act by activating or inhibiting neural modules, in order to facilitate appropriate information processing states. This proposition maps rather neatly onto the neural model of the way in which cholinergic pathways may modulate information processing capacity. One important neurochemical system that is responsible for the control of the cortical state is the ascending cholinergic pathway to the cortex (Warburton, 1975, 1981). Warburton (1981) proposed that the release of acetylcholine at the cortex increases electrocortical arousal, and hence the size of the evoked potentials, and that this improves the probability of their being distinguished from background cortical acitivity; in Norman's terms, the cholinergic pathways do not cause a cognitive operation, but change the cortical state to make the operation more accurate and more efficient.

Warburton (1990) has argued that improved information processing can be achieved by nicotine-induced stimulation of the cholinergic system, because nicotine acts to reduce fluctuations in cortical arousal as a result of sustained acetylcholine release at the cortex. This may be a consequence either of enhanced activity in the ascending cholinergic pathway or of presynaptic action at the cortex.

The ascending pathway from the nucleus basalis deteriorates in SDAT; muscarinic receptor numbers and function remain stable over the course of the disease, but there is a significant loss of nicotinic receptors in all cortical laminae (Kellar et al., 1987). At first sight, this loss would seem to preclude effective enhancement of cognitive function via this route in SDAT patients. However, there is some indication that the extent of cholinergic cell loss may have been overestimated. Lams et al. (1988) have suggested that the cholinergic neurons survive despite significant loss of acetylcholine-associated enzymes (measures of which have previously been interpreted as a measure of neuron density). In addition, recent work has suggested that instead of a reduced number of nicotinic binding sites, high affinity nicotinic binding sites are converted into low affinity sites in the course of the disease (Nordberg et al., 1988), and that this increased number of low affinity sites may actually result in enhanced functioning of residual cholinergic neurons (Sarter et al., 1990).

In healthy volunteers, the beneficial effects of nicotine on sustained attention have been consistently documented. Nicotine tablets held in the mouth for 5 min reduce the vigilance decrement which occurs over time in the Mackworth clock task (Wesnes *et al.*, 1983). Nicotine gum produces dose-related increases in the number of correct detections and decreases in reaction time to make those correct detections on the rapid visual information processing task (Rusted and Warburton, unpublished data). In an earlier study using nicotine tablets (Wesnes and Warburton, 1984), 1.5 mg nicotine produced a performance improvement on the rapid visual information processing task which closely resembled the improvement produced by smoking a single cigarette. Oral nicotine also reduces the size of the Stroop effect in both deprived smokers and non-smokers (Wesnes and Warburton, 1978), indicating enhanced selective attention for relevant information.

Of greater significance for the therapeutic potential of nicotine, Wesnes and Revell (1984b) have reported that nicotine antagonizes the scopolamine-induced deficits on the rapid visual information processing task and the Stroop task, a positive indication that nicotine may improve information processing in a deficient system.

In the light of these findings, we were interested to know whether nicotine would have any effect on patients who are in the early stages of SDAT. In a study completed at the Institute of Psychiatry in London, the effects of subcutaneous doses of nicotine on the information processing performance of patients with SDAT were examined (Sahakian *et al.*, 1989; Jones and Sahakian, 1990). Nicotine produced a dose-related improvement in performance in the detection of signals in the rapid visual information processing task, such that the performance of patients approached the performance of the healthy elderly control group. Nicotine also produced improvements in reaction times relative to baseline and placebo performances on this task.

In a critical flicker fusion test run on the same patients, nicotine produced a dose-related improvement in the frequency with which the patients saw the lights as fused. Higher resolution of flashes is interpreted as improved cortical functioning.

The authors argued that the improved attention performance in this patient sample is the behavioural consequence of improved cortical functioning. Nicotine sustains release of acetylcholine at the cortex, and consequently lapses of attention and the concomitant variations in information processing normally observed (particularly in these patients) are reduced.

These findings have implications for the role of nicotine in other cholinergically mediated deficits. Specifically, if the short-term memory difficulties in SDAT are associated with central executive dysfunction, then nicotine should promote enhanced performance on these tasks. However, Jones and Sahakian (1990) found that the dose-related improvements in attentional processing were not mirrored by improvements in a working memory task. Similarly, preliminary studies in our laboratories have not produced improvements in working memory tasks such as problem solving or visuospatial memory following nicotine gum. Both of the latter tasks show reliable decrements in performance in the elderly and in healthy volunteers administered scopolamine.

A review of the literature shows that the effects of nicotine on short-term memory have not been so robust as those of scopolamine. An early study by Andersson and Hockey (1977) provided weak evidence that smoking may enhance storage of information, but only of information intentionally encoded for recall. One interpretation of this finding is an attentional one; the group who smoked may have been more efficient at selecting the relevant information.

In contrast, Peeke and Peeke (1984), who studied the effects of smoking on immediate memory in 2-h deprived smokers, found that recall of a 50-word list was improved immediately after learning. In a complimentary study of a low and a high nicotine cigarette, the high nicotine cigarette produced improved recall while the low nicotine cigarette was less effective. We have also found improved recall relative to placebo of a 48-word list immediately after ingestion of a 1.5 mg nicotine tablet (Warburton *et al.*, 1986). However, both of these studies involve rather long word lists, and it could be argued that an attentional component is involved. We tested this hypothesis directly in a recent study involving immediate free recall of either 10- or 30-word lists following ingestion of a 1.5 mg nicotine tablet (Rusted and Eaton-Williams, in press). In accordance with the attentional hypothesis, nicotine significantly improved free recall of 30-item lists, but not of 10-item lists. More importantly, co-administration of the same dose of nicotine did not reverse scopolamine-induced recall deficits either for 10- or 30-item lists. This was in contrast to the effective reversal of scopolamine-induced deficits in a sustained attention task reported by Wesnes and Revell (1984b).

Further work is obviously needed to resolve these discrepancies. However, an interim assessment of the nicotine work to date suggests that there is only a partial overlap between the effects of scopolamine and those of nicotine. While scopolamine affects both attentional and memorial processes, the effects of nicotine seem to be limited to the advantages which can be gained by improvements in focused or selective attention. If such is the case, then additional pharmacological studies may contribute to the detailed specification of the distinctive functions of an attentional and a memorial supervisory system.

Concluding Comments

Psychological models of information processing have provided the basis for a detailed examination of the cognitive effects of cholinergic modulation. The pattern of effects reported in experimental studies with young adults, the healthy elderly and patients with SDAT is consistent with the view that cholinergic blockade or dysfunction precludes effective allocation of processing resources by the central executive mechanism of the working memory. The cholinergic system is also involved in the modulation of attention, with scopolamine-induced deficits and nicotine-induced enhancement of function reliably demonstrable. The extent to which attention and memory functions employ common or independent mechanisms of action is as yet unclear.

The impact of cognitive psychology on pharmacological studies depends upon the adoption of current models of information processing; there is at this stage little to be gained from global assessment of function. With the implementation of more sophisticated paradigms, we have the tools for a detailed examination of neurochemical correlates of information processes. By using those tools effectively, we may develop a reciprocal relationship between the disciplines, whereby psychopharmacology may contribute directly to the differentiation of processes and structures and provide a testing ground for theoretical models of memory and attention.

References

Andersson, K. and Hockey, G. R. J. (1977) Effects of cigarette smoking on incidental memory. *Psychopharmacologia*, **52**, 223–6.

Atkinson, R. C. and Shiffrin, R. M. (1968) Human memory: a proposed system and its control processes. In: Spence, K. W. and Spence, J. T. (eds) *The Psychology of Learning and Motivation: Advances in Research and Theory*, Vol. 2, pp. 89–195. New York: Academic Press.

Baddeley, A. D. (1986) *Working Memory*. Oxford: Oxford University Press.

Baddeley, A. D. and Hitch, G. J. (1974) Working memory. In: Bower, G. (ed.) *The Psychology of Learning and Motivation*, Vol. VIII, pp. 47–88. New York: Academic Press.

Baddeley, A. D. and Lieberman, K. (1980) Spatial working memory. In: Nickerson, R. (ed.) *Attention and Performance VIII*, pp. 521–539. Hillsdale, New Jersey: Erlbaum.

Baddeley, A. D., Elridge, M., Lewis, V. and Thompson, N. (1984) Attention and retrieval from long-term memory. *J. Exp. Psychol. [Gen.]*, **113**, 518–40.

Ball, M. J. (1977) Neuron loss, neurofibrillary tangles, and granulovacuolar degeneration in the hippocampus with aging and dementia. A quantitative study. *Acta Neuropathol.*, **37**, 111–18.

Bartus, R. T., Dean, R. L., Beer, B. and Lippa, A. S. (1982) The cholinergic hypothesis of geriatric memory dysfunction. *Science*, **217**, 408–17.

Caine, E. D., Weingartner, H., Ludlow, C. L., Cudahy, E. A. and Wehry, S. (1981) Qualitative analysis of scopolamine-induced amnesia. *Psychopharmacology*, **74**, 74–80.

Callaway, E. and Band, R. I. (1958) Some pharmacological effects of atropine. *Arch. Neurol. Psychiatry*, **79**, 91–102.

Cohen, N. J. (1984) Preserved learning capacity in amnesia: evidence for multiple storage systems. In: Squire, L. R. and Butters, N. (eds) *Neuropsychology of Memory*, pp. 83–103. New York: Guildford Press.

Craik, I. M. (1989) Changes in memory with normal aging: a functional view. In: Wurtman, R. J., Corkin, S., Growdon, J. H. and Ritter-Walker, E. (eds) *Alzheimer's Disease. Proceedings of the Fifth Meeting of the International Study Group on the Pharmacology of Memory Disorders associated with Aging*, Zurich.

Craik, F. I. M. and Lockhart, R. S. (1972) Levels of processing: a framework for memory research. *J. Verb. Learn. Verb. Behav.* **11**, 671–84.

Crow, T. (1979) Action of hyoscine on verbal learning in man: evidence for a cholinergic link in the transition from primary to secondary memory? In: Brazier, M. A. B. (ed.) *Brain Mechanisms in Memory and Learning: From Single Neuron to Man*, pp. 269–275. New York: Raven Press.

Crow, T. J. and Grove-White, I. G. (1973) An analysis of the learning deficit following hyoscine administration in man. *Br. J. Pharmacol.*, **49**, 322–7.

Cutler, N. and Narang, P. (1986) Cognitive enhancers in Alzheimer's disease. In: Cutler, N. and Narang, P. (eds) *Drug Studies in the Elderly*, pp. 313–332. New York: Plenum Press.

Drachman, D. (1977) Memory and cognitive function in man: does the cholinergic system have a specific role? *Neurology*, **27**, 783–90.

Drachman, D. A. and Leavitt, J. (1974) Human memory and the cholinergic system. *Arch. Neurol.*, **30**, 113–21.

Drachman, D. A., Noffsinger, D., Sahakian, B. J., Kurdziel, S. and Fleming, P. (1980) Aging, memory, and the cholinergic system: a study of dichotic listening. *Neurobiol. Aging*, **1**, 39–43.

Dunne, M. P. and Hartley, L. R. (1985) The effects of scopolamine upon verbal memory: evidence for an attentional hypothesis. *Acta Psychol.*, **58**, 205–17.

Frith, C. D., Richardson, J. T. E., Samuel, M., Crow, T. J. and McKenna, P. J. (1984) The effects of intravenous diazepam and hyoscine upon human memory. *Q. J. Exp. Psychol.*, **36A**, 133–44.

Ghonheim, M. M. and Mewaldt, S. P. (1975) Effects of diazepam and scopolamine on storage, retrieval and organizational processes in memory. *Psychopharmacologia*, **44**, 257–62.

Ghonheim, M. M. and Mewaldt, S. P. (1977) Studies on human memory: the interactions of diazepam, scopolamine and physostigmine. *Psychopharmacology*, **52**, 1–6.

Glenberg, A., Smith, S. M. and Green, C. (1977) Type rehearsal: maintenance and more. *J. Verb. Learn. Verb. Behav.*, **16**, 339–352.

Graf, P., Mandler, G. and Haden, P. E. (1982) Simulating amnesic symptoms in normal subjects. *Science*, **218**, 1243–4.

Harbaugh, R. E., Roberts, D. W., Coombs, D. M., Saunders, R. L. and Reeder, T. M. (1984) Preliminary report: intracranial cholinergic drug infusion in patients with Alzheimer's disease. *Neurosurgery*, **15**, 514–18.

Hasher, L. and Zacks, R. T. (1979) Automatic and effortful processes in memory. *J. Exp. Psychol.* [*Gen.*], **108**, 356–88.

Inglis, J. and Caird, W. K. (1963) Age differences in successive responses to simultaneous stimulation. *Can. J. Psychol.*, **17**, 98–105.

Johnson-Laird, P. N. (1983) *Mental Models*. Cambridge: Cambridge University Press.

Jones, G. and Sahakian, B. (1990) The effects of nicotine in patients with dementia of the Alzheimer type. In: Kewitz, H., Thomsen, T. and Bickel, U. (eds) *Pharmacological Interventions on Central Cholinergic Mechanisms in Senile Dementia (Alzheimer's Disease)*, pp. 82–8. Munich: Zuckschwerdt.

Kellar, K. J., Whitehouse, P. J., Martino-Burrows, A. M., Marcus, K. and Price, D. L. (1987) Muscarinic and nicotinic cholinergic binding sites in Alzheimer's disease cerebral cortex. *Brain Res.*, **436**, 62–8.

Kinchla, R. A. (1980) The measurement of attention. In: Nickerson, R. S. (ed.) *Attention and Performance VIII*, pp. 552–623. Hillsdale, New Jersey: Erlbaum.

Kopelman, M. D. (1986) The cholinergic neurotransmitter system in human memory and dementia: a review. *Q. J. Exp. Psychol.*, **38A**, 535–73.

Kopelman, M. D. (1987) Amnesia: organic and psychogenic. *Br. J. Psychiatry*, **150**, 428–42.

Kopelman, M. D. and Corn, T. H. (1988) Cholinergic 'blockade' as a model for cholinergic depletion: a comparison of the memory deficits with those of Alzheimer-type dementia and the alcoholic Korsakoff syndrome. *Brain*, **111**, 1079–110.

Lams, B. E., Isacson, O. and Sofroniew, M. V. (1988) Loss of transmitter-associated enzyme staining following axotomy does not indicate death of brainstem cholinergic neurons. *Brain Res.* **475**, 401–6.

Logan, G. D. and Cowan, W. B. (1984) On the ability to inhibit thought and action: a theory of an act of control. *Psychol. Rev.*, **91**, 295–327.

Mackworth, N. H. (1950) *Researches on the Measurement of Human Performance*. Medical Research Council Special Report, No. 268. London: HMSO.

Mash, D. C., Flynn, D. D. and Potter, L. T. (1985) Loss of M_2 muscarinic receptors in the cerebral cortex in Alzheimer's disease and experimental cholinergic denervations. *Science*, **228**, 1115–7.

McLelland, J. L. and Rumelhart, D. E. (1986) *Parallel Distributed Processing*, Vol. 2. Cambridge: MIT Press.

Mewaldt, S. P. and Ghonheim, M. M. (1979) The effects and interactions of scopolamine, physostigmine and methscopolamine on human memory. *Biochem. Behav.*, **10**, 205–10.

Mohs, R. C. and Davis, K. L. (1985) Interaction of choline and scopolamine in human memory. *Life Sci.*, **37**, 193–7.

Morris, R. G. (1984) Dementia and the functioning of the articulatory loop system. *Cogn. Neuropsychol.*, **1**, 143–57.

Morris, R. G. (1986) Short-term forgetting in senile dementia of the Alzheimer's type. *Cogn. Neuropsychol.*, **3**, 77–97.

Morris, R. G., Evenden, J. L., Sahakian, B. J. and Robbins, T. (1987) Computer-aided assessment of dementia: comparative studies of neuropsychological deficits in Alzheimer-type dementia and Parkinson's disease. In: Stahl, S. M., Iversen, S. D. and Goodman, E. C. (eds) *Cognitive Neurochemistry*, pp. 21–36. Oxford: Oxford University Press.

Naveh-Benjamin, M. and Jonides, J. (1984) Maintenance rehearsal: a two-component analysis. *J. Exp. Psychol.* [*Learn. Mem. Cogn.*], **10**, 369–85.

Nordberg, A., Adem, A., Hardy, J. and Winblad, B. (1988) Change in nicotinic receptor subtypes in temporal cortex of Alzheimer brains. *Neurosci. Lett.*, **86**, 317–21.

Norman, D. A. (1986) Reflections on cognition and parallel distributed processing. In: McClelland, J. L. and Rumelhart, D.E. (eds) *Parallel Distributed Processing*, Vol. 2, pp. 531–46. Cambridge, Massachusetts: MIT Press.

Norman, D. A. and Shallice, T. (1986) Attention to action: willed and automatic control of behaviour. In: Davidson, R. J., Schwartz, G. E. and Shapiro, D. (eds) *Consciousness and Self Regulation*, Vol. 4, pp. 1–18. New York: Plenum Press.

Ostfeld, A. M. and Aruguete, A. (1962) Central nervous system effects of hyoscine in man. *J. Pharmacol. Exp. Ther.*, **137**, 133–9.

Palacios, J. M. and Spiegel, R. (1986) Muscarinic cholinergic agonists: pharmacological and clinical perspectives. *Prog. Brain Res.*, **70**, 485–98.

Peeke, S. C. and Peeke, H. V. S. (1984) Attention, memory and cigarette smoking. *Psychopharmacology*, **84**, 205–16.

Perry, E. K., Tomlinson, B. E., Blessed, G., Bergman, K., Bigson, P. H. and Perry, R. H. (1978) Correlation of cholinergic abnormalities with senile plaques and mental test scores in senile dementia. *BMJ*, **ii**, 1457–9.

Petersen, R. C. (1977) Scopolamine-induced learning failures in man. *Psychopharmacologia*, **52**, 283–9.

Posner, M. I. and Boies, S. J. (1971) Components of attention. *Psychol. Rev.*, **78**, 391–408.

Rusted, J. M. (1988) Dissociative effects of scopolamine on working memory in healthy young volunteers. *Psychopharmacology*, **96**, 487–92.

Rusted, J. M. and Eaton-Williams, P. (in press) Distinguishing between attentional and amnestic effects in information processing: the separate and combined effects of scopolamine and nicotine on verbal free recall. *Psychopharmacology*, in press.

Rusted, J. M. and Warburton, D. M. (1988) Effects of scopolamine on working memory of healthy young adults. *Psychopharmacology*, **96**, 145–52.

Rusted, J. M. and Warburton, D. M. (1989) Effects of scopolamine on verbal memory: a retrieval or acquisition deficit? *Neuropsychobiology*, **21**, 76–83.

Sahakian, B., Jones, G., Levy, R., Gray, J. and Warburton, D. M. (1989) The effects of nicotine on attention, information processing, and short-term memory in patients with dementia of the Alzheimer type. *Br. J. Psychiatry*, **154**, 797–800.

Sarter, M., Bruno, J. P. and Dudchenko, P. (1990) Activating the damaged basal forebrain cholinergic system: tonic stimulation versus signal amplification. *Psychopharmacology*, **101**, 1–17.

Stern, Y., Sano, M. and Mayeux, R. (1987) Effects of oral physostigmine in Alzheimer's disease. *Ann. Neurol.*, **22**, 306–10.

Stroop, J. R. (1935) Studies of interference in serial verbal reactions. *J. Exp. Psychol.*, **18**, 643–61.

Tariot, P. N., Cohen, R. M., Welkowitz, J. A., Sunderland, T., Newhouse, P. A. and Murphy, D. L. (1988) Multiple dose arecoline infusions in Alzheimer's disease. *Arch. Gen. Psychiatry*, **45**, 901–5.

Tulving, E. (1972) Episodic and semantic memory. In: Tulving, E. and Donaldson, W. (eds) *Organization of Memory*, pp. 382–404. New York: Academic Press.

Tulving, E. (1983) *Elements of Episodic Memory*. Oxford: Oxford University Press.

Vallar, G. and Baddeley, A. D. (1984a) Fractionation of working memory: neuropsychological evidence for a phonological short-term store. *J. Verb. Learn. Verb. Behav.*, **23**, 151–61.

Vallar, G. and Baddeley, A. D. (1984b) Phonological short-term store, phonological processing and sentence comprehension: a neuropsychological case study. *Cogn. Neuropsychol.*, **1**, 121–41.

Warburton, D. M. (1975) *Brain, Behaviour and Drugs*. Chichester: Wiley.

Warburton, D. M. (1981) Neurochemical bases of behaviour. *Br. Med. Bull.*, **37**, 121–5.

Warburton, D. M. (1990) Psychopharmacological aspects of nicotine. In: Wonnacott, S., Russell, M. A. H. and Stolerman, I. P. (eds) *Nicotine Psychopharmacology*, pp. 77–111. Oxford: Oxford University Press.

Warburton, D. M. and Rusted, J. M. (1991) Cholinergic systems and information processing capacity. In: Weinman, J. and Hunter, J. (eds) *Memory: Neurochemical and Abnormal Perspectives*, pp. 87–103. London: Harwood Academic.

Warburton, D. M., Wesnes, K., Shergold, K. and James, M. (1986) Facilitation of learning and state dependency with nicotine. *Psychopharmacology*, **89**, 55–9.

Weingartner, H., Grafman, J., Boutelle, W., Kaye, W. and Martin, P. R. (1983) Forms of memory failure. *Science*, **221**, 380–2.

Wesnes, K. and Revell, A. (1984a) The separate and combined effects of nicotine on human information processing. *Psychopharmacology*, **84**, 55–9.

Wesnes, K. and Revell, A. (1984b) The separate and combined effects of scopolamine and nicotine on human information processing. *Psychopharmacology*, **84**, 5–11.

Wesnes, K. and Warburton, D. M. (1978) The effect of cigarette smoking and nicotine tablets upon human attention. In: Thornton, R.E. (ed.) *Smoking Behaviour: Physiological and Psychological Influences*, pp. 131–47. Edinburgh: Churchill Livingstone.

Wesnes, K. and Warburton, D. M. (1983) Effects of scopolamine on stimulus sensitivity and response bias in a vigilance task. *Neuropsychobiology*, **9**, 154–7.

Wesnes, K. and Warburton, D. M. (1984) Effects of scopolamine and nicotine on human rapid information processing performance. *Psychopharmacology*, **82**, 147–50.

Wesnes, K., Warburton, D. M. and Matz, B. (1983) The effects of nicotine on stimulus sensitivity and response bias in a visual vigilance task. *Neuropsychobiology*, **9**, 41–4.

Whitehouse, P. J., Price, D. L., Clark, A. W., Coyle, J. T. and Delong, M. R. (1981) Alzheimer's disease: evidence for a selective loss of cholinergic neurones in the nucleus basalis. *Ann. Neurol.*, **10**, 122–6.

Whitehouse P. J., Price, D. L., Struble, R. G., Clark, A. W., Coyle, J. T. and Delong, M. R. (1982) Alzheimer's disease and senile dementia: loss of neurons in the basal forebrain. *Science*, **215**, 1237–9.

2

A Comparison of the Animal Pharmacology of Nootropics and Metabolically Active Compounds

C. David Nicholson

Department of Pharmacology, Organon Laboratories Limited, Newhouse, UK

Introduction

Senile dementia of the Alzheimer type (SDAT), multi-infarct dementia and the less well-defined disorder, chronic organic brain disease, are of multifactorial aetiology. Rational therapy is complicated by the fact that symptoms can be caused either by vascular occlusion as in multi-infarct dementia or by neuronal degeneration as in SDAT. In the latter case, the symptoms are unlikely to be due to selective degeneration of a particular neuronal system (Palmer and Gershorn, 1990). Although the cognitive decline may be due primarily to cholinergic or glutamatergic degeneration, dysfunction in noradrenergic or serotoninergic neurons contribute to the non-cognitive changes in behaviour in dementia (Palmer and Gershorn, 1990). Consequently, therapy designed to specifically compensate for disruption in any one neurotransmitter system is unlikely to effectively treat all forms of senile dementia. Indeed, even if the cause of the dementia is known (vascular or degeneration of cerebral neurons), highly selective therapeutic agents are unlikely to treat all the symptoms. In recent years, it has become increasingly fashionable to attempt to develop selective therapeutic agents modulating specific neurotransmitter systems for the alleviation of the symptoms of dementia. However, to date these attempts have been unsuccessful. Agents which do not have one specific mechanism of action may prove to be more efficacious in the treatment of the symptoms of dementia. Indeed, the most commonly utilized agents for the treatment of the symptoms of senile dementia and chronic organic brain disease are still nootropics and metabolically active compounds.

Dementia: Molecules, Methods and Measures. Edited by I. Hindmarch, H. Hippius and G. K. Wilcock
© 1991 John Wiley & Sons Ltd

These agents have a diverse pharmacological profile. They are known to enhance cognition and to modulate cerebral blood flow and metabolism. It is the purpose of this review to compare the pharmacology of nootropics and metabolically active compounds in an attempt to explain their use in the treatment of age-associated mental disorders.

The therapeutic efficacy of nootropics and metabolically active compounds in the treatment of dementia is often questioned. However, it should be remembered that it is unlikely that any drug can attenuate the symptoms of the advanced stages of dementia. This is an important consideration when analysing the results obtained in clinical trials of agents of potential utility in the treatment of this disease. It is significant that nootropics and metabolically active compounds have shown positive results in trials performed with patients with chronic organic brain disease rather than with patients suffering from dementia of known aetiology. Chronic organic brain disease is of multiple aetiology and pathogenesis and usually deteriorates into more recognizable dementias (Kanowski, 1982). Hence, SDAT and vascular dementia can be regarded as severe stages of chronic organic brain disease (Kanowski, 1982). It is very possible that patients with chronic organic brain disease are more readily beneficially influenced by drug therapy than dementia patients. This is of obvious relevance when considering the pharmacology of nootropics and metabolically active compounds. Over the last few years, the evaluation of drugs for efficacy in patients suffering from dementia of known aetiology has increasingly become an absolute requirement. This is clearly necessary if we are to prove efficacy in a particular disease. However, as it may be much easier to treat the symptoms of chronic organic brain disease than dementia, there is potential danger of classifying drugs as inactive if they are only examined in clearly demonstrable cases of dementia.

Nootropics and Metabolically Active Compounds

The term nootropic is now extensively used to describe a wide range of chemically unrelated compounds with diverse pharmacological properties. It was originally introduced by Giurgea (1972, 1973) to describe the pharmacology of piracetam. For the purpose of this chapter, the term nootropic will be used to describe compounds which are either chemically related or have a very similar pharmacology to this compound. The structures of a number of nootropic agents are presented in Figure 1. Metabolically active compounds are a further diverse range of compounds used in the therapy of chronic organic brain diseases. This group of compounds includes the ergot alkaloids (Figure 2), the vinca alkaloids (Figure 3) and the alkylxanthines (Figure 4); this chapter will compare the pharmacology of these drugs as representative of this class of compound. Other drugs whose pharmacological profile is similar to the agents being reviewed here are idebenone (Moos *et al.*, 1988), bifemelane (Saito *et al.*, 1985; Schindler, 1989), indeloxazine (Schindler, 1989) and pyritinol (Martin, 1983). Although widely known as metabolic enhancers, these compounds have very diverse pharmacological activities and the extent to which these agents owe their clinical efficacy to a direct enhancement of cellular metabolism awaits clarification.

Effects on Cognition

Nootropics improve learning and memory in a variety of experimental paradigms (Moos *et al.*, 1988). In general, such effects are observed both in normal animals and in

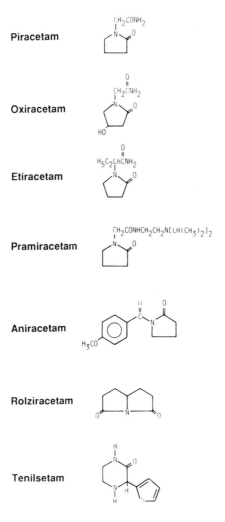

Figure 1. The chemical structure of nootropics

those in which a cognitive impairment has been induced by hypercapnia, scopolamine or cyclohexamide (Cumin *et al.*, 1982; Banfi and Dorigotti, 1984; Schindler *et al.*, 1989; Murray and Fibiger, 1986; Marriott *et al.*, 1984). Nootropics have been found to improve information acquisition, consolidation and retrieval and it is presently unclear which effect, if any, predominates. However, some reports indicate that an ability to improve information acquisition is particularly significant (Wolthuis, 1971). This is important as such results could have been influenced by effects of the compound on vigilance and attention rather than on memory formation or recall. Hence, the effects of nootropics on learning and memory still require further investigation and clarification. A hurdle in our understanding of the effect of nootropics on learning and memory is the lack of a clear hypothesis concerning their mechanism of action. However, recently the nootropics have been shown to augment long-term potentiation (LTP) of population spikes in the mossy fibres of the CA_3 system of the guinea-pig hippocampus

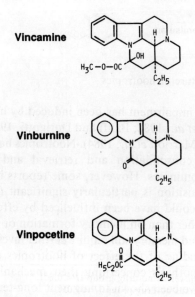

Co-Dergocrine

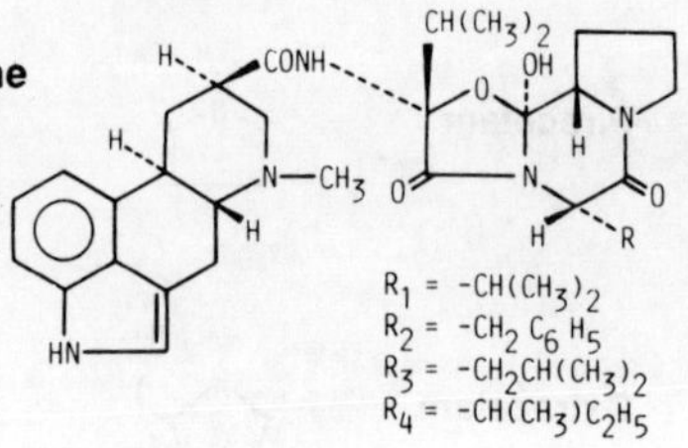

R₁ = -CH(CH₃)₂
R₂ = -CH₂C₆H₅
R₃ = -CH₂CH(CH₃)₂
R₄ = -CH(CH₃)C₂H₅

Nicergoline

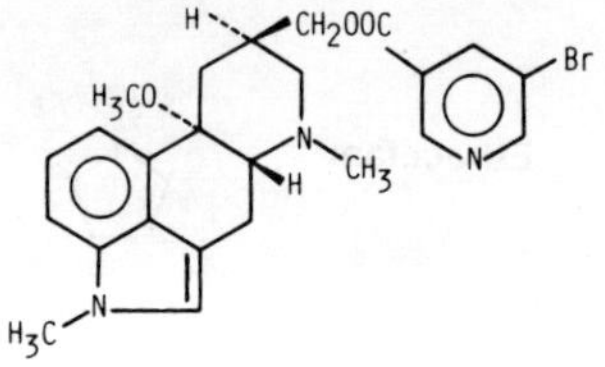

Figure 2. The chemical structure of ergot alkaloids

(Pugliese *et al.*, 1989; Satoh *et al.*, 1989; see Table 1). It is a matter of speculation how these compounds enhance hippocampal neuronal excitability. However, the fact that they do so may provide some explanation for the effect of these compounds on learning and memory. Recently aniracetam has been shown to selectively potentiate responses to AMPA (α-amino-3-hydroxy-5-methyl-4-isoxazole propionate) receptor stimulation in hippocampal slices (Ito *et al.*, 1990). Such activity will increase the responsiveness of the neurons to stimulation of other glutamate receptors such as those preferentially stimulated by NMDA (*N*-methyl-D-aspartic acid) and hence may explain the effects of nootropics on LTP.

Nootropics increase the release of dopamine from the cerebral cortex (Funk and Schmidt, 1984) and have at least an indirect potentiating effect on cholinergic function

Vincamine

Vinburnine

Vinpocetine

Figure 3. The chemical structure of vinca alkaloids

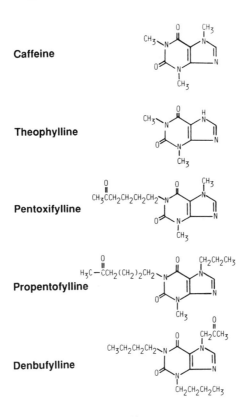

Figure 4. The chemical structure of alkylxanthines

Table 1. Effects of various drugs on the LTP of the population spike in the mossy fibre – CA_3 system of the guinea-pig hippocampus *in vitro*

Drug	Concentration (M)	Relative magnitude (No-drug group = 1.0)
Aniracetam	10^{-7}	3.1*
Piracetam	10^{-5}	3.3*
Bifemelane	10^{-6}	2.9*
Idebenone	10^{-7}	2.4*
Vinpocetine	10^{-7}	2.4*
Thyrotrophin-regulatory hormone	10^{-6}	2.0*
Imipramine	10^{-6}	1.6
Methamphetamine	10^{-6}	1.8*
Chlorpromazine	10^{-6}	1.0
Haloperidol	10^{-6}	1.0
Midazolam	10^{-9}	0.2†
Scopolamine	10^{-5}	0.0†

Note: *Significant augmentation versus no-drug group ($P < 0.05$).
   †Significant inhibition versus no-drug group ($P < 0.05$).
Source: Satoh *et al.* (1989).

24 *C. D. Nicholson*

in the brain (Poschel, 1988). As dopamine is believed to have a role in information acquisition (Iversen, 1977), enhancement of dopamine release may contribute to the beneficial effects of nootropics on memory formation. Cholinergic dysfunction is believed to play a central role in cognitive dysfunction in dementia (Bowen *et al.*, 1976; Perry, 1986; Hagen and Morris, 1988); therefore, the interplay between nootropics and the cholinergic system may also be involved in their mechanism of action.

Metabolically active compounds have been demonstrated to enhance cognition in a variety of experimental paradigms. Vinpocetine, co-dergocrine and denbufylline all enhance cognition in passive avoidance paradigms in which a learning or memory deficit has been induced by hypoxia, ischaemia or scopolamine (Schindler *et al.*, 1984; de Noble *et al.*, 1986; Nicholson *et al.*, 1989). The mechanisms of action of these compounds are not clearly understood. The results, however, indicate an effect on attention or memory formation in animal models of SDAT and multi-infarct dementia. Vinpocetine increases the turnover of brain catecholamine levels (Rosdy *et al.*, 1976; Kiss *et al.*, 1982) and enhances the increase in cortical cyclic AMP level produced by noradrenaline (Lapis *et al.*, 1979). Since it is thought that cortical dopamine and noradrenaline can modulate attention, learning and memory (Iversen, 1977), such activity, rather than a direct effect on cellular metabolism, may explain the effect of vinpocetine in passive avoidance tests.

Vinpocetine, the ergot alkaloids (including co-dergocrine) and alkylxanthines such as denbufylline reduce the rate of breakdown of cyclic nucleotides by inhibiting cyclic nucleotide phosphodiesterase isoenzymes (Table 2). Five distinct families of cyclic nucleotide phosphodiesterases have now been characterized, with differing regulatory characteristics and substrate specificities (Beavo and Reifsnyder, 1990; Nicholson *et al.*, 1990). At least three of these isoenzyme families identified are present in rat (Figure 5) and human cerebral cortex. Selective inhibitors of the different isoenzyme families have been identified and their ability to differentially modulate tissue function described (Nicholson *et al.*, 1990). The selectivity of the ergot alkaloids has been incompletely characterized; they have merely been shown to possess some selectivity for an isoenzyme

Table 2. The inhibition of cyclic nucleotide phosphodiesterase activities

Drug	IC_{50} or K_i (μM)			
	Ca^{2+}/calmodulin dependent PDE	High K_m cyclic AMP	Cyclic GMP stimulated PDE	Cyclic AMP PDE
Denbufylline*	>100		>100	0.7
Vinpocetine[†]	21		>500	>500
Co-dergocrine[‡] alkaloids:				
Dihydroergocritine		50		24
Dihydroergocornine		76		25
Dihydroergocryptine		35		0.4

Note: *Isoenzymes from rat cerebral cortex (Nicholson *et al.*, 1989).
[†]Isoenzymes from rabbit aorta (Hagiwara *et al.*, 1984).
[‡]Isoenzymes from rat hypothalmus (Venutti *et al.*, 1982). Values for low K_m cyclic AMP PDE are for a poorly resolved fraction which is probably a mixture of Ca^{2+}/calmodulin dependent PDE and cyclic GMP stimulated PDE, both of which have a high K_m for cyclic AMP in rat brain (Nicholson *et al.*, 1989).
PDE = phosphodiesterase.

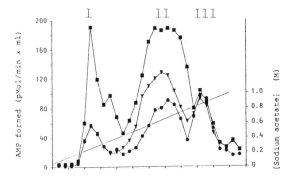

Figure 5. Separation profile of cyclic nucleotide phosphodiesterase activities from rat cerebral cortex. Fractions were assayed with 1 μmol/l cyclic AMP (●), 1 μmol/l cyclic AMP in the presence of Ca^{2+}/calmodulin (■) and 1 μmol/l cyclic GMP (▼). Peaks I and II are additionally stimulated by cyclic GMP; the activity of peak III is unaffected by both regulators. From Nicholson *et al.* (1989)

with a high affinity for cyclic AMP. In contrast, vinpocetine selectively inhibits the Ca^{2+}/calmodulin-dependent isoenzyme, whilst denbufylline selectively inhibits the cerebral cyclic AMP high affinity isoenzyme. The denbufylline-sensitive isoenzyme has been demonstrated to be an important regulator of cyclic AMP metabolism in the cerebral cortex of animals (Nicholson *et al.*, 1989; Challiss and Nicholson, 1990) and man (Wilke, 1990). The vinpocetine-sensitive isoenzyme is present in the cerebral cortex but the importance of this isoenzyme for cyclic nucleotide hydrolysis is incompletely characterized. As inhibition of these isoenzymes stimulates tyrosine hydroxylase (Tank and Weiner, 1981; Kehr *et al.*, 1985) and increases the release of noradrenaline and dopamine from brain slices (Schoffelmeer *et al.*, 1985), inhibition of cyclic nucleotide phosphodiesterase may account for the effects of these compounds on brain catecholamine turnover and cortical cyclic AMP levels. Second messenger systems, such as the one involving cyclic AMP, have been postulated to play an important role in learning and memory (Goelet *et al.*, 1986; Abrams and Kandel, 1988). Although the cellular mechanisms involved in short-term, intermediate and long-term memory formation have not been elucidated, cyclic AMP-mediated modulation of protein kinases and the expression of genes from the cell nucleus are believed to be involved (Goelet *et al.*, 1986). More extensive evaluation of the role played by second messenger systems in memory formation will clarify the role played by cyclic AMP in cognition and may prove to be a rewarding area of future research. Denbufylline has recently been demonstrated to enhance the excitability of hippocampal neurons (Sutor *et al.*, 1990). As the neuronal excitability in the hippocampus is believed to be involved in memory formation, this finding may help clarify the effects of denbufylline and other similar phosphodiesterase inhibitors such as rolipram (Moos *et al.*, 1988) and possibly vinpocetine and co-dergocrine on cognition.

Effects on Cerebral Blood Flow and Metabolism

In contrast to the metabolically active compounds, the nootropics have no marked effects on cerebral blood flow.

Metabolically active compounds do modulate tissue blood flow in animals (Nicholson, 1990). However, because vasodilator therapy is unlikely to be beneficial and may even be contraindicated in the treatment of dementia (Hachinski et al., 1974; Hossmann, 1982; Mohs and Davis, 1987), such activity is unlikely to contribute to their clinical utility. Indeed, it is important to demonstrate that compounds which possess vasodilator activity do not cause a further reduction in blood flow and nutrient supply to underperfused areas of the brain. In an animal model in which vasodilators such as nimodipine and papaverine cause such a further deterioration of flow and nutrient supply, co-dergocrine and the alkylxanthines pentoxifylline and denbufylline actually increase the oxygen tension of the oligaemic cerebral cortex (Nicholson and Angersbach, 1986); the vinca alkaloid vinpocetine has been shown not to produce a stealing of blood away from underperfused areas of brain in patients suffering from cerebrovascular disease (Heiss and Podreka, 1981). Why some vasoactive compounds cause a further deterioration of blood flow in partially ischaemic tissue, whereas others actually increase blood flow, is unknown. One possibility is that the ability of some of these compounds to improve blood rheology (Nicholson, 1990), an effect which can be expected to increase blood flow through oligaemic tissue, is important. Alternatively, because metabolic stimulation may recruit a vascular reserve not normally influenced by vasodilator drugs, the ability of some compounds to stimulate cellular metabolism could be significant.

The most direct evidence that compounds possess metabolic activity is provided by investigations examining their effect on respiratory rate in mitochondrial suspensions (MacKenzie et al., 1984). Such experiments have shown that vinca and ergot alkaloids, but not the alkylxanthine pentoxifylline, increase the mitochondrial respiratory rate in vitro. Animal experiments have shown agents such as the vinca alkaloids vinpocetine and vinburnine to increase cerebral oxygen and glucose consumption (Karpati and Szporny, 1976; Lacroix et al., 1979). In addition, vinca alkaloids, ergot alkaloids and alkylxanthines attenuate the effects of cerebral metabolic depressants such as triethyl tin (Lamar et al., 1986; Nicholson and Angersbach, 1986). Such metabolic activity may explain the ability of compounds such as co-dergocrine and vinpocetine to prolong the survival time in animals following periods of hypoxia (Lamar et al., 1986; King, 1987a,b). However, many such compounds reduce body temperature and stimulate respiration, both of which are sufficient to influence survival times in these tests (King, 1987a; Cartheuser, 1988). Consequently, data from such experiments should be extrapolated with caution to man. However, at least vinpocetine and vinburnine have been demonstrated to produce a greater prolongation of survival time following periods of anoxia in mice than can be explained by their hypothermic effects alone (King, 1987b).

The nootropics have also been reported to enhance cerebral metabolic activity (Moyersoons and Giurgea, 1974; Nickolson and Wolthius, 1976; Milanova et al., 1983). It is unknown whether the mechanism of action of the compounds in these tests is related to their effects on cognition or whether a further mechanism of action is responsible for these effects. Piracetam stimulates adenylate kinase (Nickolson and Wolthius, 1976) and thus may be expected to maintain tissue ATP levels in undernourished (ischaemic) tissue. This could explain the activity of piracetam in tests designed to show protective activity under conditions of hypoxia.

Neuronal Protection

In addition to effects on cognition and cerebral blood flow and metabolism, some, but not all, of the metabolic enhancing compounds have been demonstrated to protect hippocampal neurons from the deleterious effects of ischaemia. In particular, such effects have been reported for the alkylxanthine propentofylline (de Leo *et al.*, 1987) and the vinca alkaloid vinpocetine (Sauer *et al.*, 1988). Reports are not available on the effects of nootropics in such tests.

The mechanism of action of vinpocetine and propentofylline awaits clarification. It is, however, possibly significant that both these compounds inhibit the cellular reuptake of adenosine (Fredholm *et al.*, 1983; Stefanovich, 1983). Propentofylline has recently been shown to increase extracellular adenosine levels during cerebral ischaemia (Andine *et al.*, 1990). The excessive release of glutamate and stimulation of postsynaptic NMDA receptors, with a consequent massive influx of Ca^{2+}, is believed to be the cause of neuronal death following cerebral ischaemia (Cotman and Iversen, 1987; Marangos *et al.*, 1987). Since adenosine can inhibit the postsynaptic Ca^{2+} influx elicited by NMDA receptor stimulation (Schubert and Kreutzberg, 1987), an increase in the extracellular concentration of adenosine, induced by inhibition of cellular reuptake, would be expected to protect neurons from the effects of ischaemia. This postulate is supported by the fact that theophylline, an adenosine receptor antagonist, actually potentiates ischaemia-induced neuronal damage (Rudolphi *et al.*, 1987).

The ability of these compounds to reduce neuronal cell loss in the hippocampus is potentially useful in the treatment of vascular dementia. Furthermore, because cell loss in the hippocampus occurs during the early stages of SDAT, it may also be relevant to the use of such agents in the treatment of neuronal dementia. Neuronal protective activity may not lead to an immediate improvement in the patient's condition, but may rather attenuate the progression of the disorder. Clinical trials are normally designed to show an improvement in the patient's condition rather than a reduction in the rate of disease progression, and it is possible that neuronal protective activity is often overlooked in such trials. Such effects of vinpocetine and propentofylline have, however, only been reported in animal models in which global cerebral ischaemia is followed by reperfusion. These models may be of dubious relevance to conditions in which focal ischaemia persists. Neuronal protection under such conditions has yet to be reported.

Conclusion

In conclusion, the available data on nootropics and metabolically active compounds indicates that, in animals, they can influence cognition. However, it is more difficult to decide if this is mediated via a direct effect on the laying down or recall of memory or if it is an indirect effect produced through increased vigilance. The influence of these compounds on cognition may be explicable by their effects on cerebral neurotransmitter release or turnover. The nootropics have been described as affecting cholinergic, dopaminergic and noradrenergic transmission. The metabolically active compounds modulate aminergic transmitter release and can modulate the response to glutamatergic transmission. Potentially, inhibition of cyclic nucleotide phosphodiesterase may be involved in these effects of metabolically active compounds. Clearly, however, more detailed studies are required to analyse the relative importance of these differing activities more carefully. Effects on diverse neurotransmitter systems may beneficially influence not only cognitive dysfunction in patients with dementia but also disturbances in mood.

Many metabolically active compounds are vasodilators and increase cerebral blood flow; however, it is unlikely that this contributes to any beneficial effect of these compounds in dementia. Indeed, vasodilator activity may be contraindicated in compounds used in the treatment of dementia.

The pharmacology of nootropics and metabolically active compounds is complex. They have several mechanisms of action. Possibly because they do not have a clear mechanism of action, these agents have been discarded by many research groups as interesting lead compounds in the search for novel and more effective anti-dementia agents. It is presently fashionable to investigate increasingly selective agents (e.g. M_1 muscarinic receptor agonists or glutamatergic agents) for use in the treatment of dementia. However, dementia is a complex disease involving dysfunction of diverse neuronal circuits. It is unlikely that a very selective drug will treat all aspects of the disease. Compounds which have an ability to modulate several effector systems may prove to be the most useful agents. Research aimed at increasing our understanding of the action of the nootropics and metabolically active drugs may yet yield more effective agents for the treatment of at least the milder forms of chronic organic brain disease. In addition to effects on cognition, these compounds also protect the brain from physical and chemical damage. This activity may be a useful facet in the mechanism of action of these compounds as it may delay the progression of dementia pathology. The mechanism of action of the nootropics in such tests is unknown. However, in the case of vinpocetine and propentofylline, inhibition of the cellular reuptake of adenosine may be responsible for the neuronal protective effects.

References

Abrams, T. W. and Kandel, E. R. (1988) Is contiguity detection in classical conditioning a system or a cellular property? Learning in aplysia suggests a possible molecular site. *Trends Neurosci.*, **11**, 128–35.
Andine, P., Rudolphi, K. A., Fredholm, B. B. and Hagberg, H. (1990) Effect of propentofylline (HWA 285) on extracellular purines and excitatory amino acids in CA1 of rat hippocampus during transient ischaemia. *Br. J. Pharmacol.*, **100**, 814–18.
Banfi, S. and Dorigotti, L. (1984) Experimental behavioral studies with oxiracetam on different types of chronic cerebral impairment. *Clin. Neuropharmacol.*, **7**(1, suppl.), 768–9.
Beavo, J. A. and Reifsnyder, D. H. (1990) Primary sequence of cyclic nucleotide phosphodiesterase isozymes and the design of selective inhibitors. *Trends Pharmacol. Sci.*, **11**, 150–5.
Bowen, D. M., Smith, C. D., White, P. and Davidson, A. W. (1976) Neurotransmitter related enzymes and indices of hypoxia in senile dementia and other abiatrophies. *Brain*, **99**, 459–96.
Cartheuser, C. F. (1988) Slow channel inhibitor effects on brain function: tolerance to severe hypoxia in the rat. *Br. J. Pharmacol.* **95**, 903–13.
Challiss, R. A. J. and Nicholson, C. D. (1990) Effects of selective phosphodiesterase inhibitors on cyclic AMP hydrolysis in rat cerebral cortical slices. *Br. J. Pharmacol.*, **99**, 47–52.
Cotman, C. W. and Iversen, L. L. (1987) Excitatory amino acids in the brain – focus on NMDA receptors. *Trends Neurosci.*, **10**, 263–5.
Cumin, R., Bandle, E. F., Gamzu, E. and Haefely, W. E. (1982) Effects of the novel compound aniracetum (Ro 13-5057) upon impaired learning and memory in rodents. *Psychopharmacology*, **78**, 104–11.
de Leo, J., Toth, L., Schubert, P., Rudolphi, K. and Kreutzberg, G. W. (1987) Ischaemia-induced neuronal cell death, calcium accumulation and glial response in the hippocampus of the Mongolian gerbil and protection by propentofylline (HWA 285). *J. Cereb. Blood Flow Metab.*, **7**, 745–51.

de Noble, V., Repetti, S. J., Gelpke, L. W., Wood, L. M. and Keim, K. L. (1986) Vinpocetine: nootropic effects on scopolomine-induced and hypoxia-induced retrieval deficits of a step-through passive avoidance response in rats. *Pharmacol. Biochem. Behav.*, **24**, 1123–8.

Fredholm, B. B., Lindgren, E., Lindstrom, L. and Vernet, L. (1983) The effects of some drugs with purported antianoxic effect in veratridine-induced purine release from isolated rat hypothalamic synaptosomes. *Acta Pharmacol. Toxicol.*, **52**, 236–44.

Funk, K. F. and Schmidt, J. (1984) Changes of dopamine metabolism by hypoxia and effect of nootropic drugs. *Biomed. Biochem. Acta*, **11**, 1301–4.

Giurgea, C. (1972) Pharmacology of integrative activity of the brain. Attempt at nootropic concept in psychopharmacology. *Actual. Pharmacol.*, **25**, 115–56.

Giurgea, G. (1973) The 'nootropic' approach to the pharmacology of the integrative activity of the brain. *Cond. Reflex*, **8**, 108–15.

Goelet, P., Castellucci, U. F., Schacher, S. G. and Kandel, E. R. (1986) The long and the short of long term memory – a molecular framework. *Nature*, **322**, 419–22.

Hachinski, V. C., Lassen, N. A. and Marshall, J. (1974) Multi-infarct dementia: a cause of mental deterioration in the elderly. *Lancet*, **ii**, 207–10.

Hagan, J. J. and Morris, R. G. M. (1988) The cholinergic hypothesis of memory: a review of animal experiments. In: Iversen, L. L., Iversen, S. D. and Snyder, S. H. (eds) *Handbook of Psycho-pharmacology*, Vol. 20, pp. 237–324. New York: Plenum Press.

Hagiwara, M., Endo, T. and Hidaka, H. (1984) Effects of vinpocetine on cyclic nucleotide metabolism in vascular smooth muscle. *Biochem. Pharmacol.*, **33**, 453–7.

Heiss, W. D. and Podreka, I. (1981) *Die Wirkung von Vinpocetin auf die regionale Hirndurchblutung bei Patienten mit chronisch-Zerebrova skulaffen Erkrankungen mit der intravenosen Xenon-clearance-methode*. Report for Thiemman Pharmaceuticals.

Hossmann, K. A. (1982) Treatment of experimental cerebral ischemia. *J. Cereb. Blood Flow Metab.*, **2**, 275–97.

Ito, I., Tanabe, S., Kolnda, A. and Sugiyama, H. (1990) Allosteric potentiation of quinqualate receptors by a nootropic drug aniracetam. *J. Physiol.*, **424**, 533–43.

Iversen, S. D. (1977) Brain dopamine systems and behaviour. In: Iversen, L. L., Iversen, S. D. and Snyder, S. H. (eds) *Handbook of Psychopharmacology*, Vol. 8, pp. 333–85. New York: Plenum Press.

Kanowski, S. (1982) Clinical and pathological aspects of chronic organic brain syndrome. *Exp. Brain Res.*, suppl. 5, 223–34.

Karpati, E. and Szporny, L. (1976) General and cerebral haemodynamic activity of ethyl apovincaminate. *Arzneimittelforschung*, **26**, 1908–11.

Kehr, W., Debus, G. and Neumeister, R. (1985) Effects of rolipram, a novel antidepressant on monoamine metabolism in rat brain. *J. Neural Transm.*, **63**, 1–12.

King, G. A. (1987a) Protection against hypoxia-induced lethality in mice: comparison of the effects of hypothermia and drugs. *Arch. Int. Pharmacodyn. Ther.*, **286**, 282–98.

King, G. A. (1987b) Protective effects of vinpocetine and structurally related drugs on the lethal consequences of hypoxia in mice. *Arch. Int. Pharmacodyn. Ther.*, **286**, 299–307.

Kiss, B., Lapis, E., Palosi, E., Groo, D. and Szporny, L. (1982) Biochemical and pharmacological observations with vinpocetine, a cerebral oxygenator. In: Wauquier, A., Borgers, M. and Amery, W. K. (eds) *Protection of Tissues against Hypoxia, Vol. 7: International Symposium on Protection of Tissues against Hypoxia*, pp. 305–9. Amsterdam: Elsevier.

Lacroix, P., Quiniou, M. J., Linee, P. and Le Polles, J. B. (1979) Cerebral metabolic and haemodynamic activities of L-eburnamonine in the anaesthetized dog. *Arzneimittelforschung*, **29**, 94–101.

Lamar, J. C., Beaughard, M., Bromont, C. and Poignet, H. (1986) Effects of vinpocetine in four pharmacological methods of cerebral ischaemia. In: Krieglstein, J. (ed.) *Pharmacology of Cerebral Ischaemia*, pp. 334–9. Amsterdam: Elsevier.

Lapis, E., Balazs, Z. M. and Rosdy, B. (1979) Biochemical effects of semi-synthetic vinca alkaloids on the cyclic AMP system. Third Congress of the Hungarian Pharmacology Society, pp. 429–33.

MacKenzie, E. T., Gotti, B., Nowieki, J.-P. and Young, A. R. (1984) Adrenergic blockers as cerebral antiischaemic agents. In: Mackenzie, E. T. (ed.) *L.E.R.S.*, Vol. 2, pp. 219–43. New York: Raven Press.

Marangos, W. F., Greenamyre, T., Penney, J. B. and Young, A. B. (1987) Glutamate dysfunction in Alzheimer's disease: a hypothesis. *Trends Neurosci.*, **10**, 65–8.

Marriott, J. G., Poschel, B. P. H., Voigtman, R. E., Abelson, J. S. and Butler, D. E. (1984) Cognition actuating properties of dihydro-pyrrolizine 3,5 (2H, 6H)-dione (CI-911) in animal models. *Soc. Neurosci. Abstra.*, **10**, 252.

Martin, K. J. (1983) On the mechanism of action of Encephabol. *J. Int. Med. Res.*, **11**, 55–65.

Milanova, D., Nikolov, R. and Nikolova, M. (1983) Study on the anti-hypoxic effect of some drugs used in the pharmacotherapy of cerebrovascular disease. *Methods Find. Exp. Clin. Pharmacol.*, **5**, 407–22.

Mohs, R. C. and Davis, K. L. (1987) The experimental pharmacology of Alzheimer's and related dementias. In: Meltzer, H. (ed.) *Psychopharmacology, the Third Generation of Progress*, pp. 921–8. New York: Raven Press.

Moos, W. H., Davis, R. E., Schwartz, R. D. and Gamzu, E. R. (1988) Cognition activators. *Med. Res. Rev.*, **8**, 353–91.

Moyersoons, F. and Giurgea, C. E. (1974) Protective effect of piracetam in experimental barbiturate intoxication: EEG and behavioural studies. *Arch. Int. Pharmacodyn. Ther.*, **210**, 38–48.

Murray, C. L. and Fibiger, H. C. (1986) The effect of pramiracetam (CI-879) on the acquisition of a radial arm maze task. *Psychopharmacology*, **89**, 378–81.

Nicholson, C. D. (1990) Pharmacology of nootropics and metabolically active compounds in relation to their use in dementia. *Psychopharmacology*, **101**, 147–59.

Nicholson, C. D. and Angersbach, D. (1986) Denbufylline (BRL 30892) – a novel drug to alleviate the consequences of cerebral ischaemia. In: Krieglstein, J. (ed.) *Pharmacology of Cerebral Ischaemia*, pp. 371–96. Amsterdam: Elsevier.

Nicholson, C. D., Jackman, S. A. and Wilke, R. (1989) The ability of denbufylline to inhibit cyclic nucleotide phosphodiesterase and its affinity for adenosine receptors and the adenosine re-uptake site. *Br. J. Pharmacol.*, **97**, 889–97.

Nicholson, C. D., Challiss, R. A. J. and Shahid, M. (1991) Differential modulation of tissue function and the therapeutic potential of selective inhibitors of cyclic nucleotide phosphodiesterase isoenzymes. *Trends Pharmacol. Sci.*, **12**, 20–7.

Nickolson, V. J. and Wolthuis, O. L. (1976) Effect of the acquisition enhancing drug piracetam on rat cerebral energy metabolism. Comparison with naftidrofuryl and methamphetamine. *Biochem. Pharmacol.*, **25**, 2241–4.

Palmer, A. M. and Gershorn, S. (1990) Is the neuronal basis of Alzheimer's disease cholinergic or glutamatergic. *FASEB J.*, **4**, 2745–52.

Perry, E. (1986) The cholinergic hypothesis – ten years on. *Br. Med. Bull.*, **42**, 63–9.

Poschel, B. (1988) New pharmacological perspectives on nootropic drugs. In: Iversen, C. L. and Iversen, S. D. (eds) *Handbook of Psychopharmacology*, Vol. 20, pp. 437–69. New York: Plenum Publishing.

Pugliese, A. M., Corradetti, R. and Pepeu, G. (1989) Effect of the cognition enhancing agent oxiracetam on electrical activity of hipocampal slices. *Br. J. Pharmacol.*, **96**, 80P.

Rosdy, B., Balazs, M. and Spzorny, L. (1976) Biochemical effects of ethyl apovincaminate. *Arzneimittelforschung*, **26**, 1973–6.

Rudolphi, K. A., Keil, M. and Hinze, H. J. (1987) Effect of theophylline on ischemically induced hippocampal damage in Mongolian gerbils: a behavioral and histopathological study. *J. Cereb. Blood Flow Metab.*, **7**, 74–81.

Saito, K., Honda, S., Egawa, M. and Tobe, A. (1985) Effects of bifemelane hydrochloride (MC1 20104) on acetylcholine release from cortical and hippocampal slices. *Jpn. J. Pharmacol.*, **39**, 410–4.

Satoh, M., Ishihara, K. and Katsuki, H. (1989) A pharmacological profile of LTP in CA_3 region of guinea-pig hippocampus in vitro. *Biomed. Res.*, **10**(2, suppl.), 125–9.

Sauer, D., Rischke, R., Beck, T., Rossberg, C., Mennel, H. D., Bielenberg, C. W. and Krieglstein, J. (1988) Vinpocetine prevents ischemic cell damage in rat hippocampus. *Life Sci.*, **43**, 1733–9.

Schindler, U. (1989) Pre-clinical evaluation of cognition enhancing drugs. *Prog. Neuropsychopharmacol. Biol. Psychiatry*, **13**, S99–S115.

Schindler, U., Rush, D. and Fielding, S. (1984) Nootropic drugs: animal models for studying effect on cognition. *Drug Dev. Res.*, **4**, 567–76.

Schoffelmeer, A. N. M., Wardeh, G. and Mulder, A. H. (1985) Cyclic AMP facilitates the electrically evoked release of radiolabelled noradrenaline, dopamine and 5-hydroxytryptamine from rat brain slices. *Naunyn Schmiedebergs Arch. Pharmacol.*, **330**, 74–6.

Schubert, P. and Kreutzberg, G. W. (1987) Pre- versus post-synaptic effects of adenosine on neuronal calcium fluxes. In: Gerlach, E. and Becker, B. F. (eds) *Topics and Perspectives in Adenosine Research*, pp. 521–32. Berlin, Heidelberg: Springer.

Stefanovich, V. (1983) Uptake of adenosine by isolated bovine cortex microvessels. *Neurochem. Res.*, **11**, 1459–69.

Sutor, B., Alzheimer, C., Ameri, A. and ten Bruggencate, G. (1990) The low K_m phosphodiesterase inhibitor denbufylline enhances excitability in guinea-pig hippocampal slices. *Naunyn Schmiedebergs Arch. Pharmacol.*, **342**, 349–56.

Tank, A. W. and Weiner, N. (1981) Effect of carbachol and 56 mM potassium chloride on the cyclic AMP-mediated induction of tyrosine hydroxylase in neuroblastoma cells in culture. *J. Neurochem.*, **36**, 518–31.

Venutti, P., Ferretti, C. and Porteleone, P. (1982) Ergot alkaloids and phosphodiesterase; 'in vitro' activities in several rat 'brain areas'. *Experientia*, **38**, 601–3.

Wilke, R. (1990) The selective inhibition of cyclic nucleotide phosphodiesterase isoenzymes from human brain by denbufylline. *Eur. J. Pharmacol.*, **183**, 1367.

Wolthuis, O. L. (1971) Experiments with UCB 6215, a drug which enhances acquisition in rats: its effects compared with those of metamphetamine. *Eur. J. Pharmacol.*, **16**, 283–97.

3

New Anti-dementia Molecules

Brenda Costall and Robert J. Naylor

The School of Pharmacy, University of Bradford, UK

Historical Approaches to Preclinical Work

Batteries of animal cognitive tests based on different aspects of cognitive performance, whether the test be based on reference or working memory, with spatial cues included or not, have met with limited success in terms of the development of new anti-dementia molecules. This probably reflects the approaches taken to the development of new molecules. If one accepts that the core symptoms of cognitive disorders relate to a loss of limbic and cerebral acetylcholine function (see review by Bartus *et al.*, 1982), the past approaches of searching for compounds which will directly enhance cerebral cholinergic function would appear eminently sensible. However, such approaches have been hampered by the lack of specifity of the cholinomimetics for the central nervous system and, on the whole, peripheral side effects have thwarted the progression of potential cognitive enhancing drugs to the clinic (Giacobini, 1987; Heise, 1987; Moos *et al.*, 1988).

Clues as to new potential approaches to the enhancement of cerebral cholinergic function were derived from tests on novel compounds which could selectively influence cerebral 5-hydroxytryptamine (5-HT). It would appear that within the limbic-cortical circuitry, important for the control of mood, emotion and cognitive performance, the receptor sites linked to the 5-HT system which influence mood and emotion are of the 5-HT$_3$ subtype. Thus, 5-HT$_3$ receptor antagonists are able to reduce anxiety in animals, and are able to reduce the behavioural consequences of a mesolimbic dopamine excess designed to mimic the situation thought to pertain in schizophrenia (see review by Costall *et al.*, 1990b). The neurotransmitters involved in anxiety and schizophrenia may differ, but the 5-HT$_3$ receptor antagonists are still able to correct the disturbed neurotransmission. This has lead to the concept that antagonists at the 5-HT$_3$ receptor are able to correct disturbed limbic-cortical function without affecting normal

Dementia: Molecules, Methods and Measures. Edited by I. Hindmarch, H. Hippius and G. K. Wilcock
© 1991 John Wiley & Sons Ltd

neurotransmitter processes. It is certainly a pleasing hypothesis that drugs can be developed for mental illness which become effective only in disease, and it is not surprising that this group of 5-HT$_3$ receptor antagonists have created worldwide interest and have stimulated extensive clinical trials to establish whether or not the potential promised by the preclinical work occurs in humans. The first clinical report that a 5-HT$_3$ receptor antagonist had anxiolytic activity (Lecrubier *et al.*, 1990) has thus been met with considerable interest, and the results of other trials now nearing completeness are awaited eagerly.

What is the link with novel anti-dementia molecules? Firstly, it should be remembered that cognitive disturbances contribute to part of the symptomatology of the mental diseases for which the 5-HT$_3$ receptor antagonists have been forwarded as potential new therapy. Secondly, the brain circuitry involved with, say, anxiety and psychosis clearly has parallels with those disturbed in cognitive disorders. Hence, if 5-HT$_3$ receptor antagonists are able to correct the neuronal disturbances associated with mood/emotional disorders, is it possible that they may also influence disturbed acetylcholine function?

The concept of compounds being able to correct a disturbed limbic-cortical neuro-transmission caught the imagination of many neuroscientists, and many other approaches to that revealed via the 5-HT system have been explored. One approach emerged from clinical observations. In man, the angiotensin-converting enzyme (ACE) inhibitors have been used for the treatment of hypertension. The prototype compound, captopril, subsequently became the subject of a quality of life study in which it was compared with methyldopa and propranolol. The question was raised as to why patients taking captopril felt better than those on the more traditional treatments (Croog *et al.*, 1986). First thoughts were that the side effects of captopril were markedly less than for the older compounds. Nevertheless, there appeared to be clues that the feeling of 'well-being' associated with captopril therapy may have more important psychopharmacological implications (Etienne and Zubensko, 1987). This was subsequently shown to be the case – captopril and other ACE inhibitors were found to have anxiolytic properties in animal models (Costall *et al.*, 1990a). The subsequent stages of preclinical work addressed the question as to whether the feeling of well-being also reflected improved cognitive performance.

This chapter describes the tests which have been developed or utilized to demonstrate that both the 5-HT$_3$ receptor antagonists and the ACE inhibitors have cognitive enhancing potential. These findings fulfil the hypothesis posed above, and provide novel approaches to the treatment of cognitive disorders.

The Animal Tests

Tests have been developed which utilize mouse, rat and marmoset. The first test to be employed was a simple mouse procedure using a black and white test box. The test is based on the aversive properties of the white, brightly lit compartment of a two-compartment box in which the less aversive black, dimly lit area is simultaneously available via a door located at floor level in the partition between the two compartments. Initially, mice taken from dark home conditions, in a dark container, to the dark test room, and placed in the centre of the brightly lit compartment will move carefully around the edges of the light compartment until the doorway into the less aversive dark is located. They then enter the dark where they spend the majority of the test period time, and in which they exhibit most exploratory behaviour. The latency for the initial move from the light to the dark on the first day of test is in the order of 12 s. When placed in the box on a daily basis young adult mice slowly learn to locate the doorway to the dark more rapidly, and by the fourth and fifth day of test the latency of the initial move is reduced to some 2–3 s. This habituation pattern is impaired by scopolamine, by lesions of the nucleus basalis (the area providing cortical and limbic cholinergic innervation) and in old age (Barnes *et al.*, 1990). The questions which we have posed are whether the impairments in performance can be attenuated by 5-HT₃ receptor antagonists or ACE inhibitors. Further, could such compounds even improve the basal habituation patterns? We have analysed the actions of a wide variety of 5-HT₃ receptor antagonists and ACE inhibitors, but in this chapter we concentrate on the compounds most advanced at the clinical level – ondansetron (a 5-HT₃ receptor antagonist) and ceranapril (an ACE inhibitor). The latter compound was selected for development because it was found to penetrate the brain well (Cushman *et al.*, 1990) and subsequently it was shown that doses which caused marked functional changes in the brain were many orders of magnitude lower than those which had any influence on blood pressure (Costall *et al.*, 1989). Indeed, the safety margin is such that influence on blood pressure is not a problem to be considered as regards the activity of ceranapril on mood and emotion or on cognitive performance. The novel compound Hoe 065, which is structurally related to ACE inhibitors, has also been reported to improve learning and memory in the rodent without producing cardiovascular effects (Hock *et al.*, 1989).

To complement the mouse studies two approaches have been used in rat, one utilizing a T maze reinforced alternation task and one assessing performance in a water maze. The T maze task was essentially that described by Salamone *et al.* (1982), with some minor methodological changes. Food was withdrawn from the animals 2 days prior to testing for 23 h each day. The rats were then required to learn a task in which they ran down one arm of a T and then selected either the right or left arm of the T to gain a banana-flavoured food pellet as reward. Animals were first given a clue on the direction to move by use of a barrier. On the next run they must move opposite to the direction first indicated by the barrier, i.e. they must alternate in a random manner defined by the barrier position. Over a period of some days the animals achieve over 80% correct responses. This can be subject to impairments by agents such as scopolamine.

In the water maze task, a modification of that described by Morris (1984), rats are required to locate a submerged island in an opaque fluid by developing strategies from spatial cues. Animals are allowed to explore the pool and are then introduced to the island. In a relatively short time (1–2 days with repeated testing) rats develop a strategy for locating the island speedily regardless of the quadrant of the pool from which they start the search. This behaviour is also highly susceptible to impairment by scopolamine.

The marmoset test is somewhat more complex, but requires that an animal selects between two junk objects to gain a food reward (marmosets will work for 'tempting' food rewards without food deprivation). The rewarded object is moved from left to right in the Wisconsin Test Apparatus to a pseudo-random schedule, and the animal is required to select the correct object on six consecutive occasions. The rewarded object is then changed (same day reversal paradigm) and the marmoset must then abandon the contingency learned immediately prior, and must change strategy to select the new object to the same criterion of six consecutive correct responses. Marmosets which have been trained can perform the initial task with efficiency, but find the reversal task

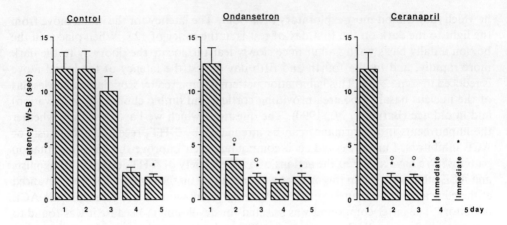

Figure 1. The abilities of ondansetron and ceranapril to improve mouse habituation performance. Young adult mice received daily injections of vehicle (control), ondansetron (10 ng/kg i.p. b.d.) or ceranapril (50 ng/kg i.p. b.d.) for 5 days and the latency of movement from the white (W) to the black (B) section of the test box recorded. Each value is the mean ±S.E.M. of five determinations. * indicates a significant reduction in latency compared with day 1 values ($P < 0.001$); ° indicates improved performance versus control values ($P < 0.001$) (one-way ANOVA followed by Dunnett's t test); 'immediate' indicates an immediate movement from the white to the black section

far more difficult, and make far more errors on the reversal task before criterion is reached (Barnes *et al.*, 1990). One can use this difficult reversal paradigm to assess the action of potential cognitive enhancers.

Preclinical Indicators of Cognitive Enhancing Potential

Using the mouse habituation paradigm it can be shown that young adult mice 'learn' to locate a less aversive environment on repeat exposure over 4 days. The initial latency to move from the white to the black compartment is reduced from 12–13 s on day 1 to 2–3 s on day 4 (Figure 1). Treatment with either ondansetron or ceranapril at subanxiolytic doses (10 ng/kg and 50 ng/kg i.p. b.d., respectively) improves habituation performance such that by day 2 animals are performing as well as normal, untreated animals on day 4 (Figure 1). This ability to rapidly locate the door to the less aversive compartment can be dramatic in that mice can move so speedily that they have located the dark compartment before activation of the remote video recorder. This is indicated on the figures as 'immediate'.

The ability of mice to habituate to the black and white box is impaired by scopolamine given twice daily at a dose which does not seriously interfere with autonomic function (measured by pupil diameter). The impairments caused by scopolamine are inhibited by both ondansetron and ceranapril, again at very low doses, such that habituation patterns are reinstated and, indeed, mice perform extremely efficiently (Figure 2). Scopolamine can also be given acutely to cause a transient impairment of habituation performance and this again can be inhibited by low doses of ondansetron or ceranapril (Figure 3). A more permanent impairment of habituation patterns is caused by lesions of the nucleus basalis magnocellularis, the cell body area providing major cholinergic

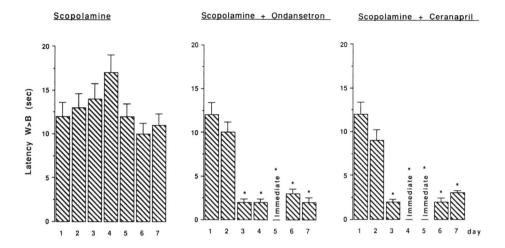

Figure 2. The abilities of ondansetron and ceranapril to inhibit chronic scopolamine impairment of mouse habituation performance. Young adult mice received daily injections of scopolamine (0.25 mg/kg i.p. b.d.) plus vehicle, ondansetron (10 ng/kg i.p. b.d.) or ceranapril (50 ng/kg i.p. b.d.) for 7 days and the latency of movement from the white (W) to the black (B) section of the test box recorded. Each value is the mean ±S.E.M. of five determinations. * indicates a significant reduction in scopolamine impairment ($P<0.001$)(one-way ANOVA followed by Dunnett's *t* test); 'immediate' indicates an immediate movement from the white to the black section

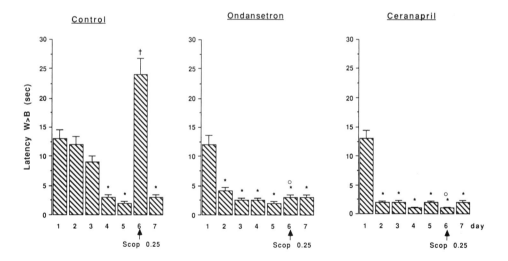

Figure 3. The abilities of ondansetron and ceranapril to inhibit an acute scopolamine impairment of mouse habituation performance. Young adult mice received injections of vehicle (control), ondansetron (10 ng/kg i.p. b.d.) or ceranapril (50 ng/kg i.p. b.d.) for 7 days; on the sixth day of treatment they also received scopolamine (Scop) (0.25 mg/kg i.p.). The latency of movement from the white (W) to the black (B) section of the test box was recorded. Each value is the mean ±S.E.M. of five determinations. * indicates a significant increase in performance relative to day 1 values ($P<0.001$); ° indicates antagonism of the scopolamine impairment relative to the control values ($P<0.001$) (one-way ANOVA followed by Dunnett's *t* test)

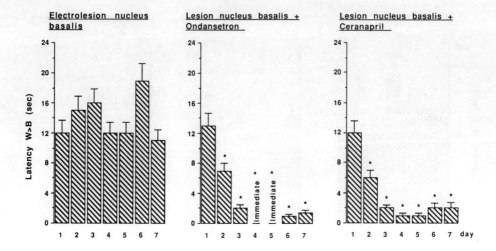

Figure 4. The abilities of ondansetron and ceranapril to inhibit impairment in mouse habituation caused by electrolesions of the nucleus basalis. Young lesioned adult mice received vehicle, ondansetron (10 ng/kg i.p. b.d.) or ceranapril (50 ng/kg i.p. b.d.) for 7 days and the latency of movement from the white (W) to the black (B) section of the test box was recorded. Each value is the mean ± S.E.M. of five determinations. * indicates a significant increase in performance relative to vehicle control ($P < 0.001$) (one-way ANOVA followed by Dunnett's t test); 'immediate' indicates an immediate movement from the white to the black section

input to cortical and limbic areas which are known to be important for cognitive function. Such lesions cause a 70–80% loss in cortical choline acetyltransferase, whether the mechanism for lesion induction is electrolesion or via neurotoxin using ibotenic acid (location of lesion: ant 2.3, lat. 2.1 from the midline, vert. − 4.5 from the skull surface – Lehmann, 1974; ibotenic acid 2 μg in 0.25 μl, electrolesion 1 mA for 10 s). The impairment in habituation can be inhibited by low doses of ondansetron or ceranapril (Figure 4 – the data given here is for electrolesion, which is indistinguishable from that obtained using ibotenic acid lesions).

It is interesting that habituation patterns can be as grossly impaired in aged animals as in animals receiving chronic scopolamine or with nucleus basalis lesions. The aged mice are aged 8–10 months and weigh 33–38 g, compared with 25–30 g for the young adult mice used at 6–8 weeks of age. The aged mice have no impairments in motor performance and do locate the opening in the partition between the light and dark compartments of the test box. However, they appear not to associate the dark with relief from the aversive white environment and fail to make the decision to move from the initial start compartment. This impairment is highly susceptible to antagonism by low doses of ondansetron or ceranapril; indeed, for both the 5-HT$_3$ receptor antagonist and the ACE inhibitor the performance of aged mice is so improved that they move so rapidly from the white to the dark compartment that this cannot be monitored by activation of the remote video system. Hence, the speed of movement has been categorized as 'immediate' (see Figure 5).

The battery of data obtained from the mouse habituation tests show that a 5-HT$_3$ receptor antagonist such as ondansetron or an ACE inhibitor such as ceranapril are able to (a) improve basal performance, (b) inhibit scopolamine impairments, (c) inhibit

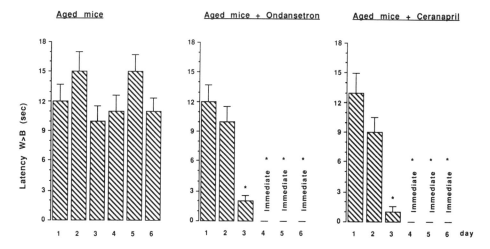

Figure 5. The abilities of ondansetron and ceranapril to improve the performance of aged mice. Aged mice received vehicle, ondansetron (10 ng/kg i.p. b.d.) or ceranapril (50 ng/kg i.p. b.d.) for 6 days and the latency of movement from the white (W) to the black (B) section of the test box was recorded. Each value is the mean ± S.E.M. of five determinations. * indicates a significant increase in performance relative to vehicle controls ($P < 0.001$) (one-way ANOVA followed by Dunnett's *t* test); 'immediate' indicates an immediate movement from the white to the black section

impairments caused by lesions of the nucleus basalis which are associated with limbic and cortical choline acetyltransferase loss, and (d) inhibit impairments associated with old age.

The question then raised is the potential extrapolation of such findings from a mouse model to rat and primate. In both species we found confirmation of the data obtained in mouse. Thus, the impairments in the performance of rats in the T maze caused by scopolamine were inhibited by ondansetron (100 ng/kg i.p. b.d.) and ceranapril (0.5 μg/kg i.p. b.d.) (Figure 6). Similarly, the impairments in T maze performance caused by lesions of the nucleus basalis magnocellularis (location of lesion: ant. 5.8, vert. − 8.2, lat. ± 2.6 – Paxinos and Watson, 1982; 2 μg ibotenic acid in 0.25 μl) were inhibited by treatment with ondansetron or ceranapril (Figure 7). In contrast, the 5-HT$_3$ receptor antagonists failed to influence the deficits in T maze performance caused by hemicholinium-3 (5 μg/day infused into the lateral ventricles) (Figure 8). Thus, reduction or prevention of cholinergic transmission at the presynaptic level does not allow the cognitive enhancing effects of agents such as ondansetron to be revealed. The underlying neurochemistry which contributes to our understanding of the mechanisms of action of agents such as ondansetron is in line with this, and will be discussed later. In the rat, as in the mouse, the findings are consistent: ondansetron and ceranapril will inhibit impairment in T maze performance associated with (a) scopolamine administration, (b) lesions of the nucleus basalis and (c) old age, but will not inhibit impairment caused by hemicholinium-3.

The abilities of ondansetron and ceranapril to inhibit scopolamine-induced impairments in cognitive performance of rats was further confirmed using a water maze test. The percentage of time spent in the correct island quadrant searching for the submerged island is reduced by scopolamine, and the latency to escape onto the island

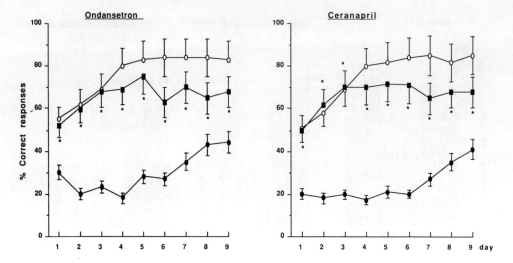

Figure 6. The abilities of ondansetron and ceranapril to inhibit scopolamine-induced deficits in the performance of a T maze reinforced alternation task in the rat. Rats received daily treatment with vehicle (○——○), scopolamine (●——●, 0.25 mg/kg i.p. b.d.), scopolamine plus ondansetron (■——■, 100 ng/kg i.p. b.d.) or scopolamine plus ceranapril (■——■, 0.5 μg/kg i.p. b.d.) and the percentage correct responses recorded. Each value is the mean ±S.E.M. of six determinations. *indicates a significant increase in choice performance compared with scopolamine-treated controls ($P < 0.01$–0.001) (two-way ANOVA followed by Dunnett's t test)

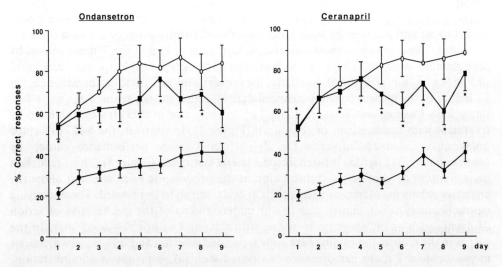

Figure 7. The effects of ondansetron and ceranapril on nucleus basalis induced deficits in performance of a T maze reinforced alternation task in the rat. Lesioned animals received daily treatment with vehicle (●——●), ondansetron (■——■, 100 ng/kg i.p. b.d.) or ceranapril (■——■, 0.5 μg/kg i.p. b.d.) for 9 days and the percentage correct responses recorded. Each value is the mean ±S.E.M. of six determinations. *indicates a significant increase in choice performance compared with lesioned vehicle controls ($P < 0.01$–0.001) (two-way ANOVA followed by Dunnett's t test); normal vehicle treated rats (○——○) were run as a reference control

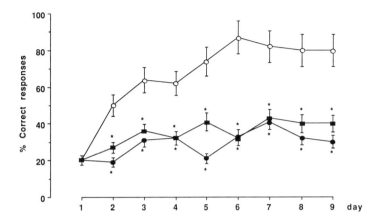

Figure 8. The effect of ondansetron in the rat on the deficits in T maze reinforced alternation performance caused by intracerebroventricular infusion of hemicholinium-3 (5 μg/day). The hemicholinium-3 infused animals received peripheral treatment with vehicle (●——●) or ondansetron (■——■ , 1.0 μg/kg i.p. b.d.); a group of non-hemicholinium infused rats were run as a control (○——○). Each value is the percentage correct responses recorded and is the mean ± S.E.M. of six determinations. * indicates a significant decrease in choice performance compared with control values ($P < 0.01-0.001$) (two-way ANOVA followed by Dunnett's t test)

is delayed. These impairments in performance were corrected by ondansetron and ceranapril (1 μg/kp i.p.) given at the same time as the scopolamine (Figure 9). Thus, in addition to improving basal performance, and improving the responding of aged animals and animals with nucleus basalis lesions, ondansetron and ceranapril have been shown to inhibit scopolamine impairments in three rodent tests involving spatial tasks: mouse habituation, T maze alternation and the Morris water maze.

The final series of tests performed have utilized a primate object discrimination reversal task. Common marmosets were used in a Wisconsin General Test Apparatus. Whilst we have subsequently shown that agents such as ondansetron are able to reverse a scopolamine impairment in marmoset cognitive performance (Jones *et al.*, 1990), the findings reported here are those which lead, in combination with the rodent findings, to the advancement of ondansetron and ceranapril to the clinic. When presented with two junk objects the marmoset is required to select the one which is food rewarded (positive stimulus) to a criterion of six consecutive correct responses. Since the animals are trained on this test paradigm, even though the objects are new to them, they are able to develop a strategy which allows selection of the first rewarded object with relative ease. For example, individual animal data is given in Figure 10 which shows that the animal made approximately 10 errors before gaining criterion. However, when the rewarded object is changed on the same test occasion to the previously unrewarded object, the marmosets find it far more difficult to abandon the learned contingency and change to the reversal task. The numbers of errors to criterion on the reversal task therefore increased to some 20–28. In the presence of ondansetron, 1 ng/kg s.c., the numbers of errors to criterion are reduced on both the initial and reversal tasks, with the improvements on the reversal task being most dramatic (20–28 errors reducing down to 3–14 errors – see Figure 10). After removal of drug treatment, performance of the marmoset returns to the level recorded before intervention with ondansetron.

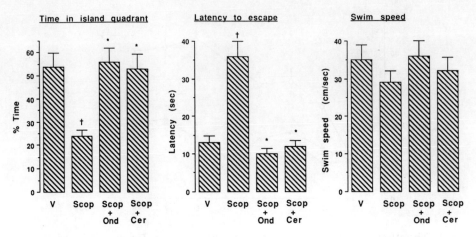

Figure 9. The abilities of ondansetron and ceranapril to inhibit scopolamine-induced impairment of rat behaviour in the water maze test. Animals received vehicle (V), scopolamine (Scop) (0.25 mg/kg i.p.) or scopolamine plus ondansetron (Ond) (1 μg/kg i.p.) or scopolamine plus ceranapril (Cer) (1 μg/kg i.p.), and the latency to escape from the water onto an island, the percentage of time spent in the island quadrant and the swim speed measured. Each value is the mean ± S.E.M. of six determinations. The significance of the scopolamine-induced impairment and the ability of ondansetron and ceranapril to inhibit the effects of scopolamine is indicated by [†] ($P<0.001$) and [*] ($P<0.001$), respectively (Dunnett's t test)

In all of the tests discussed so far it is important to note that the findings with ondansetron can be extended to other 5-HT$_3$ receptor antagonists. For example, in Figure 11 the effects of ondansetron are compared with those of zacopride, ICS205-930 and granisetron. Each of these 5-HT$_3$ receptor antagonists improved performance on both the initial and reversal tasks.

What are the Biochemical Correlates of the Cognitive Enhancing Actions of 5-HT$_3$ Receptor Antagonists and ACE Inhibitors?

There is evidence that both the 5-HT$_3$ receptor antagonists and the ACE inhibitors may facilitate cholinergic function to improve cognitive performance. 5-HT and the 5-HT$_3$ receptor agonist 2-methyl-5-HT have been shown to reduce [^{3}H]-acetylcholine release from rat entorhinal cortex in vitro and such effects are specifically antagonized by the 5-HT$_3$ receptor antagonists (Barnes et al., 1989b). The existence of such an inhibitory 5-HT tone or function in vivo could afford a mechanism of action for the 5-HT$_3$ receptor antagonists to enhance cholinergic function and cognition. This would be in agreement with the literature reporting that 5-HT depletion or a reduction in 5-HT synthesis can improve learning and memory (see Altman et al., 1990).

A similar mechanism of action may be relevant to the cognitive enhancing actions of the ACE inhibitors. Angiotensin II has been shown to inhibit [^{3}H]-acetylcholine release from the rat and human cortex, effects mediated via angiotensin II receptors (Barnes et al., 1989a). It is hypothesized that ACE inhibitors may facilitate cognitive processes through the reduced availability of angiotensin II, thus removing an inhibitory effect on the cholinergic neuron. In this respect it is of interest that patients with Alzheimer's disease are reported to have an increased ACE activity (Arregui et al., 1982).

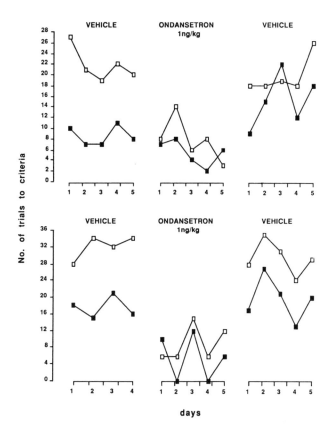

Figure 10. The ability of ondansetron (1 ng/kg s.c.) to improve the performance of individual marmosets in an object discrimination (■———■) and reversal task (□———□). The data indicates the number of trials to criteria using a 5-day vehicle treatment followed by a 5-day treatment with ondansetron with a subsequent 5-day period of vehicle administration

The hypothesis is also supported by data obtained using Hoe 065, a compound structurally related to the ACE inhibitors which is reported to facilitate learning and memory (Hock *et al.*, 1989) and to enhance the activity of choline acetyltransferase as well as the capacity of the high affinity choline uptake system (Wiemer *et al.*, 1989). It was concluded that the increased cholinergic activity caused by this drug probably reflects an enhanced release of acetylcholine.

Summary

Evidence is presented that the 5-HT$_3$ receptor antagonists and the ACE inhibitor ceranapril increase performance in behavioural tests of cognition in the rodent and primate. The compounds act in different ways to antagonize 5-HT function or to reduce the availability of angiotensin II. However, the consequence of both actions may be to enhance acetylcholine release in limbic brain systems. The behavioural and biochemical profile of action of the 5-HT$_3$ receptor antagonists and ACE inhibitors is indicative of their potential role in the treatment of cognitive impairment in man.

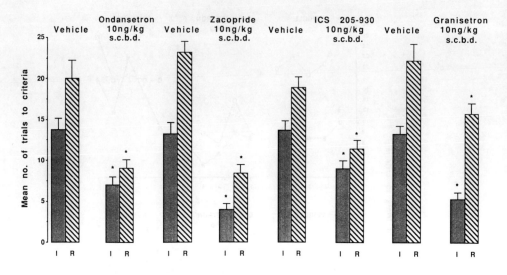

Figure 11. The ability of 5-HT$_3$ receptor antagonists to improve performance in the marmoset in an object discrimination task (I) and a reversal task (R). Each value is the mean $\pm$ S.E.M. of the number of trials to criteria. * indicates a significant increase in performance ($P < 0.05-0.01$) (paired t test)

Acknowledgements

The work reported in this chapter represents the efforts of the Neuropharmacology Research Group at Bradford directed by, in addition to the authors, Dr J. M. Barnes, Dr N. M. Barnes, Dr A. M. Domeney and Dr M. E. Kelly. The authors acknowledge the enthusiastic hard work of the team at Bradford which resulted in the discovery of new cognitive enhancing agents and gave the first indications of their mechanism of action. However, it is appreciated that the reported data would not have been possible without the provision of the correct pharmacological tools and the vision to encourage their exploitation, and the authors particularly wish to acknowledge the efforts of Dr M. B. Tyers of Glaxo Group Research and of Dr Z. P. Horovitz of The Squibb Research Institute.

References

Altman, H. J., Normile, H. J., Galloway, M. P., Ramirez, A. and Azmitia, E. C. (1990) Enhanced spatial discrimination learning in rats following 5,7-DHT-induced serotonergic deafferentation in the hippocampus. Brain Res., 518, 61–6.

Arregui, A., Perry, E. K., Rosor, M. and Tomlinson, B. E. (1982) Angiotensin converting enzyme in Alzheimer's disease: increased activity in caudate nucleus and cortical areas. J. Neurochem., 82, 1490–2.

Barnes, J. M., Barnes, N. M., Costall, B., Horovitz, Z. P. and Naylor, R. J. (1989a) Angiotensin II inhibits the release of [³H] acetylcholine from rat entorhinal cortex in vitro. Brain Res. 491, 136–143.

Barnes, J. M., Barnes, N. M., Costall, B., Naylor, R. J. and Tyers, M. B. (1989b) 5-HT$_3$ receptors mediate inhibition of acetylcholine release in cortical tissue. Nature, 338, 762–3.

Barnes, J. M., Costall, B., Coughlan, J., Domeney, A. M., Gerrard, P. A., Kelly, M. E., Naylor, R. J., Onaivi, E. S., Tomkins, D. M. and Tyers, M. B. (1990) The effects of ondansetron, a 5-HT$_3$ receptor antagonist, on cognition in rodents and primates. Pharmacol. Biochem. Behav., 35, 955–62.

Bartus, R. T., Dean, R. L., Beer, B. and Lippa, A. S. (1982) The cholinergic hypothesis of geriatric memory dysfunction. *Science*, **217**, 408–17.

Costall, B., Coughlan, J., Horovitz, Z. P., Kelly, M. E., Naylor, R. J. and Tomkins, D. M. (1989) The effects of ACE inhibitors captopril and SQ 29 852 in rodent tests of cognition. *Pharmacol. Biochem. Behav.*, **33**, 573–79.

Costall, B., Domeney, A. M., Gerrard, P. A., Horovitz, Z. P., Kelly, M. E., Naylor, R. J. and Tomkins, D. M. (1990a) Effects of captopril and SQ 29 852 on anxiety-related behaviours in rodent and marmoset. *Pharmacol. Biochem. Behav.*, **36**, 13–20.

Costall, B., Naylor, R. J. and Tyers, M. B. (1990b) The psychopharmacology of 5-HT$_3$ receptors. *Pharmacol. Ther.*, **47**, 181–202.

Croog, S. H., Levine, S., Byron, B., Bulpitt, C. J., Jenkins, C. D., Klerman, G. L., Williamson, G. H. and Testa, M. A. (1986) The effects of antihypertensive therapy on the quality of life. *N. Engl. J. Med.*, **314**, 1657–64.

Cushman, D. W., Wang, F. L., Fung, W. C., Harvey, C. M. and De Forrest, J. M. (1990) Differentiation of angiotensin-converting enzyme (ACE) inhibitors by their selective inhibition of ACE in physiologically important target organs. *Am. J. Hypertens.*, in press.

Etienne, P. E. and Zubensko, G. S. (1987) Does captopril elevate mood? *Trends Pharmacol. Sci.*, **8**, 329–30.

Giacobini, E. (1987) Models and strategies of cholinomimetic therapy of Alzheimer disease. In: Dowdall, M. J. and Hawthorne, J. N. (eds) *Cellular and Molecular Basis of Cholinergic Function*, pp. 882–901. Chichester: Harwood.

Heise, G. A. (1987) Facilitation of memory and cognition by drugs. *Trends Pharmacol. Sci.*, **8**, 65–8.

Hock, F. J., Gerhands, H. J., Wiemer, G., Stechl, J., Ruger, W. and Urbach, H. (1989) Effects of the novel compound, Hoe 065, upon impaired learning and memory in rodents. *Eur. J. Pharmacol.*, **171**, 79–85.

Jones, D. N. C., Carey, G. J., Costall, B., Domeney, A. M., Gerrard, P. A., Naylor, R. J. and Tyers, M. B. (1990) Scopolamine induced deficits in a primate object discrimination task are reversed by ondansetron. *British Association for Psychopharmacology Annual Meeting*, Cambridge, 15–18th July, Abstract 112.

Lecrubier, Y., Puech, A. J. and Azcona, A. (1990) 5-HT$_3$ receptors in anxiety disorders. *British Association for Psychopharmacology Annual Meeting*, Cambridge, 15–18th July, Abstract 19.

Lehmann, A. (1974) *Atlas Stereotaxique du Cerveau de la Souris*. Paris: Editions du Centre National de la Recherche Scientifique.

Moos, W. H., Davis, R. E., Schwarz, R. D. and Gamzu, E. R. (1988) Cognition activators. *Med. Res. Rev.*, **8**, 353–91.

Morris, R. (1984) Development of a water-maze procedure for studying spatial learning in the rat. *J. Neurosci. Methods*, **11**, 47–60.

Paxinos, G. and Watson, C. (1982) *The Rat Brain in Stereotaxic Coordinates*. London: Academic Press.

Salamone, J. D., Beart, P. M., Alpert, J. E. and Iversen, S. D. (1982) Impairment in T-maze reinforced alternation performance following nucleus basalis magnocellularis lesions in rats. *Behav. Brain Res.*, **13**, 63–70.

Wiemer, G., Becker, R., Gerhards, H., Hock, F., Stechl, J. and Ruger, W. (1989) Effects of Hoe 065, a compound structurally related to inhibitors of angiotensin converting enzyme, on acetylcholine metabolism in rat brain. *Eur. J. Pharmacol.*, **166**, 31–9.

4

Some Considerations on the Methodology of Clinical Trials with Potential Anti-dementia Compounds in Patients with Alzheimer's Disease

Klaudius R. Siegfried

Clinical Research/Neuroscience, Hoechst AG, Frankfurt and University of Frankfurt, Germany

Introduction

This chapter will deal with questions about the design and the outcome measures of clinical trials of potential anti-dementia compounds in patients with Alzheimer's disease (AD). My comments and suggestions aim to help improve the methodology of these types of trials in order to make them *more sensitive* to drug effects on the major symptoms of AD. This appears to be a very important task in view of the present situation of drug research in this field of neuropsychopharmacology. Although it cannot be ruled out that by serendipity a wonder drug is found with striking effects in a large majority of patients, it is at least not highly likely that this will happen. Therefore, we will have mostly to deal with drugs which are only efficacious in subgroups of patients with AD and have, at least in relatively short-term treatment periods, only mild to moderate effects. However, if we cannot detect the effects of such drugs due to insensitive methods, we also will not be able to give the chemists appropriate feedback which may enable them to understand whether they are on the right path with their drug designs or have selected a wrong approach. As a consequence, many promising and interesting lead substances may be unwarrantedly dropped.

In the following it is not attempted to add another test or scale to the long list of already existing assessment instruments and to propose another completely new design.

Dementia: Molecules, Methods and Measures. Edited by I. Hindmarch, H. Hippius and G. K. Wilcock
© 1991 John Wiley & Sons Ltd

The objectives will be rather to elaborate selection criteria for outcome measures and designs which seem to be sensitive to treatment effects. This will be done on the basis of a critical review of the literature on both the methodology of psychometric assessments and the nature of the cognitive deficits characteristic of AD.

Consequences of an Assumed Pharmacological Heterogeneity of AD for Drug Design

There is increasing evidence that the patient population that meets the DSM-III-R criteria of 'primary degenerative dementia of the Alzheimer type' (APA, 1987) and/or the NINCDS-ADRDA criteria of 'probable Alzheimer's disease' (McKhann *et al.*, 1984) is neuropsychologically, clinically, neuropathologically and neurochemically a heterogeneous group. If this is so, then the usual investigations of random samples of patients will *not* be very sensitive towards the effects of drugs which will probably only affect one or a few sub-groups of the patient population. This is particularly likely to happen with drugs whose design is based on a highly disease-specific hypothesis such as that of a cholinergic deficit. As a possible solution to this problem of the insensitivity of investigations of random samples of patients, a so-called 'enrichment design' is proposed. Such a type of design has recently successfully been employed in clinical trials with tacrine and velnacrine in the USA.*

Indications of the Heterogeneity of AD

Indirect and partly also direct evidence in support of the hypothesis of the pharmacological heterogeneity of AD comes from various sources of observation.

Indirect evidence: neuropsychological and clinical observations. The pattern of core symptoms in AD, i.e. of the various cognitive deficits, seems to vary within the patient population in such a way that several relatively distinct subtypes can be delineated in the early stages of the disease. In the literature, at least four different subtypes of characteristic clinical pictures are described:

1. A majority of patients are characterized by a marked impairment of *memory* functions as the dominant clinical feature (Albert *et al.*, 1989; Reisberg *et al.*, 1989; Cohen *et al.*, 1981), frequently associated with difficulties of abstract thinking.
2. There seems to be another subtype with *attentional* deficits as the dominant clinical feature (Cohen *et al.*, 1981).
3. Another type of patient is characterized by dramatic *language* problems as their prominent symptom.
4. There is also a patient group, although relatively small, with a marked impairment of *visuospatial abilities* as their most obvious early deficit (Albert *et al.*, 1989).

The variety of clinical subtypes in AD is additionally increased by psychopathological disturbances of perception, mood, drive and behaviour, such as depression, euphoria, retardation, agitation, aggressiveness and psychotic symptoms (delusions, hallucinations) (Rubin, 1990; Albert *et al.*, 1989; Berrios, 1989), which are frequently associated with

---

*I am grateful to my colleague Dr M. Murphy, PGU Neuroscience, Hoechst Roussel Pharmaceuticals Inc. for having given me the chance of discussing the pros and cons of an enrichment design.

the cognitive disorders. These psychopathological disturbances are, in turn, not only due to pure psychological reactions but seem to be also partly related to pathological neurotransmitter systems (Siegfried, 1989).

Indirect evidence: neuropathological observations. In spite of the well-known findings of similarities of the degeneration products in brains of both patients with presenile and senile dementia of the Alzheimer type, there are also indications of neuropathological differences between these two groups. Gottfries (1989) pointed out that the frequency of central atrophy is significantly lower in presenile dementia than in the senile type. Also the frequency of white matter low attenuations was found to be significantly lower in presenile than in senile patients.

Direct evidence: neurochemical observations. Whereas the above mentioned subgroups may be interpreted as indirect evidence for a pharmacological heterogeneity of AD, there are also some more direct hints. This direct evidence indicates that in subgroups of patients with AD, different neurotransmitter systems or combinations of these systems may be affected. In addition to the most consistent and well-known neurochemical finding of pathology of the central cholinergic system (Perry, 1986; Davies, 1981; Drachman and Glosser, 1981; Terry and Davies, 1980), there are also significant reductions in adrenaline, 5-hydroxytryptamine (5-HT) and perhaps also dopamine levels in subgroups of these patients (Whitehouse *et al.*, 1989; Rossor and Iversen, 1986; Arnstein and Goldman-Rakic, 1985; Bowen and Davison, 1984; Yates *et al.*, 1983, 1981; Perry *et al.*, 1981; Cross *et al.*, 1981; Gottfries, 1980; Carlsson *et al.*, 1980; Adolfssen *et al.*, 1978; Davies and Maloney, 1976).

At present, it is scarcely possible to demonstrate clear relationships between the various neuropsychological, neuropathological and neurochemical disorders described. Nevertheless, the above review suggests that it is at least not unlikely that the group of patients with AD consists of different *pharmacological* subgroups. This would mean that patients with AD will not respond uniformly to a specific pharmacological intervention. However, this problem is further enhanced by two additional difficulties. Firstly, there are hitherto no clinical diagnostic tools or biological markers to identify the assumed pharmacological subgroups reliably. Secondly, evidence from animal models suggests that learning and memory problems based upon a combined deficit of two or more transmitter systems are only responsive to pharmacological treatment if it is simultaneously directed towards all deficient transmitter systems. This must be concluded from findings in animals with combined cholinergic (nucleus basalis of Meynert) and ascending noradrenergic bundle lesions which caused memory problems that could not be improved by a cholinesterase inhibitor alone but only by combined and simultaneous treatment of both the cholinergic and the noradrenergic deficit (Davis *et al.*, 1988). The implication of this finding is that even if a test drug influences the right transmitter system, it will not have any therapeutic benefit as long as the other transmitter systems affected by the disease remain unchanged.

The Insensitivity of Usual Treatment Designs to Drug Effects
in Pharmacologically Heterogeneous Patient Samples

If the hypothesis of the pharmacological heterogeneity of patients with AD is correct, then it must have consequences for the designs of our drug trials.

First of all, the random patient samples usually chosen for such investigations may be too small to demonstrate significant treatment effects because the responder group may not be adequately represented and intra-treatment group variances will be too large (in the case of the use of traditional randomized group designs) in comparison to the treatment-induced inter-group variances. Secondly, even if some trials may be able to demonstrate treatment effects, these are likely to be underestimated. Thirdly, favourable findings obtained for the test drug in one trial will not consistently be replicated in further trials because the proportion of patients who belong to the subgroup of responders is uncontrollable and may therefore vary considerably with the patient samples.

The Enrichment Procedure

As there is no possibility of identifying the subgroup of possible responders by diagnostic procedures, there seems to be only three solutions to the above mentioned problem:

1. The patient samples must be considerably increased so that the possible responder group has an enhanced chance of being sufficiently represented in the sample. This is a very costly and time-consuming approach and the treatment effects will probably still be underestimated.
2. A way to reduce the 'noise' caused by huge inter-patient variances would be to use cross-over designs. They are known to include the risk of carry-over effects which may considerably affect their internal validity. Nevertheless, these problems can be minimized by wash-out periods of an appropriate length in between the treatment phases. An insurmountable problem of cross-over designs is, however, that they cannot be used in long-term trials (i.e. several weeks or months of treatment) in patients with progressive diseases such as AD. Short-term cross-over studies designed to measure acute or subacute effects in early phase II dose-finding trials in patients with AD can be justified because the changes in the severity of the disease occur not over a matter of days but of months. However, cross-over studies seem *not* to be appropriate for pivotal efficacy studies as these require treatment periods of several months and involve the risk of incomparable, shifting baselines.
3. As both of the above solutions have their problems, the most elegant way of designing a pivotal efficacy study which is sensitive towards drug effects occurring only in a subgroup of patients seems to be a so-called 'enrichment procedure'. Enrichment studies consist of three phases or segments (in addition to the screening period): (a) a test treatment period after which the patients are selected on the basis of their response according to a predefined criterion; (b) a subsequent wash-out period (which must be long enough to avoid carry-over effects); and (c) a usual double-blind placebo-controlled randomized group study (the so-called 'replication phase') with those patients who were selected as potential responders in the test treatment according to a predefined criterion.

Enrichment studies are sometimes criticized for being 'biased'. This is no real reproach if it only means that they are designed to be particularly sensitive to drug effects in subgroups of the patient population. If, however, the word 'biased' implies that they give a one-sided, distorted picture of reality, this is not true. It would be only true if the investigators or sponsors would later on claim they had demonstrated efficacy for *all* patients with AD. Therefore, it is very important that study reports on enrichment trials give the exact proportion of patients who were selected as potential responders and included in the replication phase. The size of this proportion will be necessary to determine the practical usefulness of the drug for the treatment of AD.

Furthermore, enrichment procedures are only relevant for clinical practice if the test treatment period is relatively short. If a patient has to be treated for many weeks or even months before any decision can be made as to whether he is a potential responder, this would be a useless procedure for clinical practice.

General Methodological Requirements of Tests and Scales used for the Assessment of Treatment Effects

At least as important as the study design is the sensitivity of the outcome measures of clinical trials towards potential drug effects on the core symptoms of AD. Outcome measures include efficacy, safety and tolerance assessments. In the following, only efficacy measures of clinical trials with anti-dementia compounds will be dealt with. I will focus on cognitive performance tests and clinical observer scales, as these are the most important efficacy measures used in such trials.

Psychometric Instruments can have Different Purposes

When discussing the question of how to select the right assessment instrument, one must first of all clearly point out the purpose of the assessment planned. Obviously, there are several quite different reasons for applying tests or scales in clinical trials. The assessments can be used for:

1. *Descriptive* reasons, i.e. to give a fairly detailed and comprehensive description of the patient's symptom patterns.
2. An estimation of the *severity* of the disease (or, which is not exactly the same, a determination of the stage of the disease).
3. *Discriminatory* purposes (i.e. to help in the differential diagnosis).
4. A *prediction* of the course of the disease (i.e. a prognosis).
5. The assessment of *changes* in the disease, e.g. changes in the spontaneous course of the disease or changes due to therapeutic intervention (McDonald, 1986).

Although there are some methodological properties that all assessment instruments, irrespective of the purpose they are used for, should have in common (e.g. high 'objectivity' and 'inter-rater reliability'; Lienert, 1961), different purposes also require different methodological standards.

There is not such a thing as *the* validity of a psychometric instrument; there are several aspects of reliability and validity (Cronbach, 1970) and not all of these are equally important for the various purposes for which assessment instruments can be used. Similarly, different purposes also require different distributions of item difficulty* indices

---

*Item difficulty is a technical term which is defined by the percentage of persons who answer an item correctly (in the case of performance tests) or give an answer indicative of the behaviour to be measured (in the case of personality questionnaires, behaviour rating scales, etc.) (Anastasi, 1972).

and total scores. It is, therefore, not advisable to use scales or tests constructed for a descriptive task or for severity estimations as instruments for measuring change (Smith, 1979; Honigfeld, 1983). A scale with a descriptive purpose must, for example, comprise all essential symptoms of the syndrome to be assessed. It therefore does not only consist of sensitive but also of very stable symptoms (or items). Similarly, for discriminatory scales, mainly items which discriminate between two or more diagnostic groups, for example between multi-infarct dementia (MID) and AD, will be selected. These items, however, are not necessarily most sensitive to change but, on the contrary, are more likely to refer to very constant features of the diseases compared.

Methodological Properties of Good Efficacy Measures

The most important selection criterion for scales and tests to be used as outcome measures in clinical trials is *sensitivity to change* in the disease tested. It is therefore essential to know which methodological properties such measuring instruments need to have.

The majority of items should be of a *moderate difficulty* for the patient population tested. One has to bear in mind that the degree of difficulty is not a constant property of items but depends on the patient population used. The patient samples used for test or scale construction must therefore have approximately the same degree of severity of the disease as the sample selected for the clinical treatment trial planned. If, for example, the original patient sample consisted of a group of patients with more severe degrees of severity, then the performance test is likely to be too 'easy' for mildly to moderately severe patients and will, therefore, be insensitive to treatment influences due to ceiling effects. On the other hand, a rating scale will be insensitive due to a 'floor effect' if it was constructed for patients with milder degrees of the disease but is used in severer patients.

The most appropriate form of *reliability* for instruments used for measuring changes is a *parallel tests reliability* determined by comparisons of two (or more) equivalent forms of the test after a short time interval. If for some reason no equivalent forms are available, then an instrument with a relatively high internal consistency and a moderately high retest reliability assessed after intervals of 2 or more weeks is acceptable. Tests or scales with a very high retest reliability, determined after intervals of several weeks, seem *not* to be ideal for measuring change, as high retest reliability is not only the result of a low error of measurement but also of the stability of the behavioural aspects assessed (see the so-called 'reliability-validity dilemma of change measures' – Petermann, 1978).

The most important *validity* aspect for change measurements is a proven *sensitivity* to changes in the disease investigated. As a rule, highly sensitive scales or tests do not contain all symptoms of the disease, but only those which are particularly sensitive to change. For such measuring instruments, it must, however, be demonstrated that the changes assessed are predictive of later changes in other symptoms of the disease. This form of predictive validity is necessary for an evaluation of the changes measured and will help to distinguish 'pseudo-sensitive' from sensitive scales (see last chapter).

The Construction of Sensitive Assessment Instruments

For sensitive instruments only those items are to be selected which in previous investigations have proven to be sensitive to change. One may say that this proposal, although a logical suggestion, is practically totally useless for the field of research on anti-dementia compounds because there is, so far, no real efficacious drug in this field and hence also no experience with the sensitivity of items and tests. This is, however, only partly true; there are some sources of indirect information which can help us to find potentially sensitive items and tests.

Firstly, one can refer to findings of longitudinal and cross-sectional studies of changes in the course of AD. These studies teach us which cognitive functions or symptoms change with the severity of the AD and which remain relatively stable. Also, findings on normal cognitive ageing can partly be of help if one considers AD to be a form of pathologically speeded ageing. Secondly, information on the sensitivity of tests or items to change is also available from studies on the acute and subacute cognitive effects of drugs such as physostigmine and arecoline on the one hand and scopolamine on the other.

Information obtained from the above mentioned sources suggests that certain tests of memory and learning, attention and language function seem to be sensitive to change in patients with AD (Albert *et al.*, 1989; Branconnier, 1986; Corkin *et al.*, 1986; Erickson and Howieson, 1986; Mohs *et al.*, 1986; Reisberg *et al.*, 1989; Cohen *et al.*, 1981).

Functions of recent memory. Recent memory is markedly affected in patients with AD and can be assessed by tasks of recognition (immediate and delayed), free recall and serial learning (Erickson and Howieson, 1986; Kaszniak *et al.*, 1986; Mohs *et al.*, 1986; Wilson *et al.*, 1983). In recognition tasks, healthy elderly people show only mild impairments compared with recall tasks, whereas patients with AD perform much worse than expected for their age (Erickson and Howieson, 1986; Kaszniak *et al.*, 1986). A longitudinal study with Alzheimer patients conducted by Mohs and co-workers (1986) demonstrated that performance in word recognition and paired-associate learning tasks showed a significant impairment over the period of 1 year and was correlated with increases in the severity of the disease. In contrast, free recall tasks proved to be too difficult to be sensitive to changes in the disease.

Recognition and serial learning tasks were also used successfully in trials with physostigmine, arecoline and scopolamine, where they were able to demonstrate acute and subacute drug effects (Wesnes and Simpson, 1988; Huff *et al.*, 1988; Blackwood and Christie, 1986; Rose and Moulthrop, 1986; Johns *et al.*, 1985; Mohs *et al.*, 1985; Harbaugh *et al.*, 1984; Muramoto *et al.*, 1984; Agnoli *et al.*, 1983; Levin and Peters, 1982; Thal and Fuld, 1983; Thal *et al.*, 1983; Davis and Mohs, 1982; Sullivan *et al.*, 1982; Christie *et al.*, 1981; Drachman and Sahakian, 1980; Davis *et al.*, 1978; Peters and Levin, 1982; Sitaram *et al.*, 1978; Petersen, 1977; Berger and Stein, 1969).

Working memory functions and attention. Primary or short-term memory appears to be mildly impaired in patients with AD when simple memory span tests such as the digit span forward (WAIS) or the Corsi test, a non-verbal spatial task, are used (Erickson and Howieson, 1986; Kaszniak *et al.*, 1986). Digit span forward performance was found to deteriorate with progression of the disease (Storandt *et al.*, 1986; Wilson and Kaszniak, 1986). In the early stages of AD, deficits and subtle changes in short-term memory functions can more easily be assessed when short-term memory tasks more complex than digit span are used. These tasks do not simply require short-time retention but in addition some information processing in the form of organizing and restructuring the informational input. This indicates that the so-called central executive of the working memory (Baddeley and Hitch, 1974; Baddeley, 1986) seems to be already impaired early in the course of the disease. Experimental trials with scopolamine, if considered as valid dementia models, support this hypothesis (Rusted and Warburton, 1988; Rusted, 1988). Deficiencies of the central executive of working memory could also account for both the encoding and retrieval problems found in AD.

As a rule, testing of working memory involves the combination of two tasks to be performed simultaneously. Baddeley et al. (see Baddeley, 1988) used, for example, a pursuit tracking task (patients had to try to keep a stylus in contact with a moving spot of light) plus a usual digit span task. These tasks are dependent on the different 'slave systems' of working memory, which is why their simultaneous performance requires the coordination capacities of the 'central executive'.

When performing both tasks simultaneously, the performance level of patients with AD was disrupted dramatically and disproportionately in comparison with age-matched healthy subjects. Follow-up investigations after intervals of 6 and 12 months demonstrated a progressive deterioration in patients with AD. The problem with such tests of working memory is that they only seem to be adequate for very mild cases of AD, as they are too difficult to be sensitive to changes in all other patient groups. This problem can be solved by taking into account that one important aspect of the central executive of working memory is attention, which, according to Kahneman (1973), must be conceived as a limited, allocatable resource. Baddeley (1981, pp. 22) himself states that 'the central executive is becoming increasingly like a pure attentional system'. If this is so, then simple tests of attention, which can easily be used in patients with AD, should be employed to measure this important aspect of working memory.

Cohen et al. (1981) pointed out that an attentional deficit is a major characteristic in a large subgroup of patients in the early stages of AD. Trials with cholinomimetics and also with scopolamine have demonstrated that changes in attention, which can be measured, for example, by digit-symbol substitution tasks (Wechsler, 1955), choice reaction time or vigilance tasks, are sensitive to acute and subacute drug effects (Huff et al., 1988; Parrott, 1986; Warburton and Wesnes, 1984). Investigations with the Mini-Mental State Examination and the 'Alzheimer's Disease Assessment Scale' (ADAS) found significant changes in the items 'attention' and 'concentration' over a period of 1 year in patients with AD (Yesavage et al., 1988). Such changes in attention are not unrelated to the above mentioned sensitive learning and memory functions because both memory encoding and retrieval are attention-demanding (Baddeley, 1986).

Language functions. Besides impairments in recent memory, working memory and attention, language deficits are also one of the early symptoms of AD (Albert et al., 1989; Branconnier, 1986; Corkin et al., 1986; Irigaray, 1973). Language functions were proven to deteriorate considerably in AD patients within 1 year (Yesavage et al., 1988).

The early problems observed are word-finding difficulties. Mohs et al. (1986) found in their longitudinal study that in the Boston Naming Test (Kaplan et al., 1978), in which subjects are asked to give the names of objects presented to them in black and white drawings, patients with AD are significantly impaired compared with healthy elderly people. The performance level in this test, however, was not particularly sensitive to increasing language disorders observed over a 1-year follow-up period. Early language deficits seem to become more apparent when the ability to generate categories of words is tested (Branconnier, 1986). This ability can be assessed by using category instance fluency tests (Benson, 1979), in which patients are asked to generate as many examples as possible from a certain category of things within a specified time limit. These findings are consistent with Warrington's (1975) notion that in dementia the language problems are due to a breakdown of the patient's conceptual networks.

Some Remarks on the use of Comprehensive Clinical Rating Scales and Clinical Global Impression Scales

Comprehensive Clinical Rating Scales

In the decisive efficacy trials (or 'pivotal studies') of late phase II/early phase III development, comprehensive clinical rating scales, and also clinical global impression scales, will have to be used as efficacy measures because only with these instruments can we demonstrate that the drug affected all essential aspects of the dementia syndrome. However, it was noted above that comprehensive scales are unlikely to be very sensitive as they are comprised of both sensitive and relatively insensitive (or stable) items. Their sensitivity can, however, be considerably enhanced by increasing the weight of sensitive items for the total scale score. This can be achieved by either giving such items higher scores or by increasing the number of such items. As a result, sensitive items will strongly determine the total scale score. An example of this strategy is the use of memory tasks in the ADAS (Rosen *et al.*, 1984); these determine a major part of the sum score of this scale and thus considerably enhance its sensitivity to drug effects.

Clinical ratings in existing dementia rating scales are either to be made on a relatively abstract construct level (e.g. rating of the general performance level of 'recent memory') or they are based on the direct observation of the patient's performance in certain clearly defined tasks (e.g. to name certain objects, to recall test instructions, etc.). Strictly performance-based ratings are preferable to ratings on a construct level. This is because in performance-based ratings the function to be observed is operationally defined, which guarantees a high inter-rater reliability. This, in turn, is an important prerequisite for a sensitive measure. Scales with low inter-rater reliabilities have a large standard error of measurement which will mask subtle drug-related changes.

Some comprehensive clinical dementia scales include not only cognitive symptoms but also symptoms of mood, drive and other psychiatric disorders. Although the non-cognitive disorders are not completely independent of the cognitive symptoms of the dementia syndrome, the intercorrelations between both areas are usually relatively low. It is therefore proposed that cognitive and non-cognitive functions should be assessed and evaluated separately and that both groups of items are not summed up to give a single total score. Otherwise, this can lead to two types of undesirable consequences.

Firstly, the total score may not indicate any changes although clear changes have occurred. This can happen if there are opposite trends in affective and cognitive areas. It is, for example, known that in the very early or even the prodromal stages of AD there is a trend for patients to become depressive. When the disease progresses (i.e. the cognitive symptoms become worse), the frequency of depression is first reduced and may in late stages of the disease again slightly increase (Siegfried, 1989). The reverse situation would be a drug-related improvement in cognitive symptoms which leads to increased mood problems because the patient may have more insight into his personal situation. The second type of undesirable consequence of a total score comprising both cognitive and non-cognitive items would be *pseudosensitivity* of the scale, that is, the total score may indicate a therapeutic improvement which is *not* due to a change in the (cognitive) core symptoms of the disease but to unspecific activation effects on mood and alertness. This weakness of some comprehensive scales such as the Sandoz Clinical Assessment Geriatric Scale (SCAG) (see Shader *et al.*, 1974) has produced in clinical trials the impression of efficacy for some drugs which in clinical practice proved to be at best only marginally effective.

Clinical Global Impression Scales

A similar, if not a more enhanced risk of pseudosensitivity is associated with the use of clinical global impression scales. Whereas in comprehensive clinical scales the weight and influence of the individual items on the total score is predefined and strictly determined by an algorithm and therefore analysable, this is not the case with a global impression score. Hence, the investigator is allowed to arbitrarily give his own weights to the various aspects of the disease, whereby the number of aspects taken into account, the kind of aspects chosen and the allocation of weights to these aspects may considerably vary from observer to observer. This more or less intuitive weight allocation is prone to typical rating errors such as the 'halo effect' and the 'generosity effect'. By 'halo effect' it is meant that the rater's general impression is strongly influenced by the exaggerated and overwhelming weight given to one specific aspect at the expense of the weight of all other aspects (Cronbach, 1970). The 'generosity effect' means the tendency to give a favourable rating. In a clinical trial, this may be due to the investigator's expecting to find favourable results. In such a case, he would give all effects he is able to detect and which in his opinion are properties of the verum drug a prominent weight, even if the effects are small and rather unspecific. The more general (or global) and less specific the ratings are, the more ambiguous the rater's interpretations can be and the more likely that halo and generosity effects will occur (Cronbach, 1970; Campbell *et al.*, 1973).

A combination of both these effects can lead to a high 'pseudosensitivity' for clinical global impressions. I therefore consider a general statement which maintains that 'the effectiveness of nootropics is more easily demonstrated through global clinical measures' than through any other type of assessments as problematic (see Amaducci *et al.*, 1990).

The consequence of the weaknesses of global impression assessments cannot be to no longer employ such scales in further clinical trials. This advice would ignore the valuable aspects of this sort of assessment. Global impression scales allow some aspects of the pharmacodynamic profile of a test compound which nobody has thought of before and which otherwise would have been overlooked to be taken into consideration. This means they can have a heuristic value. Furthermore, global impressions of efficacy, when consistent with the observations made through other assessment instruments, can be considered as indicators of the clinical relevance of the drug effects under investigation. The only consequence to be drawn from the above mentioned risks of judgement errors must be to not give global impressions the role of ultimate outcome measures but to use them as additional supportive information to comprehensive clinical scales, psychometric performance tests and perhaps also scales of (instrumental) activities of daily living. This would at least permit the analysis and explanation of the global impression and thus distinguish results due to pseudosensitivity from true efficacy.

References

Adolfsson, R. C. G., Gottfries, L., Orland, B. E. *et al.* (1978) Reduced levels of catecholamines in the brain and increased activity of monoamine oxidase in platelets in Alzheimer's disease; therapeutic implications. In: Katzman, R., Terry, R. D. and Bick, K. L. (eds) *Alzheimer's Disease; Senile Dementia and Related Disorders*, pp. 441–51. New York: Raven Press.

Agnoli, A., Martucci, N., Manna, V., Conti, L. and Fioravanti, R. (1983) Effect of cholinergic and anticholinergic drugs on short-term memory in Alzheimer's dementia: a neuropsychological computerised electroencephalographic study. *Clin. Neuropharmacol.*, 6, 311–23.

Albert, M. S., Moss, M. and Milberg, W. (1989) Memory testing to improve the differential diagnosis of Alzheimer's disease. In: Iqbal, K., Wilsniewski, H. M. and Windblad, B. (eds) *Alzheimer's Disease and Related Disorders*, pp. 55–69. New York: Alan R. Liss.

Amaducci, L., Angst, J., Bech, P., Benkert, O., Bruinvels, J., Engel, R. R., Gottfries, C. G., Hippius, H., Levy, R., Lingjaerde, O., Lopez-Iborj, J. J., Orgogozo, J. M., Pull, C., Saletu, B., Stoll, D. and Woggon, B. (1990) Consensus conference on the methodology of clinical trials of 'nootropics', Munich, June 1989. Report of the Consensus Committee. *Pharmacopsychiatry*, 23, 171–5.

Anastasi, A. (1972) *Psychological Testing*, 3rd edn. London: Macmillan.

APA (1987) *Diagnostic and Statistical Manual of Mental Disorders*, 3rd edn revised. Washington, D.C.: American Psychiatric Association.

Arnstein, A. F. T. and Goldman-Rakic, P. S. (1985) Alpha 2-adrenergic mechanisms in prefrontal cortex associated with cognitive decline in aged human primates. *Science*, 230, 1273–6.

Baddeley, A. D. (1981) Reading and working memory. *Bull. Brit. Psychol. Soc.*, 35, 414–7.

Baddeley, A. (1986) *Working Memory*. Oxford: Clarendon Press.

Baddeley, A. (1988) Cognitive psychology and human memory. *Trends Neurosci.* 11(4), 176–81.

Baddeley, A. and Hitch, G. J. (1974) Working memory. In: Bower, G. (ed.) *Recent Advances in Memory and Motivation*, Vol. VIII, pp. 47–90. New York: Academic Press.

Benson, D. F. (1979) Neurologic correlates of anomia. In: Whitaker, H. and Whitaker, H. A. (eds) *Studies in Neurolinguistics*, Vol. 2, pp. 293–328. New York: Academic Press.

Bereiter, C. (1962) Using tests to measure change. *Pers. Guid. J.* 6–11.

Berger, B. D. and Stein, L. (1969) An analysis of the learning deficits produced by scopolamine. *Psychopharmacologia*, 14, 271–83.

Berrios, G. E. (1989) Non-cognitive symptoms and the diagnosis of dementia – historical and clinical aspects. *Br. J. Psychiatry*, 154(4, suppl.), 11–66.

Blackwood, D. H. R. and Christie, J. E. (1986) The effects of physostigmine on memory and auditory P300 in Alzheimer-type dementia. *Biol. Psychiatry*, 21, 557–60.

Branconnier, R. J. (1986) A computerised battery for behavioural assessment in Alzheimer's disease. In: Poon, L. W. (ed.) *Handbook for Clinical Memory Assessment of Older Adults*, pp. 189–96. Washington, D.C.: American Psychological Association.

Bowen, D. M. and Davison, A. N. (1984) Dementia in the elderly: biochemical aspects. *J. R. Coll. Physicians Lond.*, 18, 25–7.

Campbell, J. P., Dunnette, M. D., Arvey, R. D. and Hellervik, C. V. (1973) The development and evaluation of behaviourally based rating scales. *J. Appl. Psychol.*, 57, 15–22.

Carlsson, A., Adolfsson, R., Aquilonius, S. M., Gottfries, R. G., Oreland, L., Svennerholm, L. and Windblad, B. (1980) Biogenic amines in human brain in normal aging, senile dementia and chronic alcoholism. In: Goldstein, M., Calne, D. B., Lieberman, A. and Thorner, M. O. (eds) *Ergot Compounds and Brain Function: Neuroendocrine and Neuropsychiatric Aspects*. New York: Raven Press.

Christie, J. E., Phil, M., Shering, A., Ferguson, J. and Glen, A. M. (1981) Physostigmine and arecoline: effects of intravenous infusions in Alzheimer presenile dementia. *Br. J. Psychiatry*, 138, 46–50.

Cohen, D., Eisdorfer, C. and Walford, R. L. (1981) Histocompatibility antigens (HLA) and patterns of cognitive loss in dementia of the Alzheimer type. *Neurobiol. Aging*, 2(4), 277–80.

Corkin, S., Growden, J. H., Sullivan, E. V., Nissen, M. J. and Huff, F. J. (1986) Assessing treatment effects: A neuropsychological battery. In: Poon, L. W. (ed.) *Handbook for*

Clinical Memory Assessment of Older Adults, pp. 156–67. Washington, D.C.: American Psychological Association.

Cronbach, K. J. (1970) *Essentials of Psychological Testing*, 3rd edn. New York: Harper and Row.

Cross, A. J., Crow, T., Perry, J. A., Blessed, G. and Tomlinson, B. E. (1981) Reduced dopamine-beta-hydroxylase activity in Alzheimer's disease. *BMJ*, **282**, 93–4.

Cunningham, W. R. (1986) Psychometric perspectives: validity and reliability. In: Poon, L. W. (ed.) *Handbook for Clinical Memory Assessment of Older Adults*, pp. 27–31. Washington, D.C.: American Psychological Association.

Davies, P. (1981) Theoretical treatment possibilities for dementia of the Alzheimer type: The cholinergic hypothesis. In: Crook, Th. and Gershon, S. (eds) *Strategies for the Development of an Effective Treatment for Senile Dementia*. New Canaan: Mark Powley Associates.

Davies, P. and Maloney, A. F. J. (1976) Selective loss of central cholinergic neurons in Alzheimer's disease. *Lancet*, **ii**, 1403 (letter).

Davis, K. L. and Mohs, R. C. (1982) Enhancement of memory processes in Alzheimer's disease with multiple-dose intravenous physostigmine. *Am. J. Psychiatry*, **139**, 1421–4.

Davis, K. L., Mohs, R. C., Tinklenberg, J. R., Pfefferbaum, A., Hollister, L. E. and Kopell, B. S. (1978) Physostigmine: Improvement of long-term memory processes in normal subjects. *Science*, **201**, 272–4.

Davis, K. L., Vahramharoutunian, M. D. and Kanof, P. (1988) Therapeutics of Alzheimer's disease for clinical and preclinical issues. *J. Psychopharmacol.*, **2**(2).

Drachman, D. A. and Glosser, G. (1981) Pharmacologic strategies in aging and dementia: the cholinergic hypothesis. In: Crook, Th. and Gershon, S. (eds) *Strategies for the Development of an Effective Treatment for Senile Dementia*, pp. 35–51. New Canaan: Mark Powley Associates.

Drachman, D. A. and Sahakian, B. J. (1980) Memory and cognitive functions in the elderly: a preliminary trial of physostigmine. *Arch. Neurol.*, **37**, 674–5.

Erickson, R. C. and Howieson, D. (1986) The clinician's perspective: measuring change and treatment effectiveness. In: Poon, L. W. (ed.) *Handbook for Clinical Memory Assessment of Older Adults*, 69–80. Washington, D.C.: American Psychological Association.

Eysenck, M. W. (1984) *A Handbook of Cognitive Psychology*. London: Lawrence Erlbaum Association.

Ferris, St. H., Crook, Th., Flicker, Ch., Reisberg, B. and Bartus, R. T. (1986) Cognitive impairment and evaluating treatment effects: psychometric performance tests. In: Poon, L. W. (ed.) *Handbook for Clinical Memory Assessment of Older Adults*, 139–48. Washington, D.C.: American Psychological Association.

Gottfries, C. G. (1980) Amine metabolism in normal aging and in dementia disorders. In: Roberts, P. J. (ed.) *Biochemistry of Dementia*, Ch. 10. Chichester: John Wiley and Sons.

Gottfries, C. G. (1989) Alzheimer's disease – one, two or several. *J. Neural Transm. Park. Dis. Dement. Sect.*, **1**, 22.

Guilford, J. P. (1954) *Psychometric Methods*. New York: McGraw-Hill.

Harbaugh, R. E., Roberts, D. W., Coombs, D. W., Saunders, R. L. and Reeder, T. M. (1984) Preliminary report: intracranial cholinergic drug infusion in patients with Alzheimer's disease. *Neurosurgery*, **15**, 514–18.

Honigfeld, G. (1983) Psychopathology rating scales for use by nursing personnel. In: Crook, J., Ferris, S. and Bartus, R. (eds) *Assessments in Geriatric Psychopharmacology*, pp. 81–96. New Canaan: Mark Powley.

Huff, F. J., Michel, S. F., Corkin, S. and Growdon, J. H. (1988) Cognitive functions affected by scopolamine in Alzheimer's disease and normal aging. *Drug Dev. Res.*, **12**, 271–8.

Irigaray, L. (1973) *Le Langue des Déments*. The Hague: Mouton.

Johns, C. A., Haroutunian, V., Greenwald, B. S., Mohs, R. C., Davis, B. M., Kanof, P., Horvath, T. B. and Davis, K. L. (1985) Development of cholinergic drugs for treatment of Alzheimer's disease. *Drug Dev. Res.*, **5**, 77–96.

Kahneman, D. (1973) *Attention and Effort*. Englewood-Cliffs: Prentice-Hall.

Kaplan, E., Goodglass, H. and Weintraub, S. (1978) *The Boston Memory Test*. Boston: Kaplan and Goodglass.

Kaszniak, A. W., Poon, L. W. and Riege, W. (1986) Assessing memory deficits: an information processing approach. In: Poon, L. W. (ed.) *Handbook for Clinical Memory Assessment of Older Adults*, pp. 168–88. Washington, D.C.: American Psychological Association.

Levin, H. S. and Peters, B. H. (1982) Long-term administration of oral physostigmine and lecithin improve memory in Alzheimer's disease. Notes and letters. In: Corkin, S., Davis, K. L., Growdon, J. H., Usdin, E. and Wartman, R. J. (eds) *Alzheimer's Disease: A Report of Progressed Aging*, Vol. 19. New York: Raven Press.

Lienert, G. A. (1961) *Testaufbau und Testanalyse*. Weinheim: Beltz-Verlag.

McDonald, R.Sc. (1986) Assessing treatment effects: behaviour rating scales. In: Poon, L. W. (ed.) *Handbook for Clinical Memory Assessment of Older Adults*, pp. 129–38. Washington, D.C.: American Psychological Association.

McKhann, G., Drachman, D., Folstein, M., Katzman, R., Price, D. and Stadlan, E. M. (1984) Clinical diagnosis of Alzheimer's disease. Report of the NINCDS-ADRDA Work Group under the Auspices of Department of Health and Human Services Task Force on Alzheimer's Disease. *Neurology*, 34, 939–44.

Mohs, R. C., Davis, B. M., Mathe, A. A., Rosen, W. G., Johns, C. A., Greenwald, B. S., Horvath, T. B. and Davis, K. L. (1985) Intravenous and oral physostigmine in Alzheimer's disease. *Interdiscipl. Top. Gerontol.*, 20, 140–51.

Mohs, R.C., Kim, Y., Johns, C. A., Dunn, D. P. and Davis, K. L. (1986) Assessing changes in Alzheimer's disease: memory and language. In: Poon, L. W. (ed.) *Handbook for Clinical Memory Assessment of Older Adults*, pp. 149–55. Washington, D.C.: American Psychological Association.

Muramoto, O., Sugishita, M. and Ando, K. (1984) Cholinergic system and constructional praxis: a further study of physostigmine in Alzheimer's disease. *J. Neurol. Neurosurg. Psychiatry*, 47, 485–91.

Parrott, A. C. (1986) The effects of transdermal scopolamine and four dose levels of oral scopolamine (0.15, 0.3, 0.6 and 1.2 mg) upon psychological performance. *Psychopharmacology*, 89, 347–54.

Perry, E. K. (1986) The cholinergic hypothesis – ten years on. *Br. Med. Bull.*, 42(1), 63–9.

Perry, E. K., Blessed, G., Tomlinson, B. E., Perry, R. H., Crow, T. J., Cross, A. J., Dockray, G. J., Dimaline, R. and Arregui, F. (1981) Neurochemical activities in human temporal lobe related to aging and Alzheimer type changes. *Neurobiol. Aging*, 2, 251–6.

Petermann, I. (1978) *Veränderungsmessung*. Stuttgart: Kohlhamer.

Peters, B. H. and Levin, H. S. (1982) Chronic oral physostigmine and lecithin administration in memory disorders of aging. In: Corkin, S., Davis, K. L., Growdon, J. H. *et al.* (eds) *Alzheimer's Disease: A Report of Progress*. Aging, Vol. 19, pp. 421–6. New York: Raven Press.

Petersen, R. C. (1977) Scopolamine induced learning failures in man. *Psychopharmacology*, 52, 283–9.

Reisberg, B., Ferris, St. H., Deleon, M.J., Kluger, A., Franssen, E., Borenstein, J. and Alba, R. C. (1989) The stage specific temporal course of Alzheimer's disease: functional and behavioural concomitants upon cross-sectional and longitudinal observations. In: Iqbal, K., Wisniewski, H. M. and Windblad, B. (eds) *Alzheimer's Disease and Related Disorders*, pp. 23–41. New York: Alan R. Liss.

Rose, R. P. and Moulthrop, M. A. (1986) Differential responsivity of verbal and visual recognition memory to physostigmine and ACTH. *Biol. Psychiatry*, 21, 538–42.

Rosen, W. G., Mohs, R. C. and Davis, K. L. (1984) A new rating scale for Alzheimer's disease. *Am. J. Psychiatry*, 141, 1356–64.

Rossor, M. and Iversen, L. L. (1986) Non-cholinergic neurotransmitter abnormalities in Alzheimer's disease. *Br. Med. Bull.* 42(1), 70–4.

Rubin, E. H. (1990) Psychopathology of senile dementia of the Alzheimer type. In: Wurtmann, A. J., Corkin, S., Growdon, J. H. and Ritter-Walker, E. (eds) *Alzheimer's Disease*, pp. 53–60. New York: Raven Press.

Rusted, J. M. (1988) Dissociative effects of scopolamine on working memory in healthy young volunteers. *Psychopharmacology*, 96, 487–92.

Rusted, J. M. and Warburton, D. M. (1988) The effects of scopolamine on working memory in healthy young volunteers. *Psychopharmacology*, 96, 145–51.

Shader, R. I., Harmatz, J. S. and Salzman, C. (1974) A new scale for clinical assessment in geriatric populations: Sandoz Clinical Geriatric (SCAG). *J. Am. Geriatr. Soc.*, 22, 101–13.

Siegfried, K. (1989) Depression and dementia of the Alzheimer type: implications for psycho-pharmacological research. *Human Psychopharmacol.*, 4, 237–45.

Sitaram, N., Weingartner, H. and Gillin, J. C. (1978) Human serial learning: enhancement with arecoline and impairment with scopolamine correlated with performance on placebo. *Science*, **201**, 274–6.

Smith, J. (1979) Nurse and psychiatric aide rating scales for assessing psychopharmacology in the elderly: a critical review. In: Raskin, A. and Jarvik, L. F. (eds) *Psychiatric Symptoms and Cognitive Loss in the Elderly*. New York: Halsted Press.

Storandt, M., Botwinick, J. and Danziger, W. L. (1986) Longitudinal changes: patients with mild SDAT and matched healthy controls. In: Poon, L. W. (ed.) *Handbook for Clinical Memory Assessment of Older Adults*, pp. 277–84. Washington, D.C.: American Psychological Association.

Sullivan, E. V., Shedlack, K. J., Corkin, S. and Growdon, J. H. (1982) Physostigmine and lecithin in Alzheimer's disease. In: Corkin, S., Davis, K. L., Growdon, J. H. *et al.* (eds) *Alzheimer's Disease: A Report of Progress*. Aging, Vol. 19, pp. 361–8. New York: Raven Press.

Terry, R. D. and Davies, P. (1980) Dementia of the Alzheimer type. In: Cowan, W. M., Zach, W. H. and Kandel, E. R. (eds) *Annual Review of Neuroscience*, Vol. 3, pp. 77–95. Palo Alto: California Annual Reviews.

Thal, L. J. and Fuld, P. A. (1983) Memory enhancement with oral physostigmine in Alzheimer's disease. *N. Engl. J. Med.*, **308**, 720.

Thal, L. J., Feld, P. A., Masur, D. M. and Sharpless, N. S. (1983) Oral physostigmine and lecithin improve memory in Alzheimer's disease. *Ann. Neurol.*, **13**, 491–6.

Warburton, D. M. and Wesnes, K. (1984) Drugs as research tools in psychology: cholinergic drugs and information processing. *Neuropsychobiology*, **11**, 121–32.

Warrington, E. K. (1975) The selective impairment of sematic memory. *Q. J. Exp. Psychol.*, **27**, 635–57.

Wechsler, D. (1955) *The Measurement and Appraisal of Adult Intelligence*. Baltimore: Williams and Wilkins.

Wesnes, K. A. and Simpson, P. A. (1988) Can scopolamine produce a model of the memory deficits seen in aging and dementia? In: Gruneberg, M. M., Morris, P. E. and Sykes, R. N. (eds) *Practical Aspects of Memory: Current Research and Issues*, Vol. 2, pp 236–41. Chichester: John Wiley and Sons.

Whitehouse, P. J., Gambetti, P., Harik, S. I., Kalaria, R. N., Perry, G., Younkin, S. I., Tabaton, M. and Unnerstall, J. R. (1989) Neurochemistry of dementia: establishing the links. In: Iqbal, K., Wisniewski, H. W. and Winblad, B. (eds) *Alzheimer's Disease and Related Disorders*, pp. 131–142. New York: Alan R. Liss.

Wilson, R. S., Kaszniak, A. W. (1986) Longitudinal changes: progressive idiopathic dementia. In: Poon, L. W. (ed.) *Handbook of Clinical Memory Assessment of Older Adults*, pp. 285–93. Washington, D.C.: American Psychological Association.

Wilson, R. S., Bacon, L. D., Fox, J. H. and Kaszniak, A. W. (1983) Primary memory and secondary memory in dementia of the Alzheimer type. *J. Clin. Neuropsychol.*, **5**, 337–44.

Yates, C. M., Ritchie, I. M., Simpson, J., Maloney, A. F. J. and Gordon, A. (1981) Noradrenaline in Alzheimer-type dementia and Down's syndrome. *Lancet*, **ii**, 39–40(letter).

Yates, C. M., Simpson, J., Gordon, A., Maloney, A. F. J., Allison, Y., Ritchie, I. M. and Urquhart, A. (1983) Catecholamines and cholinergic enzymes in presenile and senile Alzheimer type dementia and Down's syndrome. *Brain Res.*, **280**, 119–26.

Yesavage, J. A., Poulsen, S. L., Sheikh, J. and Tanke, E. (1988) Rates of change of common measures of impairment in senile dementia of the Alzheimer's type. *Psychopharmacol. Bull.*, **24**(4), 531–4.

5

Scientific Basis for Therapeutic Developments in Alzheimer's Disease

G. K. Wilcock

Department of Care of the Elderly, University of Bristol, UK

Essentially there are two approaches to developing new treatments for Alzheimer's disease: re-evaluating previously characterized compounds which appear to exhibit a property that might indicate potential efficacy by, for example, treating the neurotransmitter deficits discovered in Alzheimer's disease, or on the other hand developing new molecules targeted directly at more fundamental aspects of the disease process itself. Both these approaches have their advantages and disadvantages, and examples are included in this chapter. We must also hope that in the longer term it will be possible to prevent Alzheimer's disease from occurring, or that the techniques of modern medical and scientific research will isolate the underlying cellular abnormalities and lead to the ability to arrest it. This is probably a longer term goal, albeit an essential one.

The Heterogeneity of Alzheimer's Disease

Is Alzheimer's disease a single condition? This is of course one of the most important fundamental questions to answer, and when new developments in treatment are considered it is usually tacitly assumed that Alzheimer's disease is in fact a single disease entity. If it is not, then it may well be that we should be taking into account the relevance of clinical subgroups when evaluating the efficacy of any new therapy.

The Age Effect

It is now well established that Alzheimer's disease in younger and older subjects is qualitatively and quantitatively different. In an early study, Rossor and colleagues (1984) examined the neurochemical correlates of early and late onset types of Alzheimer's

Dementia: Molecules, Methods and Measures. Edited by I. Hindmarch, H. Hippius and G. K. Wilcock
© 1991 John Wiley & Sons Ltd

disease in 49 subjects and 54 control brains. As one would expect, the Alzheimer's group as a whole showed a significant reduction in the activity of cholinergic marker enzymes, and also of cortical concentrations of noradrenaline, gamma-aminobutyric acid and somatostatin. When subgrouped by age, however, it was apparent that the older subjects had a biochemical deficit that was largely limited to a reduction in cholinergic marker enzymes, which was predominantly confined to the temporal lobe and hippocampus. There was also a reduced level of somatostatin, again confined to the temporal cortex. Younger subjects, on the other hand, had more widespread cholinergic deficiency which was also greater than that in the older subjects. In addition, the non-cholinergic neurotransmitter deficits apparent in the group as a whole were largely concentrated in the younger subjects. This research team used the age of 80 years as the watershed between older and younger people, and their neurochemical findings had been substantiated by others. In addition, examination of the extent of the neuronal loss and of senile plaque and neurofibrillary tangle formation has shown that this parallels the neurochemical differences between older and younger subjects (Rothschild and Kasansin, 1936; Corsellis, 1962; Hubbard and Anderson, 1981).

Differences in the clinical manifestations of Alzheimer's disease in early and late onset forms have also been reported, although the age at which patients were divided into early and late onset forms was 65 years rather than 80 years as in the neurochemical and neuropathological studies. In particular, early onset cases have been reported to have a possible heightened selective vulnerability of the left hemisphere, while older subjects may have psychological evidence of a predominantly right hemisphere nature (Filley *et al.*, 1986; Seltzer and Sherwin, 1983). As the disease progresses, which usually happens more rapidly in younger than in older subjects, these different patterns are lost and the later middle and end stages of the dementia are in many ways indistinguishable, irrespective of the age of onset. It is therefore apparent from studies of several different parameters that Alzheimer's disease in younger and late onset forms may be subject to different mechanisms, and possibly have differing aetiological bases.

Other Evidence for Heterogeneity

There are now many studies in the literature at both a clinical and basic science level indicating that heterogeneity may extend beyond the simple age-defined categorization reported above. Mayeux *et al.* (1985) studied 121 consecutive patients with dementia of the Alzheimer's type, following many of the subjects over 4 years. They were able to identify four separate subgroups: those with little or no progression, whom they grouped together as 'benign'; a 'myoclonic' group exhibiting myoclonic jerks and also characterized by severe intellectual decline and frequent mutism, often after a younger age of onset; a group with extrapyramidal abnormalities, marked by severe intellectual and functional decline and frequent psychotic symptoms unrelated to the prescription of phenothiazines; and, of course, a typical group exhibiting a gradual progressive decline, both intellectually and functionally. Only those with myoclonus were on average younger. A similar study by Chui and colleagues (1985) of 146 individuals indicated that the presence of myoclonus and extrapyramidal disorders was associated with the greatest severity of dementia, and that this was not related to the prescription of phenothiazines. As well as showing differences that were not related to the age of onset of the disorder, this study also showed that language disorders were more prevalent and severe in younger subjects, which of course also strengthens the hypothesis that age of onset itself may define subgroups, as already discussed.

Further differences are also apparent at a clinical level. Friedland *et al.* (1988) has reviewed some of the available evidence, including the apparent ability of positron emission tomography (PET) to identify subjects with predominantly left or right temporoparietal hypometabolism, who have impaired constructional ability when carrying out simple tasks such as drawing a house. Those whose hypometabolism is predominantly left-sided, in comparison, show constructional abilities that are significantly less affected (Goodglass and Kaplan, 1972).

The levels of various neurotransmitter metabolites, in particular homovanillic acid, hydroxyindoleacetic acid and biopterin concentrations in cerebrospinal fluid, also differ depending upon whether or not the subjects exhibit myoclonus or extrapyramidal disorders. In addition, at a neuroanatomical level, the degree of neuronal loss and neurofibrillary tangle formation in the various subcortical nuclei similarly differentiates subgroups, and in one study a group of elderly subjects with clinical and histologically confirmed Alzheimer's disease were shown to have normal levels of cholinergic marker enzymes and no diminution of neurons in the basal nucleus of Meynert, despite significant dementia. They showed, however, a loss of neurons from noradrenergic and, to a lesser extent, serotoninergic subcortical sites (Wilcock *et al.*, 1988).

In summary, there is therefore important evidence to indicate that subjects with Alzheimer's disease may be segregated into subgroups when a variety of different parameters are considered. These include clinical, neurochemical and neuropathological criteria, and, in the older age group, it would appear that there is even a subgroup who do not have a significant cholinergic deficit. All these factors must be taken into account when developing and evaluating new therapeutic strategies.

Cholinergic Strategies

Many strategies aimed at improving cholinergic function have been evaluated in the treatment of Alzheimer's disease, with disappointing results. Although initially rejected as being of little clinical benefit, anticholinesterases have enjoyed a resurgence of interest since the study of tacrine hydrochloride (THA) published by Summers *et al.* in 1986. The ensuing controversy has led to attempts to reevaluate several different cholinergic strategies that act on the cholinesterase pathways, including a re-examination of the role of physostigmine, particularly in slow release form. As far as THA is concerned, the feelings emerging now that the results of several studies are available can at best be described as cautiously optimistic, although many would feel that it holds little promise, if any. It is too early, at the time of writing, to comment meaningfully on this, or on the position with respect to physostigmine, but the latter may well follow the pattern of activity reported for THA.

Evaluation of these results has been hampered by many clinical problems, including the possibility of heterogeneity and the questionable accuracy of the diagnosis of Alzheimer's disease, although in the best centres this is probably of the order of 85% when verified against autopsy confirmation.

In addition to clinical factors such as these, it is also important not to forget the complexity of the cholinergic system itself, particularly with respect to the various receptor subtypes. Until relatively recently all muscarinic receptors were thought to be alike, but we now know there are at least three different pharmacologically identifiable subtypes, and probably five different molecular forms. It has become apparent that there is a selective alteration in the density of presynaptic muscarinic receptors, often referred to as M_2 receptors, in cortical areas and in the hippocampus. It is possible that stimulation of these, either by cholinergic agonists or by increasing the amount of acetylcholine available through the use of anticholinesterases, may actually have a negative feedback on the cell, thus switching off the system rather than enhancing it, whatever effect the acetylcholine may have on the postsynaptic receptors. Even this is a simplistic analysis, and the situation is further complicated by the knowledge that nicotinic receptors are also selectively impaired in cortical areas and the hippocampus. The physiology is thus complex, and it is not surprising that simplistic models of cholinergic replacement or agonist therapy fail to yield the anticipated results. Indeed, to some extent it is remarkable that they have proved to be of any benefit at all.

Several centres are now studying the possibility of using nicotine in various forms as a therapeutic agent, and it may well be that a combination of this approach together with muscarinic agonist activity may prove more useful than either alone. A further step in the evolution of cholinergic therapy might be to use a compound or compounds that stimulate postsynaptic M_1 receptors, block M_2, and have a stimulatory effect on the nicotinic receptors as well (Goyal, 1989; Araujo *et al.*, 1988). However, as cholinergic receptors are not simply on/off switches, but rather fulfil a neuromodulatory function, even this approach would probably fall short of producing significant symptomatic relief.

Despite the complexities of this issue it seems possible that modulation of the cholinergic pathways in Alzheimer's disease may hold some hope for those with a predominantly cholinergic deficit, i.e. particularly the elderly and also others who are early in the course of their disease, before other neurotransmitter deficits have arisen to an extent that significantly impairs function. In the latter circumstance, we may well have to design multiple neurotransmitter enhancement strategies.

The Development of Trophic Factors as Potential Therapeutic Agents

It has been known for some time that certain types of neuron require externally derived trophic factors in order to maintain their integrity and to function normally. One of the best known examples of these has coincidentally been found to play a potentially important role in the integrity of the cholinergic system, and possibly therefore also in the treatment of Alzheimer's disease. It was established in the 1930s that nerve growth factor (NGF) was essential for the developing sympathetic nervous system (for review see Levi-Montalcini, 1987). We now know that NGF receptors are present on cholinergic cells in the basal nucleus of Meynert (Allen *et al.*, 1989) and that the level of messenger RNA for the NGF receptor in the same region of the brain is not diminished in Alzheimer's disease in this region (Goedert *et al.*, 1989). This implies that it might be possible to maintain the viability of cholinergic cells in Alzheimer's disease, and for that matter in other conditions where there is a similar defect. Human NGF is present in the human brain in such small quantities that it has been difficult to assay, and it is proving equally difficult to synthesize sufficient quantities of pure human NGF for use in clinical trials. It probably will not be long, however, before small scale pilot studies of NGF will be undertaken, using a system that delivers NGF directly into the ventricular system within the brain, as it will almost certainly not pass the blood-brain barrier.

Although the potential use of NGF is an exciting new development in the war against Alzheimer's disease, there are fears that it might actually be detrimental rather than therapeutically useful. Some researchers believe that there is already abnormal neuritic outgrowth, hence the development of argyrophilic plaques, and that this could be aggravated by trophic factors. One can only say that at the moment there is no evidence to support this hypothesis in the studies that have been undertaken in rats or primates, although the majority of these have been relatively short-term studies. The toxicological aspects of NGF also require consideration despite the fact that it is a normal constituent of neurological tissue.

Much interest is also being shown in other potential neurotrophic factors, including epidermal growth factor, brain-derived neurotrophic factor, neurotrophin 3 and several gangliosides. If successful, such approaches may provide a means of arresting the neuronal decline in Alzheimer's disease rather than attempting to remedy the biochemical deficits that result from the death of such cells. Thus if Alzheimer's disease subjects are caught early enough in the course of their illness, there is the possibility that the disease could be slowed or arrested, resulting in a significant improvement in the quality and duration of life for the sufferer.

A4 Protein, Amyloid and the Treatment of Alzheimer's Disease

The centrally placed component of the argyrophilic or senile plaque that is found within the brain in Alzheimer's disease consists of the protein beta-amyloid. The material found in these plaques is synthesized from a larger precursor protein, which is widely conserved in different animal and even insect species, and in different tissues within the body. The beta-amyloid precursor protein, also known as the A4 protein, is very likely therefore to have an important function in the nervous system. It is a transmembrane protein, i.e. a portion lies within the membrane of the neuron, and there is a large extracellular component. The beta-amyloid segment of this precursor protein contains a little over 40 amino acids, and this fragment is somehow assembled to make the beta-amyloid itself. Modern research techniques from a number of fields have provided a wealth of information about this protein and its various forms that is very difficult to assimilate. It was originally hoped that our increasing understanding of the nature and mechanism of formation of the amyloid substance might result in the possibility of ameliorating the condition at a fundamental biochemical level. This has so far proved disappointing, despite the fact that protease inhibitors have been found as part of the precursor protein or in close association with it. In particular, the precursor protein can be made with or without an insert known as the Kunitz-type protease inhibitor, implying that its presence may either hinder the formation of plaque formation or help prevent it, depending upon whether or not the protease inhibitor is normally a component of the precursor protein. One potential therapeutic hypothesis could be that there is an alteration in proteolysis that is important in the pathogenesis of Alzheimer's disease, and that this may be amenable to pharmacological modification.

Summary

There are several avenues to the development of new therapeutic compounds for treating chronic degenerative disorders such as Alzheimer's disease. It may be that the most profitable way forward is to apply insight gained into the basic pathological processes to the development of new approaches, whether or not these involve rescreening old compounds or the synthesis of novel substances. Whichever approach is adopted, it is essential that clinical trials are undertaken in the full light and knowledge of the difficulties in interpreting the results, otherwise we may be in danger of jettisoning treatments that would be of benefit to at least a proportion of sufferers.

References

Allen, S. J., Dawbarn, D., Spillantini, M. G., Goedert, M., Wilcock, G. K., Moss, T. M. and Semenenko, F. M. (1989) Distribution of B-nerve growth factor receptors in the human basal forebrain. *J. Comp. Neurol.*, **289**, 626–40.

Araujo, D. M., Lapchak, P. A., Robitaille, Y., Gauthier, S. and Quirion, R. (1988) Differential alteration of various cholinergic markers in cortical and subcortical regions of human brain in Alzheimer's disease. *J. Neurochem.*, **50**, 1914–23.

Chui, H. C., Teng, E. L., Henderson, V. W. and Moy, A. C. (1985) Clinical subtypes of dementia of the Alzheimer type. *Neurology*, **35**, 1544–50.

Corsellis, J. A. N. (1962) *Mental Illness and the Ageing Brain*. Maudsley Monograph No. 9. Oxford: Oxford University Press.

Filley, O. M., Kelly, J. and Heaton, R. K. (1986) Neuropsychologic features of early- and late-onset Alzheimer's disease. *Arch. Neurol.*, **43**, 574–6.

Friedland, R. P., Koss, E., Haxby, J. V., Grady, C. L., Luxenberg, J., Schapiro, M. B. and Kaye, J. (1988) Alzheimer disease: clinical and biological heterogeneity. *Ann. Intern. Med.*, **109**, 298–311.

Goedert, M., Fine, A., Dawbarn, D., Wilcock, G. K. and Chao, M. V. (1989) Nerve growth factor receptor mRNA distribution in human brain: normal levels in basal forebrain in Alzheimer's disease. *Brain Res. Mol. Brain Res.*, **5**, 1–7.

Goodglass, H. and Kaplan, E. (1972) *The Assessment of Aphasia and Related Disorders*. Philadelphia: Lea and Febiger.

Goyal, R. K. (1989) Muscarinic receptor subtypes: physiology and clinical implications. *N. Engl. J. Med.*, **321**(15), 1022–9.

Hubbard, B. M. and Anderson, J. M. (1981) A quantitative study of cerebral atrophy in old age and senile dementia. *J. Neurol. Sci.* **50**, 135–45.

Levi-Montalcini, R. (1987) The nerve growth factor 35 years later. *Science*, **237**, 1154–61.

Mayeux R., Stern, Y. and Spanton, S. (1985) Heterogeneity in dementia of the Alzheimer type: evidence of subgroups. *Neurology*, **35**, 453–61.

Rossor, M. N., Iverson, L. L., Reynolds, G. P., Mountjoy, C. Q. and Roth, M. (1984) Neurochemical characteristics of early and late onset types of Alzheimer's disease. *BMJ*, **288**, 961–4.

Rothschild, D. and Kasansin, J. (1936) Clinicopathologic study of Alzheimer's disease: relationship to senile condition. *Arch. Neurol. Psychiatry*, **36**, 293–321.

Seltzer, B. and Sherwin, I. (1983) A comparison of clinical features in early- and late-onset primary degenerative dementia. One entity or two? *Arch. Neurol.* **40**, 143–6.

Summers, W. K., Majovski, L. V., Marsh, G. M., Tachiki, K. and Kling, A. (1986) Oral tetrahydroaminoacridine in long term treatment of senile dementia, Alzheimer's type. *N. Engl. J. Med.*, **315**, 1241–5.

Wilcock, G. K., Esiri, M. M., Bowen, D. M. and Hughes, A. O. (1988) The differential involvement of sub-cortical nuclei in senile dementia of Alzheimer's type. *J. Neurol. Neurosurg. Psychiatry*, **51**, 842–9.

6

The Predictive Value of Volunteer Studies with Anti-dementia Drugs

René Spiegel

Clinical Research, CNS Department, SANDOZ Pharma Ltd, Basel, Switzerland

Introduction

This chapter deals with drug experiments performed in healthy volunteers, i.e. in young or old subjects who do not suffer from the disorders which may eventually be treated with the drugs tested on them. I have previously discussed the topic of drug experiments in normal subjects with regard to neuroleptics, antidepressants and other established central nervous system (CNS) compounds (Spiegel, 1980; 1989, Chs 3 and 4) and will therefore concentrate on those issues specific for anti-dementia drugs.

Clinical development of novel CNS-active compounds usually begins with single-dose studies in volunteers. Such trials concentrate on the tolerability and safety of the compound in question and are recommended in all existing guidelines for clinical drug testing for the following reasons: (a) normal volunteers are readily available and are more homogeneous psychopathologically than psychiatric patients; (b) they are screened to be physically healthy and do not take other medication which might interact with the experimental drug; and (c) they can give truly informed consent and will take an emotionally more neutral attitude towards a drug experiment than patients who need active treatment.

On the other hand, three fundamental problems limit the freedom to perform and the conclusions to be drawn from drug experiments in healthy volunteers: (a) there are ethical concerns as to whether an unknown and therefore potentially harmful compound should be given to persons who cannot possibly benefit from it; (b) normal volunteers may differ in a number of important aspects from mentally disturbed or impaired patients, a fact rendering the interpretation of experimental results difficult; and (c) single-dose administration, which is typically performed in this type of trial, may not adequately represent the clinical situation, where chronic drug administration is more characteristic.

Dementia: Molecules, Methods and Measures. Edited by I. Hindmarch, H. Hippius and G. K. Wilcock
© 1991 John Wiley & Sons Ltd

The second issue, concern about the predictive value of volunteer studies, was extensively discussed at the 1989 European Consensus Conference on the Methodology of Clinical Trials of 'Nootropics'. The final report of the Consensus Committee (Engel *et al.*, 1990) lists a number of models used in the past for testing 'nootropic' drugs:

1. Subjects studied under conditions of hypoxia.
2. Subjects studied under mentally stressful conditions.
3. Subjects with a drug-induced memory deficit, e.g. due to scopolamine.
4. Elderly volunteers with some memory deficit.
5. Subjects with impaired vigilance as documented by the electroencephalogram (EEG).

All these 'models' have in common an element of impairment, either through manipulation of basically unimpaired subjects or through selection of slightly impaired, although non-pathological individuals. Having acknowledged that interesting pharmacodynamic information can be collected in volunteer studies, the report of the Consensus Committee then concludes with the following, essentially negative, statement: 'It was nevertheless clearly spelled out during the discussion that the predictive value of preclinical [i.e. human volunteer] models used with nootropics has been low in the past and that it would be premature to stop the development of a theoretically useful drug because of negative results in studies with human volunteers.'

While there is little controversy about the value of volunteer trials as regards single-dose tolerability and pharmacokinetics, many authors disagree about the predictive value of such studies with respect to pharmacodynamic and potential therapeutic properties of CNS-active drugs. In order to contribute to the on-going discussion, I will concentrate on findings from studies performed in our laboratories, some of them unpublished and more than 10 years old. Initially, these investigations were prompted by the hope of better characterizing the compounds used in the treatment of dementia syndromes (called 'senile cerebral insufficiency' at that time) and to understand their mechanism of action. The examples chosen are volunteer studies with Hydergine® (co-dergocrine mesylate), bromvincamine and piracetam. Further experiments concerned the alpha-2 agonists clonidine and guanfacine and two muscarinic agonists (RS 86 and BOP 086) which, based on mechanistic considerations, were of interest for the treatment of Alzheimer's disease.

All the trials described here were performed under double-blind conditions, all were placebo-controlled single-dose experiments and used randomized, balanced allocation (usually Latin squares) of treatments to subjects. All studies were performed in young (20–40 years) and, with one exception, male subjects, mostly students. The participants were medically screened before inclusion, they were fully informed about the planned experiments and received a fee for their participation. After completion of the experiments, they were informed about the most important findings.

Studies with Cerebral Metabolism Enhancers and Nootropics

Studies with Hydergine®

In the 1970s and early 1980s Hydergine was considered to be the prototype drug for the treatment of senile cerebral insufficiency (Fanchamps, 1983). Among the many studies undertaken to elucidate this compound's profile and mechanism of action, two should be mentioned in the present context: one trial performed in waking and one in sleeping subjects.

Study in waking subjects. Participants: eight healthy male subjects, 20–35 years old. Treatments: Hydergine 5 mg, 10 mg or placebo in balanced order. Parameters assessed: blood pressure, pulse rate, subjective symptoms, semantic differential (Spiegel, 1989, p. 55), reaction times and quantified EEG. The study commenced between 0800 and 0900, with assessments at baseline, and then 1, 2, 4 and 6 h after drug administration.

Both doses of Hydergine were found to slightly decrease blood pressure. The lower dose (5 mg) produced subjective stimulation in three out of the eight subjects and sedation in three subjects. Three subjects experienced nasal congestion. In the quantified EEG under resting and eyes-closed conditions, total spectral power was increased, and the absolute and relative power in the alpha band was also increased (nominally significant at $P < 0.05$). The higher dose (10 mg) produced headache or a feeling of pressure in the head in five out of the eight subjects, four subjects reported nasal congestion, and three tiredness and less drive and initiative. The quantified EEG did not show clearcut effects under eyes-closed conditions, while total power and alpha power were increased under eyes-open conditions.

It was concluded from these findings that the effects of single-dose Hydergine on subjective and objective psychometric variables in normal volunteers were unclear. The effects of 5 mg Hydergine on EEG parameters were somewhat similar to those described in patients with senile cerebral insufficiency on chronic Hydergine treatment (Matejcek *et al.*, 1979), whereas the effects of 10 mg of the drug appeared difficult to interpret.

Study in sleeping subjects. Participants: two groups of six healthy male subjects, 20–30 years old. Treatments: Hydergine 3 mg, 6 mg or placebo given 30 min before the start of sleep recordings between 2200 and 2230. Subjects spent two consecutive nights for adaptation in the sleep laboratory, then one night on either Hydergine or placebo. The first 7½ h of sleep recordings were analysed by means of conventional methods (see Rechtschaffen and Kales, 1968), providing 39 polygraphic and morning questionnaire parameters.

The main findings of this trial are displayed in Figure 1 and indicate, along with the other polygraphic and subjective data collected, that single-dose Hydergine 3 or 6 mg had no significant effects on either objective or subjective sleep parameters in normal volunteers.

Studies with Bromvincamine

This derivative of vincamine was clinically tested in the late 1970s for its effect on cognitive and mental symptoms in patients with senile cerebral insufficiency. It was shown to be significantly superior to placebo at daily doses of 60–120 mg and was later introduced in Japan under the brand name Sabromin®. Two volunteer studies were performed in our laboratories: one in waking and one in sleeping volunteers.

Study in waking subjects (Aebi and Spiegel, 1977, unpublished data). Participants: 12 healthy subjects, eight male, four female, aged 20–35 years. Treatments: bromvincamine 20 mg, 40 mg or placebo in balanced order (Latin squares). Parameters assessed: d-2

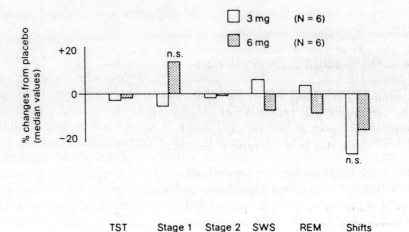

Figure 1. Hydergine at single oral doses of 3 mg and 6 mg had no significant effects on polygraphic sleep parameters. The figure shows median values of changes on active drug from individual placebo values. Note that the small variations are not statistically significant (n.s.) (3-way ANOVA with subsequent Tukey tests) and are not dose related (from Spiegel, 1982). TST = total sleep time; SWS = slow wave sleep; REM = rapid eye movement sleep; Shifts = changes from sleep stage 2 and SWS to awake and stage 1

concentration test, KLT concentration-performance test (see Spiegel, 1989, p. 51 ff.), learning of word lists and series of graphic signs, semantic differential and subjective symptoms. Assessments were performed at baseline (between 0800 and 0900) and 2, 4 and 6 h after drug administration.

The results of this study were remarkable in that up to 6 h after drug administration no differences whatsoever between the three treatments were noticed, i.e. bromvincamine in the doses tested did not have any effects on subjective and objective measures in normal volunteers.

Study in sleeping subjects (Nüesch and Spiegel, 1977, unpublished data). Participants: 12 healthy male subjects, 20–35 years. Treatments: bromvincamine 20 mg, 40 mg or placebo in balanced order (Latin squares); two adaptation nights, 7½ h of sleep analysed (methods as in sleep trial described above).

Like the study in waking subjects, this trial did not reveal any effects of the compound on objective (polygraphic) and subjective parameters of sleep in normal volunteers.

Study with Piracetam

Piracetam (brand names Nootropil®, Normabrain®) is one of the few compounds accepted by certain European drug regulatory authorities, e.g. in Germany, for the treatment of senile cerebral insufficiency. Having been introduced as the first 'nootropic drug', piracetam was studied in a polygraphic sleep investigation (Spiegel, 1982) with the same methodology as in the sleep investigations described above. Single doses of 1200 mg, 2400 mg and placebo were administered. As shown in Figure 2, piracetam at the doses given did not affect any of the polygraphic sleep parameters in a significant manner. Subjective sleep parameters were not altered either.

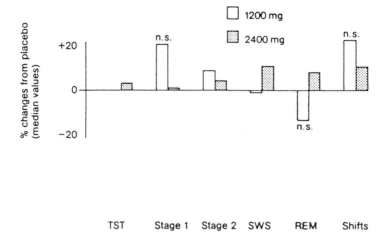

Figure 2. Piracetam at single oral doses of 1200 mg and 2400 mg had no significant effects on polygraphic sleep parameters. Methods and presentation of findings as in Figure 1 (from Spiegel, 1982)

In summary, none of the three cerebral metabolism enhancers or nootropics tested in our laboratories – Hydergine, bromvincamine and piracetam – showed clearcut effects after single-dose administration to healthy young volunteers.

Studies with Alpha-2 Agonistic Drugs

Interest in alpha-2 agonists was stimulated by a paper by Arnsten and Goldman-Rakic (1985) describing the effects of very low doses of clonidine on learning performance in aged animals. In a low (μg/kg) dose range, this compound improved learning performance in monkeys with prefrontal cortical lesions subjected to a spatial memory test. The effective dose range was narrow and showed high inter-individual variation, lower doses producing no effects and slightly higher doses leading to adverse effects on learning. Similarly positive animal results were subsequently reported for guanfacine, another alpha-2 agonist (Arnsten *et al.*, 1988).

As we had performed some studies with clonidine and guanfacine in normal volunteers years before the animal findings of Arnsten and Goldman-Rakic (1985) were published, it is of interest to briefly review these older data in view of potential indications of positive drug effects on performance and CNS effects in the subjects tested (for details see Spiegel and Devos, 1980).

Study in waking subjects. Participants: 10 healthy, normotensive male subjects, aged 20–40 years. Treatments: clonidine 0.15 or 0.30 mg, guanfacine 1.0 or 2.0 mg, or placebo; all treatments in balanced order (Latin squares) on 5 non-consecutive days. Parameters assessed: blood pressure, pulse rate, reaction time to acoustic stimuli and hand grip strength. Assessments were performed before and 1, 2, 4 and 6 h after drug administration.

Blood pressure was dose-dependently reduced after clonidine. Subjects experienced strong and dose-dependent tiredness, dryness of the mouth and dizziness after clonidine.

Neither reaction time nor hand grip strength were improved after clonidine; in fact all the (not significant) differences pointed to impaired performance after this drug. Guanfacine displayed a qualitatively similar pattern of effects; however, the action of this drug set in later, did not reach the same maximum levels, and peaked later than that of clonidine (4–6 h instead of 2 h after administration).

Evidently neither of these two alpha-2 agonists led to an improvement in visuomotor and motor performance at the doses tested.

Studies in sleeping subjects. Two polygraphic sleep studies, both involving six normotensive subjects, were carried out using the same design and methods as in the previous sleep studies. After two nights in the sleep laboratory, in order to enable the subjects to adapt to the experimental conditions, clonidine 0.15 mg, 0.30 mg or placebo in the clonidine trial, and guanfacine 1.0 mg, 2.0 mg or placebo in the guanfacine trial, was administered on three consecutive nights. The order of their administration was balanced by means of a Latin square design, and drugs were given 30 min before lights were turned off and recordings begun.

The effects of clonidine on sleep in normal volunteers were strong and dose-dependent (Figure 3): rapid eye movement (REM) sleep was significantly reduced after both doses, the mean reduction after 0.30 mg attaining more than 80%. Stage 2 sleep showed a dose-dependent increase, and the number of shifts to light sleep (stage 1) and waking as well as the percentage of stage 1 sleep showed increases. Again, the effects of guanfacine 1.0 and 2.0 mg were qualitatively similar but less pronounced than those of clonidine (details in Spiegel and Devos, 1980).

In summary, the experiments with clonidine and guanfacine show that these two alpha-2 agonists have strong and dose-dependent CNS and peripheral effects in healthy volunteers. Sedation of an unpleasant character was reported after clonidine and no indication of a positive effect on visuomotor and motor performance was present. Learning and memory were not assessed in this study. Guanfacine had qualitatively similar, although weaker effects, including its action on sleep, where clonidine, at the doses tested, almost abolished REM sleep. Clonidine is one of the most potent REM sleep suppressants (Spiegel, 1989, Ch. 4).

Studies with Muscarinic Drugs

According to the 'cholinergic hypothesis of geriatric memory dysfunction' (Bartus et al., 1982), drugs which facilitate cholinergic neurotransmission should be of symptomatic benefit in Alzheimer's disease and other disorders affecting cognitive functions in old age. Since the drugs available around 1980 to test this hypothesis suffered from serious drawbacks (cardiotoxicity, hepatotoxicity, unfavourable pharmacokinetic properties; see Palacios and Spiegel, 1986), we decided to perform a series of pharmacodynamic and pilot clinical trials with the Sandoz compound RS 86 (2-ethyl-8-methyl-2,8-diazaspiro-(4.5)-decane-1.3-dione hydrobromide; see Palacios et al., 1986). RS 86, which is well tolerated and has a better pharmacokinetic profile than other cholinergic drugs then available, was not foreseen for formal clinical development or registration, but served as a tool to study a variety of methodological and logistic issues.

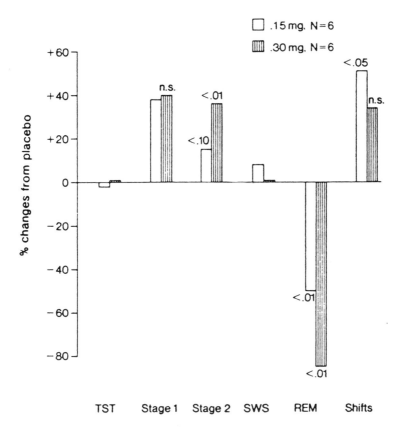

Figure 3. Clonidine at single oral doses of 0.15 and 0.30 mg had significant and dose-dependent effects on polygraphic sleep parameters: REM sleep was decreased and stage 2 sleep increased, whereas SWS was unchanged. Stage 1 (= drowsiness) and shifts from deeper sleep to drowsiness were slightly increased. Methods and presentation of findings as in Figure 1 (from Spiegel and Devos, 1980)

Studies with RS 86 in Waking Volunteers

Five experimental studies in a total of 59 healthy male volunteers, aged 20–35 years, were performed. The dose range tested was 0.25 to 2.5 mg, and the following issues were investigated: (a) tolerability, including effects on blood pressure, pulse rate and respiration, and subjective symptoms; (b) effects on psychomotor speed, memory performance and quantified EEG; and (c) interactions with the (central and peripheral) muscarinic antagonist scopolamine and the (peripheral) M_1 antagonist pirenzepine.

The results of these studies, which have been published in more detail (see Azcona *et al.*, 1986), can be summarized as follows:

1. Up to 1.5 mg, RS 86 produced few significant vegetative or subjective effects; pulse rate was slightly increased, and some subjects experienced mild tiredness. Doses of 2.0 mg or more were followed by hypersalivation, sweating, disturbed visual accommodation, shivering and occasionally by nausea.
2. Performance on a number of attention and memory tasks (reaction time, picture recognition) was not altered after single doses of 0.75 and 1.5 mg of RS 86.

3. Scopolamine administration (0.25 or 0.5 mg given subcutaneously) was followed by marked sedation, reduction of blood pressure, slowing of pulse rate, dryness of mouth, and disturbed visual accommodation and equilibrium; these effects were neither antagonized nor attenuated by RS 86 at well-tolerated doses.
4. Salivation, the most obvious peripheral action of RS 86, was completely blocked by scopolamine, and an attenuation of salivation was also seen in the experiment with RS 86 plus pirenzepine.

It was concluded from these trials in normal volunteers that RS 86 had effects partly similar to and partly different from those of other cholinergic drugs such as the cholinesterase inhibitor physostigmine. Specifically, RS 86 did not improve cognitive performance in volunteers and was not found to antagonize the effects of the muscarinic antagonist scopolamine; both effects are seen with physostigmine.

Study with RS 86 in Sleeping Subjects

Cholinergic agonists such as physostigmine, arecoline and pilocarpine have characteristic effects on polygraphic sleep parameters in man: REM sleep latency is decreased, and the percentage of REM sleep is increased in the first few hours of sleep if such compounds are administered immediately before subjects retire to bed. It was therefore of interest to study RS 86 in this respect. Two polygraphic sleep studies, each with 12 healthy male subjects aged 21–30 years, were performed (Spiegel, 1984). Design and methods corresponded to those of the sleep studies reported above, the doses tested being 0.25 or 0.5 mg of RS 86 in the first trial, 0.75 or 1.5 mg in the second, compared with placebo after two adaptation nights.

While 0.25 and 0.50 mg of RS 86 had no significant effects on electrophysiological correlates of sleep, 0.75 and 1.5 mg of the compound altered polygraphic sleep parameters in a dose-dependent fashion (Figure 4): the REM latency was shortened, REM sleep in the first third of the sleep period increased, and slow wave sleep was reduced in the first and the second third of the sleep period (data not shown). Pulse rate was dose-dependently and significantly increased after RS 86, but subjective sleep experience and the condition of the subject in the morning were not altered.

The findings of this trial were later replicated using a larger subject sample (Riemann *et al.*, 1988), and it is of interest that another muscarinic agonist, BOP 086, which is chemically related to RS 86, was also found to decrease REM sleep latency and to increase REM sleep in the first hours of sleep (Berger, unpublished data). However, the development of BOP 086 has been discontinued owing to tolerability problems.

Discussion

The findings presented in the previous section can be summarized as follows:

1. The three nootropics or cerebral metabolism enhancers tested in our laboratories – Hydergine, bromvincamine and piracetam – did not show clearcut effects, no common pattern of activity emerging after the administration of single doses of these compounds to normal young volunteers. Bromvincamine and piracetam had no discernible effects at the doses used, whereas Hydergine showed some subjective

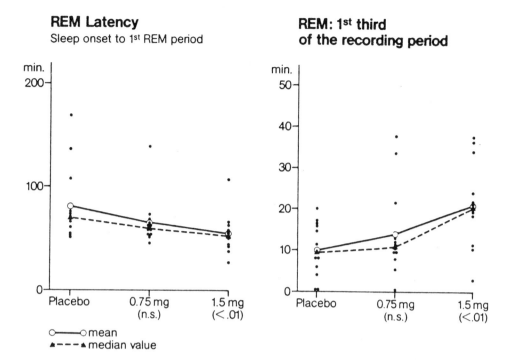

Figure 4. RS 86 reduced mean REM latency (= time from sleep onset to the appearance of the first REM period) in a significant and dose-dependent fashion. The duration of REM sleep in the first third of the recording period was significantly and dose-dependently increased (from Spiegel, 1984). n.s. = not significant

and objective action which, however, is difficult to subsume under a general concept such as increased vigilance or enhancement of cognitive functions. While this may not come as a surprise in well-functioning young volunteers, further conclusions from our experiments are not possible because none of the three compounds tested is generally accepted as an effective treatment of dementia. Although there are dozens of controlled clinical studies with Hydergine and also a number of such trials with piracetam indicating that these drugs can be of use in senile mental decline (see Nicholson, 1990), no unequivocal trials demonstrate their efficacy in patients suffering from dementia.

2. In contrast to nootropics, alpha-2 agonists like clonidine and guanfacine have clearcut and dose-dependent effects on both waking and sleeping healthy volunteers: they lower blood pressure and produce marked sedation and a number of peripheral effects. REM sleep is reduced in a dose-dependent fashion. No positive effects on motor and visuomotor performance were noted in our experiments and, to my knowledge, no favourable effects on cognitive functions have been reported by other authors using lower doses of these compounds. Again, conclusions with regard to the predictive value of volunteer trials are difficult to draw because neither clonidine nor guanfacine has so far been demonstrated to be of any therapeutic value in patients with dementia. Preliminary trials with clonidine (Mohr *et al.*, 1989) and with guanfacine (Schlegel *et al.*, 1989) in Alzheimer's disease produced negative results, and further studies with guanfacine are reported to be on-going (McEntee and Crook, 1990). It is of

course possible that the doses used in both our experiments and in the preliminary clinical trials quoted were too high and that the dose range of alpha-2 agonists having positive effects on memory function is as narrow and individual in man as it is in animals (Arnsten and Goldman-Rakic, 1985). However, until confirmatory information on the efficacy of guanfacine or clonidine in dementia becomes available, little can be deduced from our experiments regarding the predictive value of studies in healthy volunteers in the sense discussed in this paper.

3. Cholinergic drugs like physostigmine, arecoline and pilocarpine have strong central and peripheral effects in normal volunteers, and a similar spectrum of effects was evident in our experiments with the postsynaptic muscarinic agonist RS 86. With regard to its peripheral effects, RS 86 resembled other cholinergic compounds and its action on REM sleep latency also corresponded to that of other cholinergics. On the other hand, RS 86, unlike physostigmine, did not antagonize the effects of the muscarinic antagonist scopolamine and, in contrast to arecoline, it suppressed rather than augmented slow wave sleep. Thus, different cholinergic agonists display partly similar and partly different profiles of activity, and trials in healthy volunteers should be useful for characterizing cholinergic drugs qualitatively and quantitatively. Here again, however, the question of whether such experiments will predict the therapeutic value of individual compounds in dementia must remain open, because the efficacy of cholinergic drugs in this condition is still controversial; some positive findings have been reported for physostigmine in Alzheimer's disease (Thal *et al.*, 1989) and a few positive effects were also seen with RS 86 (Wettstein and Spiegel, 1984; Hollander *et al.*, 1987), but the clinical relevance of these observations is still open to question. The controversy about the utility of tacrine, probably the most widely tested cholinergic agent in Alzheimer's disease, is still on-going (see Eagger *et al.*, 1991; Levy, 1990; Byrne and Arie, 1990).

Taking all these findings and considerations together, it seems safe to say that the predictive value of volunteer studies with anti-dementia drugs is limited at present. Important pharmacodynamic and pharmacokinetic properties of CNS-active drugs can be studied and described in healthy volunteers, but predictions regarding a compound's likely therapeutic effect in demented patients would appear unfounded at present. The situation may, however, change in the near future: many drug companies are currently engaged in development programmes with cholinergic, adrenergic, serotoninergic and other agents, and I have little doubt that one or more of these principles will afford at least symptomatic benefit to groups or subgroups of patients with dementia. Then, as soon as such compounds with confirmed clinical efficacy are available, it will also be possible to give a clear answer to the main question posed in this chapter.

References

Arnsten, A. F. T. and Goldman-Rakic, P. S. (1985) Alpha-2 adrenergic mechanisms in prefrontal cortex associated with cognitive decline in aged non-human primates. *Science*, **230**, 1273–6.

Arnsten, A. F. T., Cai, J. X. and Goldman-Rakic, P. S. (1988) The alpha-2 adrenergic agonist guanfacine improves memory in aged monkeys without sedative or hypotensive side effects: evidence for alpha-2 subtypes. *J. Neurosci*, **8**, 4287–98.

Azcona, A., Roth, S. and Spiegel, R. (1986) Effects of the muscarinic agonist RS 86 in healthy volunteers. *Pharmacopsychiatry*, **19**, 323–5.

Bartus, R. T., Dean, R. L., Beer, B. and Lippa, A. S. (1982) The cholinergic hypothesis of geriatric memory dysfunction. *Science*, **217**, 408–17.

Byrne, E. J. and Arie, T. (1990) Are drugs targeted at Alzheimer's disease useful? 2. Insufficient evidence of worthwhile benefit. *BMJ*, **300**, 1132–3.

Eagger, S. A., Levy, R. and Sahakian, B. J. (1991) Tacrine in Alzheimer's disease. *Lancet*, **337**, 989–92.

Engel, R. *et al.* (1990) Consensus Conference on the Methodology of Clinical Trials of 'Nootropics', Munich, June 1989. Report of the Consensus Committee. *Pharmacopsychiatry*, **23**, 171–5.

Fanchamps, A. (1983) Dihydroergotoxine in senile cerebral insufficiency. In: Agnoli, A. *et al.* (eds) *Aging Brain and Ergot Alkaloids*. Aging, Vol. 23, pp. 311–22. New York: Raven Press.

Hollander, E., Davidson, M., Mohs, R. C., Horvath, T. B., Davis, B. M., Zemishlany, Z. and Davis, K. L. (1987) RS 86 in the treatment of Alzheimer's disease: cognitive and biological effects. *Biol. Psychiatry*, **22**, 1067–78.

Levy, R. (1990) Are drugs targeted at Alzheimer's disease useful? 1. Useful for what? *BMJ*, **300**, 1131–2.

Matejcek, M., Knor, K., Piguet, P. V. and Weil, C. (1979) Electroencephalographic and clinical changes as correlated in geriatric patients treated for three months with an ergot alkaloid preparation. *J. Am. Geriatr. Soc.*, **27**, 198–202.

McEntee, W. J. and Crook, T. (1990) Age-associated memory impairment: a role for catecholamines. *Neurology*, **40**, 526–30.

Mohr, E., Schlegel, J., Fabbrini, G. *et al.* (1989) Clonidine treatment of Alzheimer's disease. *Arch. Neurol.*, **46**, 376–8.

Nicholson, C. D.(1990) Pharmacology of nootropics and metabolically active compounds in relation to their use in dementia. *Psychopharmacology*, **101**, 147–59.

Palacios, J. M. and Spiegel, R. (1986) Muscarinic cholinergic agonists: pharmacological and clinical perspectives. *Prog. Brain Res.*, **70**, 485–98.

Palacios, J. M., Bolliger, G., Closse, A., Gmelin, G. and Malanowski, J. (1986) The pharmacological assessment of RS 86 (2-ethyl-8-methyl-2,8-diazaspiro-(4,5)-decan-1,3-dion hydrobromide). A potent, specific muscarinic acetylcholine receptor agonist. *Eur. J. Pharmacol.*, **125**, 45–62.

Rechtschaffen, A. and Kales, A. (eds) (1968) *A Manual of Standardized Terminology, Techniques and Scoring Systems for Sleep of Human Subjects*. Washington, D.C.: Public Health Service, U.S. Government Printing Office.

Riemann, D., Joy, D., Höchli, D., Lauer, C., Zulley, J. and Berger, M. (1988) The influence of the cholinergic agonist RS 86 on sleep with regard to gender and age. *Psychiatry Res.*, **24**, 137–47.

Schlegel, J., Mohr, E., Williams, J., Mann, U., Gearing, M. and Chase, T. N. (1989) Guanfacine treatment of Alzheimer's disease. *Clin. Neuropharmacol.*, **12**, 124–8.

Spiegel, R. (1980) On predicting therapeutic usefulness of psychotropic drugs from experiments in healthy persons. *Rev. Pure Appl. Pharmacol. Sci.*, **1**, 215–91.

Spiegel, R. (1982) Aspects of sleep, daytime vigilance, mental performance and psychotropic drug treatment in the elderly. *Gerontology*, **28**(1, suppl.), 68–82.

Spiegel, R. (1984) Effects of RS 86, an orally active cholinergic agonist, on sleep in man. *Psychiatry Res.*, **11**, 1–13.

Spiegel, R. (1989) *Psychopharmacology – An Introduction*, 2nd edn. Chichester: Wiley.

Spiegel, R. and Devos, J. E. (1980) Central effects of guanfacine and clonidine during wakefulness and sleep in healthy subjects. *Br. J. Clin. Pharmacol.*, **10**, 165–8S.

Thal, L. J., Masur, D. M., Blau, A. D., Fuld, P. A. and Klauber, M. R. (1989) Chronic oral physostigmine without lecithin improves memory in Alzheimer's disease. *J. Am. Geriatr. Soc.*, **37**, 42–8.

Wettstein, A. and Spiegel, R. (1984) Clinical trials with the cholinergic drug RS 86 in Alzheimer's disease (AD) and senile dementia of the Alzheimer type (SDAT). *Psychopharmacology*, **84**, 572–3.

7

European Approaches to the Design of Drug Trials in Dementia

Rolf R. Engel, H. Hippius and W. Satzger

Psychiatric Department, University of Munich, Germany

Introduction

Research into the causes of the various forms of dementia has considerably increased within the last two decades. The pathophysiology of dementia of the Alzheimer's type has received particular attention and has stimulated the development of new drugs influencing attention, cognition and memory. Because of the growing number of demented patients, these disorders and possible therapeutic strategies have become a major focus of public health considerations. The definition of internationally accepted methodological standards in that field was hampered, however, by at least two facts. Firstly, different approaches towards drug treatment for symptoms of dementia have traditionally been used. In Germany or Italy, for instance, many nootropic drugs are marketed for a rather broad indication, whereas in the United Kingdom they play a limited role. In the United States only one drug is marketed for symptoms of dementia. In Japan, vasodilators, cerebrocirculatory and metabolic enhancers are in use. Secondly, at present, no effective reference substance exists. Therefore, while methodological standards for performing drug trials with neuroleptics or anti-depressants are well established and most trials are performed along similar lines, such standards for anti-dementics are far less elaborated.

Several attempts were undertaken in the last few years to standardize the methodology in drug trials for anti-dementics. Guidelines and recommendations of expert groups (McKhann *et al.*, 1984; Kanowski *et al.*, 1990; Dahlke *et al.*, 1990) were published and national conferences on anti-dementics were held in Japan, the United Kingdom and Germany, to list only a few (Amaducci *et al.*, 1990). Two conferences concentrated on methodology. In June 1989 a conference of the CNS Drugs Advisory Board of the Food

Dementia: Molecules, Methods and Measures. Edited by I. Hindmarch, H. Hippius and G. K. Wilcock
© 1991 John Wiley & Sons Ltd

and Drug Administration (FDA) on anti-dementia drug assessment took place in Rockville, Maryland, where protocol requirements for typical phase three studies were discussed (FDA, 1989). Aspects of external and internal validity, assessment instruments and benefit–risk analysis were discussed at a high level. In July 1989 a Consensus Conference on the methodology of clinical trials of 'nootropics' took place in Munich with clinicians, scientists and drug experts from 14 European countries (Amaducci et al., 1990). The conference focused on the classification of nootropic drugs, the value of animal models and preclinical human studies, problems in design and patient characteristics, clinical, psychometric and biological assessment instruments and statistical analyses, administrative regulations and ethical problems. Thus the whole spectrum of open questions in nootropic drug studies was covered. In contrast to the FDA conference, no detailed recommendations for single outcome measures were given. The following discussion is based mainly on the results of the Consensus Conference, but it also extends and updates some of the suggestions and compares them with other statements published in between.

Terminology

The conferences mentioned above all focused on drugs intended to improve attention, cognition and memory in patients suffering from symptoms of dementia. These drugs have traditionally been called by a variety of terms (for a discussion see Amaducci et al., 1990). Within this chapter the terms 'nootropics' in the broad clinical sense, which covers drugs for impaired brain function in old age (a term used by the German health authority) and 'anti-dementics', a term that is becoming more common in the United States, are used interchangeably.

Diagnostic Criteria and Selection of Patients

The selection of a patient for a nootropic drug trial is usually a stepwise procedure. In the first step, patients with dementia as a *syndrome* are included. In the second step, patients with possible *secondary causes of dementia* are excluded. There is broad agreement that both steps should be based on the Diagnostical and Statistical Manual of the American Psychiatric Association (DSM-III-R) or the tenth edition of the International Classification of Diseases (ICD-10) and additionally on the NINCDS-ADRDA criteria for Alzheimer's disease (Amaducci et al., 1990). In order to standardize the diagnostic process, structured instruments such as the SIDAM (Strukturiertes Interview für die Diagnose der Demenz van AlzheimerTyp, der Multimfarkt-Demenz und Demenzen anderer Ätiologie mach DSM-III-R und ICD-10) (Zaudig et al., 1990) or the CAMDEX (Cambridge Examination for Mental Disorders of the Elderly) (Roth et al., 1986) can be used. Clinical diagnoses of dementia have often been criticized in the past as being notoriously unreliable. Several reports have shown that reliability can be improved to a great extent by using new standardized procedures instead of old theoretical concepts (Macfadyen and Henderson, 1986; Morris et al., 1988; Forette et al., 1989).

In addition to (but not as a substitute for) the diagnostic classification, clinical, psychometric and biological measures may be used to select particular groups of patients. This includes rating scales and tests for cognitive and non-cognitive functions (for reviews see Israel et al., 1984; van Riezen and Segal, 1988), imaging techniques, electrophysiological measures and laboratory screening. Recently, the hope for laboratory screening tests for dementia of the Alzheimer's type with a monoclonal antibody to paired helical filaments (Iqbal *et al.*, 1989) or with amyloid beta-protein deposits in non-neural tissues (Joachim *et al.*, 1989; Selkoe, 1990) was born.

In the third step, the *exclusion criteria* of the specific study have to be considered. Examples are the exclusion of severely demented patients unable to understand test instructions, of multimorbid patients, of patients receiving special concomitant medication or special CNS active drugs, or patients whose compliance and cooperation cannot be assured. In any case, the purpose of patient selection is to collect a homogeneous group of patients representing best the syndrome or the diagnostic group that the drug is aimed at. Information about the *recruiting strategy* of the patients may also be of interest and should be mentioned.

The *degree of dementia* should be documented to allow comparisons across studies and to allow critical examination of the adequacy of the outcome measures. For documentation of severity, instruments such as the Mini-Mental State (MMS) (Folstein *et al.*, 1985), the Sandoz Clinical Assessment – Geriatric (SCAG) (Venn *et al.*, 1986) or the Global Deterioration Scale (GDS) (Reisberg *et al.*, 1982) are in use. Sometimes a fixed upper limit, e.g. MMS score less than 24, is also used as an inclusion criterion (Dahlke *et al.*, 1990). This is not without problems. The results of a rather short and coarse 10-min test like the MMS should not be allowed to override diagnostical decision. Strict upper and lower limits in the MMS cannot guarantee a study population that is homogeneous from a diagnostical point of view. A low MMS score can also be present in patients with a congenital intellectual impairment or major depression, while patients with an early dementia may still score in the normal range of the MMS, if their premorbid intelligence was high.

The current method of patient inclusion bears still more problems. One concerns the *representativeness* of the study. The current practice is to use narrow inclusion criteria and, at the same time, to exclude many patients with secondary diseases or concomitant medication. Thus nootropic drug studies consider mainly patients whose general health status is above average. When the drug is later used, it will be given to multimorbid patients. The only solution to this problem is to emphasize the importance of well-organized and coordinated drug monitoring in phase IV studies. The safety data generated in the clinical trials may simply be unrepresentative of the population that will later use the drug.

Another problem concerns the *comparability* of studies. Virtually all of the older studies suffer from diagnostic criteria that are not in accordance with our current knowledge. Almost all of them have been conducted with patient samples that, according to current knowledge, were composed of many aetiologically different groups, and the 'narrow' inclusion criteria of today will probably be cut into still smaller pieces tomorrow. Thus, studies with the same drug are hard to compare over time. Presently many experts are convinced that new drugs may differentially influence the various forms of primary dementia. Nevertheless, for most drugs this has never been shown. If only select groups of patients are studied, this conviction can never be scrutinized. The use of *large* groups of patients under *broad* inclusion criteria with later *stratification* according to *prospectively* collected diagnostic measures would be a better solution.

Design of Trials

There was broad agreement on the principal design aspects of nootropic drug trials at the Rockville FDA symposium as well as at the Munich Consensus Conference. A placebo-controlled parallel group trial is the design of choice in most cases. Cross-over designs may be appropriate in some cases, since they reduce the possible heterogeneity of treatment groups. But for cross-over designs it has to be demonstrated that (a) the condition does not change without treatment during the trial duration and (b) the wash-out periods are long enough to exclude treatment transfer effects. Both requirements are hard to fulfil in most anti-dementic drug trials. As long as there is no reference drug, new drugs can and must be evaluated against *placebo*. For some acute subgroups of organic mental syndromes, e.g. the alcohol-induced organic mental disorder, trial duration may be short. In studies with drugs intended for use in chronic degenerative dementias, the length of the trial may vary between 3 months and 1–2 years, depending on the focus of the study.

Attrition is a severe problem in long-term trials with anti-dementia drugs. Due to the greater age of the patients, mortality and morbidity rates are higher than in most studies with other psychotropic drugs. Adequate patient handling may reduce the problem, at least in outpatient studies. A related problem is that of *concomitant medication*. Due to the high multimorbidity seen in this age group, most prospective study patients take other drugs as well. Detailed proposals exist regarding which CNS-active medications are acceptable during a nootropic drug trial (Dahlke *et al.*, 1990). Nevertheless, Amaducci *et al.* (1990) emphasize that the establishment of efficacy of a new drug is best (and most safely) demonstrated in a trial that is not contaminated by concomitant medication.

The calculation of an adequate *sample size* for a trial does not pose special problems in trials with anti-dementics. It is necessary to define the acceptable limits of type I and II errors, to define a clinically relevant difference, and to estimate the variability of the outcome criterion (Amaducci *et al.*, 1990). The definition of a 'clinically relevant difference', however, is less clear in trials with anti-dementics than with other psychotropic drugs; this will be discussed in the next section. Kanowski *et al.* (1990) pointed out that the choice of the main outcome variable and of the statistical methods should be made *a priori* in accordance with the hypothesized effects of a drug.

As in the case for other disorders, *multicentre trials* are often the only way to achieve adequate numbers of patients in nootropic drug trials. In this case one faces the problem of an additional source of error variance – the differences between the centres. Amaducci *et al.* (1990) suggest that joint rater training sessions before and during the multicentre trial are one way to reduce error variance. A comprehensive training programme would cover not only the rating of psychopathological symptoms, but also global clinical judgement of the severity of a syndrome, clinical judgement of improvement, assessment of side effects and clinical diagnosis.

In most clinical drug trials a single *fixed dose* or multiple fixed doses are used. Some cholinergic drugs that are currently under trial have a very limited dose range that may even vary from subject to subject. In these cases the adequate dose can be individually specified in a pretrial dose-finding phase and later be used in the double-blind phase (Amaducci *et al.*, 1990).

Outcome Measures

The selection of the appropriate *outcome measures* is usually one of the main topics of controversy in planning a nootropic drug study. Before discussing some of the measures in detail, three points should be addressed.

Instrumental sensitivity for change measurements. Instruments that are coarse enough to describe the degree of illness over a wide range of variation are usually not sensitive enough to describe small changes (Amaducci *et al.*, 1990). For the ideal outcome measure, change sensitivity is essential. This means that information about the effects of age, of disease, of drugs and of test repetition should be available. Instruments sensitive to dementia of the Alzheimer's type must not be identical to instruments sensitive to deterioration of the disease or sensitive to test repetition (Storandt *et al.*, 1986).

Besides change sensitivity, an ideal outcome measure must possess many other attributes. It should be objective, reliable, valid and one-dimensional. Norms for the elderly should be available. The measure should be relevant for everyday behaviour and non-specific to gender. International compatibility would be desirable. The range of the measurement scale should be large enough to avoid floor and ceiling effects. The measure should not only be based on a deficit model, but should assess adaptation and coping mechanisms as well. As it was stated at the Rockville FDA symposium, it's quite clear that no single outcome measure exists that meets all these requirements (FDA, 1989). A lot of theoretical and empirical work remains to be done in this field.

Problems of multifactorial measurement. It has become popular to assess drug effects by measuring simultaneously at different levels – by psychopathology, e.g. Clinical Global Impression (CGI), by objective testing, e.g. Alzheimer's Disease Assessment Scale (ADAS) (Rosen *et al.*, 1984) and by activities of daily living (ADL) scales, e.g. Nurses' Observation Scale for Geriatric Patients (NOSGER) (Spiegel, 1989). Each measure is usually rated by different and independent investigators (psychiatrist, psychologist, nurse, relative) (Kanowski *et al.*, 1990; Dahlke *et al.*, 1990). There are, however, some objections against the use of multifactorial measurement as a standard procedure. Firstly, in using multiple measures the type I error has to be corrected with Bonferroni-type procedures, thus making each single measure more insensitive (Amaducci *et al.*, 1990). Secondly, while a word-list, for instance, is a very sensitive measure for drug-induced changes even in an acute study, changes in ADL and instrumental ADL (IADL) scales are probably seen only over several months. Thus, it is theoretically unlikely that one would detect *uniform* changes among different outcome measures in a given trial with a fixed duration. In the investigation of drugs with only moderate therapeutic effects, the most sensitive approach is to select just *one* main outcome variable that nevertheless should represent the *whole* spectrum of the symptoms.

Which change is relevant? Not every statistically significant drug effect is of clinical relevance. There have been suggestions for an operationalization of clinical relevance. The drug effect should be greater than half of the standard deviation of the main variable. There should be simultaneous changes in two or more levels of measurement (e.g. CGI, neuropsychological tests, ADL scales). The number of improved patients should be greater than a predefined threshold. The devastating course of the illness should be slowed down or stopped and quality of life should be preserved. In multicentre studies the same drug effects should be noticed in different centres (Kanowski *et al.*, 1990). Thus, given the uncertainty of our diagnoses, the *minimal* challenge is that significantly more patients improve to a clinically relevant degree under the drug than under placebo.

The selection of appropriate outcome measures depends therefore on the stage of drug development, on the severity of dementia in the patients, on the length of the trial and on the availability of change-sensitive instruments. In the following the main groups of outcome measures are discussed in more detail.

Biological Measures

According to Amaducci *et al.* (1990) and Kanowski *et al.* (1990) biological measures are sensitive and valid measures, but they should not be used for assessing the clinical efficacy of a nootropic drug, since their correlation to other clinical behavioural outcome measures is rather low. Thus, while structural measures such as computerized tomography or magnetic resonance imaging, functional measures of cerebral blood flow or electro-encephalography (EEG) can help to make the differential diagnoses between dementia of the Alzheimer's type and multi-infarct dementia, single photon emission computerized tomography, positron emission tomography, EEG brain mapping and evoked potentials and magnetic resonance spectroscopy can be of help in preclinical research to test hypotheses about specific drug effects.

Global Clinical Measures

The effectiveness of nootropics is most easily demonstrated in global clinical measures (Amaducci *et al.*, 1990), of which the CGI achieves the greatest integration. These measures may be subjectively biased, however, and it is somewhat open to question exactly what they measure.

Neuropsychological Tests and Rating Scales

These are more objective and reliable than global clinical measures. At the Rockville FDA symposium the cognitive part of the ADAS (Rosen *et al.*, 1984) and tests requiring the learning of new verbal information were emphasized as being sensitive for assessing nootropic drug effects (FDA, 1989). The change sensitivity of the ADAS is not yet proven, however, and a direct comparison of the sensitivity of the many different types of verbal memory tests is still missing. In Europe several standardized tests have been developed in the last few years for healthy and demented aged subjects on a national (very often non-English language) level (Erzigkeit, 1986; Gatterer, 1990; Kessler *et al.*, 1988; Oswald, 1986; Oswald and Fleischmann, 1986; Wilson *et al.*, 1985). Automated testing procedures (Crook *et al.*, 1986; Morris *et al.*, 1987) may be of some value in future studies, especially in cases of early dementia of the Alzheimer's type or selective memory loss.

ADL Scales

ADL (simple daily activities and activities of physical maintenance) and IADL (more complex social and financial activities outside of institutions) scales have high face validity, but they are less change-sensitive and require long-term observation. They have not been used as the main outcome measure in nootropic drug trials. The NOSGER (Spiegel, 1989) is an example of a 30-item ADL scale that is non-specific to gender, culture or outpatient status, is available in three different languages, is easy to administer and includes items that assess both competence and deficits. The value of *self-rating instruments* must be viewed with caution, since most patients will not be able to assess themselves according to certain instructions (Amaducci *et al.*, 1990). The need for the assessment of affective and emotional symptoms was stated, since non-cognitive factors may be essential for the clinical outcome and they may go unnoticed when focusing on cognitive symptoms alone (Amaducci *et al.*, 1990).

Ethical Protection of Patients

As Amaducci *et al.* (1990) pointed out, investigations with psychiatric disorders involving disturbed thinking run into the following ethical dilemma: the same mental functions that the patient needs to decide whether or not to participate in a clinical trial are usually affected by the illness. Demented patients therefore require special protection against unethical research. Besides the usual guidelines as written down in the Helsinki (1964) and Tokyo (1975) declarations, Amaducci *et al.* (1990) regard the following three problems as most relevant to drug trials with anti-dementics:

1. A local ethical committee should review the trial protocol as well as the procedure used to obtain informed consent from the patient.
2. If necessary, the authorized legal guardian, the closest family member or the ward where an institutionalized patient is cared for must consent to the patient's participation in the research.
3. The freedom to withdraw from the study and procedures that are beyond routine clinical investigation and bear special risks should be clearly explained to the patient.

Continuous adequate study monitoring, on-line verification of data and interim reports for long-lasting studies further protect the patient against deviations from the authorized protocol.

Concluding Remarks

In the last few years several Anglo-American, European and national committees have contributed to the question of how to conduct clinical trials with cognition-enhancing drugs. They have more or less reached a consensus on the basic guidelines and have described what one could call the present state-of-the-art in anti-dementia research. Nevertheless, many points exist where there may be disagreement between conference participants. The Munich Consensus Conference, for example, deliberately decided *not* to recommend a particular rating scale or memory test in its report because the participants did not believe that there was a firm factual base for such a recommendation. The field of dementia and especially that of the Alzheimer's type is still rapidly progressing. Several hypotheses concerning the efficacy of drugs in demented patients, for example, and most of the outcome measures used in the 1960s and 1970s are no longer valid today. Further advances in methodology can be expected in several areas: the diagnosis of dementia should be improved by means of laboratory measures, new drugs should be more effective than they are now, and new or improved outcome measures should be developed that are sensitive indices for clinically relevant aspects of dementia.

References

Amaducci, L., Angst, J., Bech, P., Benkert, O., Bruinvels, J., Engel, R. R., Gottfries, C. G., Hippius, H., Levy, R., Lingjaerde, O., López-Ibor Jr., J. J., Orgogozo, J. M., Pull, C., Saletu, B., Stoll, K. D. and Woggon, B. (1990) Consensus Conference on the Methodology of Clinical Trials of 'nootropics', Munich, June 1989. Report of the Consensus Committee. *Pharmacopsychiatry*, **23**, 171–5.

American Psychiatric Association (1987) *Diagnostic and Statistical Manual of Mental Disorders*, 3rd edn revised (DSM-III-R). Washington, D.C.: American Psychiatric Association.

Crook, T., Salama, M. and Gobert, J. (1986) A computerized test battery for detecting and assessing memory disorders. In: Bès, A., Cahn, J., Cahn, R., Hoyer, S., Marc-Vergnes, J. P., and Wisniewski, H. M. (eds) *Senile Dementias: Early Detection*, pp. 79–85. London: John Libbey.

Dahlke, F. *et al.* (1990) Recommendations for clinical drug trials in dementia. Clinical research working group from the pharmaceutical industry on dementia. *Dementia*, **1**, 292–5.

Erzigkeit, H. (1986) *Syndrom-Kurz-Test*. 2, Revised edn. Ebersberg: Vless.

FDA (1989) *Transcript of the antidementia drug assessment symposium*, June 1989. Rockville: Food and Drug Administration.

Folstein, M., Anthony, J. C., Parhad, I., Duffy, B. and Gruenberg, E. M. (1985) The meaning of cognitive impairment in the elderly. *J. Am. Geriatr. Soc.*, **33**, 228–35.

Forette, F., Henry, J. F., Orgogozo, J. M., Dartigues, J. F., Pere, J. J., Hugonot, L., Israel, L., Loria, Y., Goulley, F., Lallemand, A. and Boller, F. (1989) Reliability of clinical criteria for the diagnosis of dementia. A longitudinal multicenter study. *Arch. Neurol.*, **46**, 646–8.

Gatterer, G. (1990) *Alters-Konzentrations-Test (AKT)*. Göttingen: Hogrefe.

Iqbal, K., Wang, G. P., Grundke-Iqbal, I. and Wisniewski, H. M. (1989) Laboratory diagnostic tests for Alzheimer's disease. *Prog. Clin. Biol. Res.*, **317**, 679–87.

Israel, L., Kosarevic, D. and Sartorius, N. (1984) *Source Book of Geriatric Assessment*, Vols 1 and 2. Basel: Karger.

Joachim, C. L., Mori, H. and Selkoe, D. J. (1989) Amyloid β-protein deposition in tissues other than brain in Alzheimer's disease. *Nature*, **341**, 226–30.

Kanowski, S., Ladurner, G., Maurer, K., Oswald, W. D. and Stein, U. (1990) Empfehlungen zur Evaluierung der Wirksamkeit von Nootropika. (Recommendations for the efficacy evaluation of nootropic drugs.) *Z. Gerontopsychol. Psychiatrie*, **3**, 67–79.

Kessler, J., Denzler, P. and Markowitsch, H. J. (1988) *Demenztest*. Weinheim: Beltz.

Loeb, C. and Gandolfo, C. (1983) Diagnostic evaluation of degenerative and vascular dementia. *Stroke*, **14**, 399–401.

Macfadyen, D. M. and Henderson, J. (1986) Dementia in later life: research and action. In: Häfner, H., Moschel, G., and Sartorius, N. (eds) *Mental Health in the Elderly. A Review of the Present State of Research*, pp. 174–81. Berlin: Springer.

McKhann, G., Drachman, D., Folstein, M., Katzman, R., Price, D. and Stadlan, E. M. (1984) Clinical diagnosis of Alzheimer's disease: report of the NINCDS-ADRDA Work Group under the auspices of Department of Health and Human Services Task Force on Alzheimer's Disease. *Neurology*, **34**, 939–44.

Morris, R. G., Evenden, J. L., Sahakian, B. J. and Robbins, T. W. (1987) Computer-aided assessment of dementia: comparative studies of neuropsychological deficits in Alzheimer-type dementia and Parkinson's disease. In: Stahl, M., Iversen, D., and Goodman, C. (eds) *Cognitive Neurochemistry*, pp. 21–36. Oxford: Oxford University Press.

Morris, J. C., McKeel, D. W. Jr, Fulling, K., Torack, R. M. and Berg, L. (1988) Validation of clinical diagnostic criteria in senile dementia of the Alzheimer type. *Ann. Neurol.*, **24**, 17–22.

Oswald, W. D. (1986) Der Zahlen-Verbindungs-Test im höheren Lebensalter. In: Daumenlang, K. and Sauer, J. (eds) *Aspekte Psychologischer Forschung*, pp. 377–88. Göttingen: Hogrefe.

Oswald, W. D. and Fleischmann, U. M. (1986) *Das Nürnberger-Alters-Inventar (NAI)*. Stuttgart: Hogrefe.

Reisberg, B., Ferris, S. H., de Leon, M. J. and Crook, T. (1982) The Global Deterioration Scale for assessment of primary degenerative dementia. *Am. J. Psychiatry*, **139**, 1136–9.

Rosen, W. G., Mohs, R. C. and Davis, K. L. (1984) A new rating scale for Alzheimer's disease. *Am. J. Psychiatry*, **141**, 1356–64.

Roth, M., Tym, E., Mountjoy, C. Q., Huppert, F. A., Hendrie, H., Verma, S. and Goddard, R. (1986) CAMDEX: a standardised instrument for the diagnosis of mental disorder in the elderly with special reference to the early detection of dementia. *Br. J. Psychiatry*, **149**, 698–709.

Selkoe, D. J. (1990) Deciphering Alzheimer's disease: the amyloid precursor protein yields new clues. *Science*, **248**, 1058–60.

Spiegel, R. (1989) *The NOSGER (Nurses' Observation Scale for Geriatric Patients)*. Basel: Clinical Research, CNS Department, Sandoz A. G.

Storandt, M., Botwinick, J. and Danziger, W. L. (1986) Longitudinal changes: patients with mild SDAT and matched healthy controls. In: Poon, L. W. (ed.) *Handbook for Clinical Memory Assessment of Older Adults*, pp. 277–84. Washington, D.C.: American Psychological Association.

Van Riezen, H. and Segal, M. (1988) *Comparative Evaluation of Rating Scales for Clinical Psychopharmacology*. Basel: Elsevier.

Venn, R. D., Hamot, H. B. and Shader, I. (1986) Sandoz Clinical Assessment – Geriatric. In: *Collegium Internationale Psychiatriae Scalarum: Internationale Skalen für Psychiatrie*. Weinheim: Beltz.

WHO (1989) *Tenth Revision of the International Classification of Diseases*, Ch. V (F): Mental, Behavioural and Certain Developmental Disorders. Clinical Descriptions and Diagnostic Guidelines. Geneva: World Health Organization, Division of Mental Health.

Wilson, B., Cockburn, J. and Baddeley, A. (1985) *The Rivermead Behavioural Memory Test*. Reading: Thames Valley Test Company.

Zaudig, M., Mittelhammer, J. and Hiller, W. (1990) *SIDAM – Strukturiertes Interview für die Diagnose der Demenz vom Alzheimer Typ, der Multiinfarkt-Demenz und Demenzen anderer Ätiologie nach DSM-III-R und ICD-10*. Munich: Logomed.

8

International Development of Anti-dementia Drugs

*B. Musch and †J.-L. Robin

*The Upjohn Company, Brussels, Belgium and †Rhone-Poulenc Rorer, Research and Development, Paris, France

Generalities

The need for the discovery and development of new pharmacological entities is still very great in many fields of medicine; on the other hand, drug research and development are becoming more challenging, more time consuming and more demanding in terms of scientific effort, regulatory requirements and resources. The following factors appear to be critical in developing new drugs: (a) the predictive value of preclinical research, (b) the feasibility of clinical research, (c) timing and (d) the cost. These factors are particularly relevant in the field of drug candidates for the treatment of neurological and psychiatric diseases and they influence their development.

The predictive value of animal pharmacology is still low, despite the outstanding achievements in many areas of neuro- and psychopharmacology, due to the fact that neurological and psychiatric diseases are particularly difficult to reproduce in animals. Many animal models are still based on the effects of clinically active reference drugs or on very hypothetical neurobiological changes. Drug candidates for dementias or for all kinds of impairment of the highest functions in human brain do not escape these constraints.

The feasibility of clinical research also appears to be low because of many methodological and practical hindrances, particularly in the area of dementia, as it will be discussed later in this chapter.

The time to achieve meaningful results tends to be long in this area of clinical research, due not only to methodological issues and the clinical characteristics of the diseases, but also to regulatory constraints. The above mentioned factors will ultimately influence costs and the allocation of resources.

Dementia: Molecules, Methods and Measures. Edited by I. Hindmarch, H. Hippius and G. K. Wilcock
© 1991 John Wiley & Sons Ltd

Before going into the specific discussion of the international development of anti-dementia drugs, one should ask why and if further research is needed in this area. The answer is quite obvious, based on the following issues: (a) the increased morbidity, (b) the unknown causes and pathogenesis, and (c) the lack of efficacious therapy.

There are two kinds of strategies in the approach to the discovery and development of new therapeutic agents for dementia: research and drug development. In the first case, the possible strategies are:

1. Serendipity or the hazardous finding of an unknown property of a drug. This appears to be quite unrealistic in the present scientific, clinical and regulatory environment.
2. The understanding of the pathogenetic mechanism. This represents at present a major challenge in the field of dementias because of the complexity of the disease and because of the possible implication of multiple system alterations.
3. Similarity with other active drugs. This appears not to be appropriate in an area where no recognized and proved therapeutic treatment exists.

In terms of drug development, two strategies seem to compete: one which aims to achieve a curative treatment, the other which searches for symptomatic relief. In the first case the heterogeneity of the clinical picture (which dementia?) represents a major challenge, and in the second case the difficulty in demonstrating proof of a significant effect leads to many methodological problems for which solutions are far from being found.

Drug development is a global process which originates with the identification of chemical leads from which are selected drug candidates through a complex and comprehensive pharmacotoxicological evaluation of their potential to produce therapeutic effects and the establishment of their safety. On average only one out of 10 000 chemical entities reaches the stage of evaluation in humans. As stated above, the decision to test a drug candidate for dementia in humans is particularly difficult due to the low predictive value of the existing animal models for this clinical condition. It is also clear that even the preliminary clinical pharmacology, needed to establish potential effects in patients, does not bring solid evidence of activity because of the discrepancy between the normal functioning of the higher cognitive functions and the clinical conditions of dementia. Nevertheless, phase I studies still maintain their value in providing a better knowledge of the drug in terms of general safety, metabolic and pharmacokinetic characteristics, and cognitive and behavioural toxicology, the latter being particularly relevant in the clinical situation in which the drug will be evaluated, and keeping in mind the age of the patient population to be treated.

Specific pharmacokinetic issues also imply the need for using the drug in patients, to provide information on possible drug interactions and the impact of reduced renal and liver function on the pharmacokinetic characteristics, all common conditions in elderly patients suffering from dementia. It is true that pilot, exploratory clinical trials in small groups of patients can help in getting some 'feeling' about the drug, but dementia is far from being an easy condition to study in a small population and without a control group.

Phase II studies should show evidence of a therapeutic effect, either in the 'curative' sense or in the 'symptomatic' one. It has to be mentioned that the lack of an established pharmacological treatment and the severity of the disease will tend to push towards an early evaluation of drug candidates in patients.

Dementia, of any origin, represents a very difficult challenge for the evaluation of drug-related effects. Furthermore, the high risks and high costs characteristic of this kind of clinical research and development mean that early studies can play a critical role in the decision to move further into extensive, time-consuming and highly demanding clinical trials. Therefore such early studies cannot be just explorative, but need to be conducted as controlled studies.

As far as studies in dementia are concerned, the critical issues that characterize trials in neurological diseases apply:

1. Dementia represents a progressively deteriorating clinical condition with a frequently unpredictable course.
2. Clinical parameters are difficult to measure.
3. There is no established disease mechanism.
4. Only partially effective and not completely established therapies exist.
5. Control groups are difficult to obtain and to maintain in the trials.
6. Study design can be a major methodological problem, because of the difficulty in defining the end-points, the duration of the study and the number of patients needed.

In fact, the definition of 'acceptable evidence of effect' is particularly cumbersome in a condition such as dementia, as well as the definition of the clinical end-points. Whether to look for a 'global' effect or an improvement in symptom clusters or target symptoms is matter of debate, and should take into account the pharmacological characteristics of the drug under evaluation. No matter which type of end-points are chosen, it is advisable that they are well established in the study protocol, and not chosen '*a posteriori*'. End-points should be considered not only for their content but also for their timing, e.g. time needed to achieve an effect, or effect at a given time. This issue is particularly relevant if one considers the influence of the natural course of the dementia on the outcome of the therapeutic response.

Motivational Issues

The way of conducting research and development of new drugs is influenced not only by specific chemical, pharmacological, clinical, social and regulatory issues, but also by the role played by the different parties involved.

Researchers, inside and outside the pharmaceutical industry, sponsors, clinical trials organizations, clinical investigators and regulatory agencies all have an important role to play in transforming a drug candidate into a therapeutic agent, but their goals can differ and can even conflict. Thus, any kind of strategy in the development of new drugs should take into account not only the specific characteristics of the clinical condition to be treated and the related medical needs, but also the heterogeneity of the 'players' involved.

This consideration is not so trivial as it can appear. Motivation of the various 'actors' in the play of drug development can influence the way a drug is studied and developed and, therefore, its success or failure. If it is true that an active and safe drug should always ultimately be registered and marketed, this is not without the risk that bad organization of resources, a lack of efficient project management or a badly conceived research and development plan could prevent the properties of a drug from being revealed. Under the label 'sponsor', for example, many different functions and organizations of a pharmaceutical company are involved. Preclinical research, clinical research, marketing and corporate management need to find an efficient way to work together on a project and to avoid conflicting positions.

The way patients participate in a study and the level and kind of motivation of the patient, the family and the family's doctor (who is not the Study Investigator in most cases) can influence the outcome of the study. This issue is particularly relevant in studies dealing with demented patients, especially in an outpatient setting. It is important in this respect that the study rationale, objectives and methodology are extensively explained to all parties directly or indirectly involved. We feel that it is particularly important to stress the involvement of the patient's physician, in cases when he is not the Study Investigator, to help in maintaining patients in the trial and to ensure compliance.

As far as the patient is concerned, it is important to mention that important differences exist between countries, for example in health care systems, in reimbursement systems and in doctor referral systems, especially if one takes into account European countries on the one hand and the United States or Japan on the other. These differences cannot be ignored in multicentre, multinational studies, and need particular attention.

The way the Investigator participates in the study is also a relevant factor to be considered, again especially when multicentre studies are needed. A well-designed study should prevent personal interpretation or 'free choices' by the Investigators, and should have an agreed protocol. All possible difficulties, bias, misinterpretations and misunderstandings should be extensively reviewed and discussed before the study begins. It is always worthwhile to stress that the time spent discussing and agreeing upon a protocol is never wasted, and it could save a lot of time, resources and money once the study is started. An understanding of and complete adherence to the protocol by the Investigator is a key step for the success of a trial.

The Investigator's skill and experience in conducting clinical trials and specifically in handling the measurement instruments involved appropriately is another critical issue in anti-dementia drug trials, because of the need for good clinical observation, close monitoring and an accurate evaluation of the patient's status. Unfortunately, well-established and commonly used instruments for assessing demented patients are lacking or still not validated (especially in the different languages needed for a multinational trial) and have not been widely tested. Consequently it is mandatory that the medical staff involved in anti-dementia drug trials are sufficiently trained before the study and that the efficacy trial itself is not used to test or validate a new instrument.

Investigator homogeneity is also a critical issue. Inter-rater reliability should be specifically assessed before each trial involving several Investigators, not only for rating scales but also for diagnostic criteria. It could even be recommended that patients' admission to the study is reviewed by an independent board to check adherence to the diagnostic criteria.

The feasibility of the patient's assessment must also be taken into account; too many variables or too many measurements do not add, in most cases, any further accuracy to a study. Another important factor is the choice of the study site. It is highly advisable that not only considerations about the Investigator's skill and experience, but also the capability of the study site to recruit the adequate number of appropriate patients in the time allotted to the study is taken into account. A review of the study site records of patient referral should take place before finally selecting the site.

Definitions

The increasing interest in anti-dementia drugs now occurring in modern neuro-psychopharmacology is due to the high market attractiveness and the great medical need for this class of drugs. This interest is stimulating a very active debate among scientists, clinicians and regulatory bodies to try to figure out guidelines and principles which could regulate the development of anti-dementia drugs.

Because of the factors already discussed, it appears that a consensus on these guidelines will not be an easy goal to achieve. However, a comprehensive review of this debate allows at least the identification of controversial issues and general agreements and can provide some recommendations.

First of all it is important to establish a definition of the disease in order to reach a consensus on the nature of acceptable anti-dementia drug claims. Although in terms of causes it should be more correct to talk about 'dementias', it has to be taken into account that the so-called senile dementia of the Alzheimer type (SDAT) is by far the most frequent type of dementia, and that guidelines for SDAT will apply equally well to other types of chronic dementing illnesses such as multi-infarct dementia. The need for the inclusion of homogeneous groups of patients in clinical trials has always to be taken into account, but it is possible to consider a common definition of 'dementia' as a neurological condition of unknown aetiology that ordinarily causes a progressive, irreversible decline in intellectual and cognitive abilities.

The other key principle which demands a consensus is the establishment of the nature of acceptable anti-dementia claims. In this respect the difference between 'curative' treatment and 'symptomatic' treatment of dementia is critical. Considering that the understanding of the real pathogenetic mechanism underlying the disease will not be achieved easily in the near future, the difference will be based on whether a drug really affects the main or 'core' phenomena of dementia or whether it influences another aspect of the dementing process. In the first instance there is a general agreement among experts that a drug cannot be considered to possess 'anti-dementia' properties unless it improves or positively affects the patient's ability to learn new and retrieve previously learned information. Of course, drugs that exert their effects on other signs or symptoms of the dementing process can also be developed, but their claim will not be of the same nature as in the case of drugs affecting the 'core' phenomena; furthermore it is reasonable to think that health authorities will regard very critically claims for actions artificially linked to dementia (so-called 'pseudospecific claims').

Early Decisions

During the development of a new drug, some key steps in the decision-making can be easily recognized.

We have already mentioned the difficulties linked to the selection of a drug candidate for dementia due to the low predictive value of animal pharmacology in this area. It is important that the available information on the animal toxicology and pharmacology is adequate and sufficient to justify the evaluation of the drug for a specific indication in a specific population and to minimize the related risk. In this respect, if it is true that the lack of effective treatment for dementia justifies higher risk, it should not be forgotten that the population to be exposed to the drug will be necessarily large in number and particularly 'at risk' because of the average age; therefore, not only will the animal data have to be as exhaustive as possible, but also the early testing in healthy volunteers has to be as informative as possible. Unfortunately early phase I studies cannot give solid information concerning clinical efficacy in the case of anti-dementia drugs, as we have already mentioned. Also information concerning the potential dose range to be used in early clinical trials will be very vague.

Phase I studies, as is usual, should provide as much information as possible in terms of safe doses and safe plasma drug concentrations both in single doses and in repeated dosing conditions. Age-matched healthy volunteers should be also exposed to the drug, and specific pharmacokinetic, drug interaction and safety data should be collected in this population.

Phase I studies in healthy subjects should not be regarded just as safety studies. A drug that can exert some effect in a patient undergoing a dementing process may produce no effect in a normally functioning brain. Nevertheless, it is important to use all available instruments and techniques to establish the clinical and pharmacological profile of the drug, possibly in a population which should resemble, as far as age range is concerned, the patient population to be admitted to the clinical trials. Accurate measurement of the possible effects of the new drug on cognitive functions and psychomotor performances, as well as the possible effects on electrophysiological signals (electro-encephalographic brain mapping and evoked potentials), should be extensively and exhaustively pursued.

Human models for conditions of impaired functioning of higher cognitive functions need to be better developed, and research in this field should not be neglected or seen as less important than large population clinical trials. These models could provide fundamental information concerning the choice of dose for the clinical trials, the selection of the population to be considered and the duration of the drug effect. With the present lack of established human models for dementia, there are only two possible strategies for choosing the doses of a potential anti-dementia drug for the first clinical trials. One, the more empirical, will consider that the best dose to employ is the one considered to be the maximum tolerated dose in the phase I study; this strategy implies that there is a monotonic positive correlation between dose and effect, and that healthy subjects and patients have the same sensitivity to the drug. Both these implications far from correspond with reality, particularly in a condition such as dementia. The second strategy will base the choice of doses on a series of assumptions about comparative absorption, disposition, metabolism and elimination, and about the correlation between species of receptor sensitivity and the predictive value of preclinical models.

Phase II Studies

In the present debate about guidelines for the development of anti-dementia drugs, there seems to be general agreement about discouraging uncontrolled use of the investigational drug to assess its efficacy in phase II studies, because the spontaneous variability in its course in any patient which is characteristic of this disease prevents open label studies from being effectively informative. The need for controlled trials and thus the need to involve sufficiently large populations, on the one hand, and concerns about exposing patients to ineffective but potentially harmful compounds on the other, should lead to attentively conceived phase II studies with maximum efficiency (using the smallest possible number of patients to test the proposed null hypothesis).

The only answer to this is to control the sources of variances that could interfere with drug effects. Phase II studies should enrol patients who are possibly free from concomitant medical illness and less severely impaired than the average demented patient, and may even involve criteria which allow the enrolment of patients more likely to respond to treatment.

Achieving an adequate selection of patients will rely on finding Investigators capable of ensuring adherence to the protocol and homogeneity of approach to patient selection and evaluation. At the same time, increasing the patient recruitment by increasing the number of Investigators should be avoided in order not to jeopardize patient characteristics and the objectivity of the assessment.

Phase III Studies

These studies are supposed to provide information about the use of a drug, for which phase II studies have established its efficacy, under conditions representative of those which are likely to be encountered once the drug is on the market. The principal aim of phase III studies will be in fact to gain experience with the drug to complete the information necessary to provide a documented drug data sheet to guide the use of the drug and reduce the risks of unknown phenomena in more vulnerable subgroups. This is particularly important in the case of demented patients, where patients with concomitant illness and treatment or with renal or hepatic failure are quite common.

It is important to note that there is a recent tendency to merge phases II and III in order to accelerate the development of a new drug. Nowadays large multicentre trials enrolling hundreds of patients are becoming more and more common to collect definitive evidence of efficacy and safety. These studies can be followed by extension protocols, where the same patients continue to be administered with the experimental drug. The advantages of this strategy are evident, but it should be underlined that in such cases the drug is in fact administered to a selected population, represented by those patients who have tolerated and preferred the drug. Consequently the need for conducting specific phase III studies still exists, and this phase should represent an important section of the final registration file.

General Considerations about Design and Methodology

Evidence of anti-dementia efficacy should be based on a significant difference between the experimental drug and an internal control in a well-conducted clinical trial. This means that each study intended to provide evidence of efficacy for an anti-dementia drug should involve an internal control; in fact, the high variation and spontaneous fluctuations among samples of demented patients prevent the use of an external control. The use of an internal control is highly recommended and almost mandatory in the case of efficacy studies for diseases characterized, like dementia, by heterogeneity in severity, symptoms and course. Because of the lack of well-established efficacious anti-dementia drugs, there is a general consensus to consider placebo the internal control in studies assessing the efficacy of a potential anti-dementia drug.

Considering that phase II studies should not only establish the efficacy of a drug but also the relationship between dose and both the therapeutic response and adverse events, the question about the advantages of the various study designs (fixed dose versus flexible dose regimens) should be raised. A general agreement exists among experts that randomizing the patients to two or more fixed dose levels should better accomplish the task of establishing clear dose–response effects. To avoid a marked drop-out rate among the patients treated with the higher doses, the final full predetermined dose can be reached progressively over a short period of time, according to drug safety characteristics, possibly established in early phase I studies. In any case, 'fixed dose' group comparisons should be preferred to studies in which patients are progressively titrated to a final dose according to their clinical response. These considerations about treatment design are particularly relevant in the case of anti-dementia drugs.

Another matter of debate is represented by the choice between parallel and cross-over designs. In the case of anti-dementia treatments, parallel designs are considered to be more appropriate. Of course, advantages exist for using cross-over designs (i.e. fewer patients, reduction in variance) and they should not be excluded 'a priori', especially for drugs aiming to have a 'symptomatic' effect. A cross-over design study should, in any case, be conducted in a way that will eliminate biases such as carry-over, withdrawal and treatment by period interaction. Specifically it is necessary to demonstrate with this type of design that patients entering any period of the study other than the first have returned to the baseline clinical state, i.e. the clinical state prior to the start of the first period.

Where to conduct a study (inpatients versus outpatients) must also be considered. It is true that ideally phase II trials in demented patients should be carried out within the hospital in inpatients to ensure a medically supervised environment. But it is also true that there is a certain reluctance to admit ambulatory demented patients to hospital for the sole purpose of participating in a study. In addition the patient may not be willing to leave his usual environment and this could interfere with the outcome of the study results. Incidentally, the attitude towards hospital admission for a clinical trial varies from country to country due to health care system characteristics and medical practice.

A reasonable compromise could be to admit the patients in the first part of the trial and leave the possibility of discharge in the late part of the trial, provided that medical supervision and assessment continues at frequent intervals. An alternative could be to test more severe patients in the phase II trials, patients that, because of their impaired functions, are already institutionalized or admitted to a hospital. The risk in this approach is that the drug can fail to show an effect because of the severity of the clinical condition. However, it can be argued that even if a trial in severely affected demented patients does not show definitive evidence of efficacy, even positive trends in such a patient population can be considered informative in terms of the potential therapeutic effect of the experimental drug; furthermore, safety data can also be collected in this type of patient population. The information resulting from these studies can then allow the initiation of trials in outpatients with less severe clinical states. These patients appear to be more appropriate for early evaluation for two reasons: firstly they are more likely to show drug-induced improvement and secondly because they are more likely to adhere to the protocol in terms of compliance and cooperation with the assessment procedures. More severe demented patients, who are more representative of the population who will be treated with the drug once it is on the market, will be enrolled in a more advanced stage of development.

Diagnosis and Severity of Illness

One of the major pitfalls of several trials in demented patients is the lack of precise and documented diagnostic criteria for patient selection. In a progressive illness such as dementia, diagnostic criteria should not only refer to well-established diagnostic systems such as that based on the Diagnostical and Statistical Manual of the American Psychiatric Association (the DSM-III-R), but should also assess and identify the stage and severity of the dementia process for each patient.

Special attention has to be paid to all inclusion and exclusion criteria in the case of demented patients. It has to be documented, and not only stated, that a patient does not suffer from any condition that may be misdiagnosed as dementia. In particular, patients should be assessed for and documented as not suffering from conditions such as retarded depression, delirium, normal pressure hydrocephalus, Parkinson's disease or brain tumour.

With regard to the assessment of the severity and stage of the dementia, this issue is still controversial, as no standard system exists or at least no consensus exists on which system should be regarded as sufficiently reliable. The main recommendation in this respect is that, whatever system is chosen, it should be used for all the clinical trials in the development programme for a given drug. It seems as if a general consensus has now been reached among experts and regulatory bodies on the fact that clinical studies in demented patients should provide, apart from the diagnostic definition according to a diagnostic system (DSM-III-R), the definition of each patient's stage of dementia according to an instrument such as the Reisberg's Global Deterioration Scale (Reisberg *et al.*, 1988) and a measure of each patient's performance on some tests of cognitive function. The following comprehensive tests are sufficiently recognized and accepted by the scientific community:

1. Alzheimer's Disease Assessment Scale (Rosen *et al.*, 1984).
2. Mini-Mental State Examination (Folstein *et al.*, 1975).
3. Dementia Rating Scale of Mattis (Coblentz *et al.*, 1973).
4. Memory Information Test (Blessed *et al.*, 1968).

Efficacy Assessment

It is not within the scope of this chapter to deal in detail with the specific instruments of efficacy assessment; these are discussed elsewhere in this volume. However, we shall consider some general issues related to the assessment of drug effects.

First of all it is important to keep in mind that to obtain recognition as a treatment for dementia, evidence should be provided that the drug has a significant and meaningful effect and exerts this effect on the 'core' symptoms of dementia. It is this type of evidence that appears to guide regulatory authorities in evaluating potential anti-dementia drugs. This evidence of an anti-dementia effect should be based on the fact that the experimental drug shows superiority to placebo both on a global assessment and on a performance assessment of cognitive functions. This was the conclusion of the FDA Anti-dementia Drug Assessment Symposium (Ad Hoc FDA Dementia Assessment Task Force, 1989), and it appears to be a well-taught approach to establish on the one hand the need for evidence of a clinically meaningful effect (global assessment) and on the other the need for evidence of a significant effect upon the 'core' manifestations of dementia (assessment of cognitive functions). Examples of adequate evaluations of cognitive functions have been already given for the assessment of the severity of the dementing process. The definition of an adequate instrument for a global assessment is more controversial.

Two types of global assessments are commonly used in clinical trials to evaluate the overall status of patients. The first is represented by the 'clinical global improvement rating', which should measure the overall amelioration or deterioration occurring in the patient's status since a baseline evaluation as perceived by the Investigator. The second type, the 'absolute global severity assessment', is meant to evaluate the absolute severity of the clinical condition in relation to the full range of severity exhibited by patients suffering from the disease for which the experimental drug is being evaluated. These types of global assessments depend on the rater's experience with this kind of rating, his training and his clinical skills. Nevertheless, these global ratings are usually standardized, e.g. on a seven point scale, where 4 represents no change, 1 indicates marked improvement and 7 marked deterioration; this to limit the options when recording an assessment.

It appears that the global assessment based on absolute severity of illness is the most likely to show greater inter-rater reliability. For this reason global improvement ratings are to be preferred, although they are not devoid of problems. For instance, the assessment has to be made by the same rater, and it is difficult to train raters in a condition such as dementia where patients showing improvement are rare. Finally, global improvement ratings can only assess major changes and therefore they are less sensitive to small clinical events. Despite all these limitations, global ratings, either of absolute severity or of global improvement, are a fundamental part of a clinical trial to assess the effects of an anti-dementia drug, and should always be used. However, their use should be accompanied by the testing of cognitive functions and of behavioural aspects.

The last general methodological issue to consider is the study duration. Although short-term trials should also be considered, it seems a study duration of at least 3 months is required to be judged as adequate to support an anti-dementia claim. Long-term trials will also be essential once that a drug has shown to possess anti-dementia properties.

Conclusion

The development of anti-dementia drugs appears to be one of the most fascinating and challenging fields of drug development. A very active debate is going on at present to better identify the content and methods of study for discovering new entities and for understanding the disease mechanism, but also to fix the principles and guidelines for developing new drugs and for guiding clinical researchers in the definition and conception of adequate clinical trials capable of showing evidence of an anti-dementia effect. Although the ultimate consensus on how to develop a new anti-dementia drug is far from being reached, it is already possible to concentrate efforts and resources on trials that, by taking into account some basic principles and their related caveats, can provide the necessary information to help in the strategic devices and in the evaluation of the potential for a drug to interfere with the dementing process.

References

Ad Hoc FDA Dementia Assessment Task Force (1989) *FDA Antidementia Drug Assessment Symposium, June 15–16*. Submitted for publication/transcript available through freedom of information requests.

Blessed, G., Tomlinson, B. E. and Roth, M. (1968) The association between quantitative measures of dementia and of senile change in the cerebral gray matter of elderly subjects. *Br. J. Psychiatry*, **114**, 797–811.

Coblentz, J. M., Mattis, S., Zingesser, H., Kasnof, S. S., Wisniuwski, H. M. and Katzman, R. (1973) Presenile dementia. *Arch. Neurol.*, **29**, 299–308.

Folstein, M. F., Folstein, S. E. and McHugh, P. R. (1975) Mini Mental State: a practical method for grading the cognitive state of patients for the clinician. *J. Psychiatr. Res.*, **12**, 189–98.

Poon, L., Crook, T., Davis, K., Eisdorfer, C., Gurland, G., Kaszniak, A. and Thompson, L. (1986) *Clinical Memory Assessment of Older Adults*. Washington, D.C.: American Psychological Association.

Reisberg, B., Ferris, S. H., de Leon, M. J. and Crook, T. (1988) The Global Deterioration Scale (GDS). *Psychopharmacol. Bull.*, **24**, 661–3.

Rosen, W., Mohs, R. and Davis, K. (1984) A new rating scale for Alzheimer's disease. *Am. J. Psychiatry*, **141**, 1356–64.

Spitzer, R. and Williams, J. (1987) *Diagnostic and Statistical Manual of Mental Disorders*, 3rd edn revised. Washington, D.C.: American Psychological Association.

9

The Development of the SKT Project

Hellmut Erzigkeit

Psychiatric Department, University of Erlangen-Nuremberg, Erlangen, Germany

With my utmost respect and sincerity, it is my great pleasure to dedicate this contribution to Professor E. Lungershausen on his sixtieth birthday

The history of the construction of the SKT – a short cognitive performance test – is a series of more or less accidental steps which led to the development of a test procedure to facilitate the measurement of cognitive disturbances caused by brain disorders such as dementia. In the capacity of a clinical psychologist in a psychiatric hospital, I had to administer all kinds of available psychometric tests for the assessment of, for example, cognitive deficits or treatment effects in order to describe clinical pictures of organic mental diseases. Since, in the course of clinical routine and research programmes, frequent tests and retests were sometimes necessary, I started to work on the problem of how to shorten existing tests or subtests and to make them more practicable. I then studied the literature to look for information on test procedures with sufficient internal or face validity which had already been elaborated upon in clinical practice. In my view, they only had to be adapted to clinical practice to make them easier to administer.

The aim was simple enough, and I was sure that it could be realized within a short time; indeed, after 2 or 3 years a first version of the test was available. For the most part, the SKT was used in clinical studies concerned with the evaluation of the treatment effects of so-called nootropic drugs. Letters from study authors as well as the great number of published study results almost forced me to leave the production of the SKT to the professionalism of a publishing company. So, in 1977, I published the test with a preliminary manual, hoping to have done my part and being sure that the interest in the SKT would soon diminish. My personal aim had been reached; the SKT was fairly well accepted by those administering the test and by the patients. The whole test procedure took just 10 to 15 minutes and yielded a result that served for an interpretation of

Dementia: Molecules, Methods and Measures. Edited by I. Hindmarch, H. Hippius and G. K. Wilcock
© 1991 John Wiley & Sons Ltd

disturbances of memory and attention. With the additional information of the total score, which could be calculated using norm values, the severity of the disease in terms of clinical descriptions could be estimated. This was sufficient for our clinical practice.

The preliminary manual contained no information on reliability and validity and I was quite surprised that this version was accepted by so many users and authors. It was probably the published results of clinical trials within which SKT scores served as measurements for the therapeutic efficacy of investigated drugs which were the cause of users and authors yet again forcing me to continue working on the SKT. They demanded information on the reliability and validity in order that the drug effects demonstrated by SKT results could become more widely accepted. So, with the help of friends, I collected data and was able to finish the construction with a final manual almost 10 years later. This was in 1986.

Reliability scores computed by, for example, Arnold (1983) were mostly higher than 0.86 for the parallel forms of the SKT. There are five parallel forms – called A to E – available. The results of clinical trials not only revealed the 'drug sensitivity' of the SKT, but also provided information on aspects of its validity. The SKT has often proven to be a sensitive test for the assessment of treatment effects. At the moment, we are working on a literature documentation of clinical trials in which SKT results were used for the evaluation of the treatment effects of so-called nootropic drugs or cognition enhancers. This documentation will be published with the next manual in 1992.

General Considerations Concerning the Test Construction

Concerning the construction in general, I think it is worth mentioning once again that the SKT was not meant to be a psychometric instrument to measure the cognitive performance of healthy subjects. It was constructed merely for the purpose of measuring cognitive disturbances in patients suffering from different degrees of organic mental disorders. Therefore, it has to be taken into consideration that with regard to the 'classical' psychological test procedures, the more a 'subject' turns into a 'patient' with cognitive deficits, certain variables – which are not of practical relevance in general psychology – become more and more important.

For example, it is obvious that patients suffering from diseases like dementia are generally less motivated to pass psychological tests or to do their best to obtain good results. Problems also arise concerning the interdependencies of the level of (premorbid) intelligence, cognitive performance and, for example, the severity of the dementia. Although these are common experiences with which every psychiatrist, psychologist or clinician is familiar, they are often neglected in norm values of psychometric tests. Their clinical relevance is evident: as we all know, a young, intelligent and well-educated patient with only mild to moderate cognitive disturbances, for instance, will still be able to perform memory tasks as well as, or even better than, an elderly, healthy person who is less educated and of lower intelligence. This should be taken into account by calculated norm tables of psychometric tests. Once in a while, we find among our patients someone well-educated or who has enjoyed professional success, perhaps a university graduate or a top manager, who may reveal how difficult differential diagnosis and estimation of cognitive disturbances can be, and how easily young and inexperienced physicians or psychologists can be fooled; these patients know how to behave, how to care for themselves and to play their role – they have often learned to converse using the very best 'small talk' in order to appear friendly, polite and well. In other words, they have learned to hide symptoms such as deficits in memory and attention or their inability to learn something new.

Not only in these cases are rating scales for the estimation of the severity of cognitive impairments a less suitable choice. To test mild, moderate and moderate to severe cognitive disturbances, performance tests are adequate instruments. In more severe stages, they definitely lose their practicability and validity. In my opinion, the diagnosis of patients suffering from severe stages of dementia can be classified without the use of psychometric tests; a diagnosis of this type can be better classified using, for example, neurological variables. At these stages rating scales are adequate instruments to estimate the severity of the dementia or its course. Personality factors – and the premorbid level of intelligence – are no longer variables which sufficiently describe the severity of the impairment because neurological symptoms predominate and the extreme cognitive deficits seem to level out or almost extinguish interpersonal differences.

The choice of performance tests or rating scales to measure cognitive deficits in demented patients is highly dependent upon the severity of the disease. Self-ratings are more influenced by personality factors and the patient's ability to describe the symptoms. Interfering problems arise due to personal use of terms and semantic inaccuracy. In our clinical experience and as, for example, Arnold and Heerklotz (1980) or Witkowski (1983) have shown, there is, to a large extent, almost no correlation between the diminution of cognitive functions and the patient's own ratings of the perceived impairments.

This is similar to the problems which arise when observer rating scales are used. Ratings of the severity of cognitive impairments are dependent upon the experience of the rater and are therefore sometimes not sufficiently comparable and cause a loss of reliability. From this point of view, the advantage of performance tests may be seen in *a more direct measurement* of cognitive functions and fewer error components are caused by inaccuracy of speech or other verbal or semantic factors.

Requirements of a Psychometric Test for Application in Clinical Practice

Regarding the test situation in clinical practice, we have to bear in mind certain aspects which are relevant for the construction of a psychometric test:

1. The test situation cannot be standardized as is usually demanded in test psychology (Michel, 1964); tests sometimes have to be administered on the wards, with patients occasionally being unable to get out of bed for the test procedures. Disturbances by room-neighbours, nurses or others cannot be completely avoided.
2. Patients are sometimes not motivated to cooperate in a psychological test.
3. Many tests, for example paper-and-pencil tests, are too difficult for the patient to perform; tremor, drug-induced disturbances of accommodation, impaired motor abilities or simply the forgetting of a pair of spectacles sometimes make it impossible to test a patient.
4. We found that the attractiveness of test material and its *character*, such as toys or games with aspects of competition, ensured the best compliance (Lehrl and Erzigkeit, 1977; Kirkilonis, 1978; Fuchs, 1979).

5. The test procedure should not last for more than approximately 10 to 15 min because, as we have shown, reliability and validity may decrease dramatically during longer testing times (Lehrl and Erzigkeit, 1977).
6. The test should not be too sensitive to influences such as noise or other disturbances, but should be highly sensitive to changes in the indicator or target variables.
7. The test should be suitable for frequent retests; therefore learning effects must be low and parallel tests are necessary.
8. The test procedure should be easy to administer and the instructions should be clear enough to ensure its correct administration by nurses as well as medical assistant personnel; this is particularly important when the test is to be used frequently within the clinical routine, and of course in clinical studies.
9. The test results should be objective and sufficiently reliable and valid.
10. The test scores or norm values should allow an estimation of the severity of the impairment and yield some information supporting the *validation* of the clinical diagnosis.
11. Last but not least, the test procedure and materials should aim to be as 'culture fair' as possible, thus allowing translation into other languages.

What Should the Test Measure?

I would like to state that psychometric tests are not a must in clinical practice and in many cases an experienced physician or psychologist is able to evaluate his therapeutic strategies and their efficacy without the help of such tests. However, these tests are of help in cases when we expect, for instance, communication problems, when we would like to describe a patient's cognitive disturbances with objective data in standardized clinical terms. Apart from this, if therapeutic effects are not expected to be obvious, we need to measure cognitive performance with a sensitive instrument. Tests, therefore, are useful in basic research, to study, for example, the course of the disease or changes in the clinical picture of demented patients. More often, they serve for the documentation of therapeutic effects in the clinical trials of the so-called nootropic drugs. Tests are also to be applied when medical opinion or evidence is required concerning forensic aspects.

Any psychometric test which measures cognitive functions is in principle also *apt for measuring cognitive decline*, which implies that basically any of these tests could be used to measure cognitive deficits in demented patients. Due to the characteristics of cognitive impairments in demented patients, we always find deficits in memory, attention or speed of information processing; therefore, a test should be suitable for measuring these variables. As we know, these variables most definitely cannot substitute for the diagnosis or describe the whole of the clinical picture of the disease, but there are some characteristic indicator variables amongst the variety which makes up the complex clinical picture. However, it is very important that the test procedure in clinical practice should not be the same as the standardized test situation demanded in general test psychology, as described by, for example, Michel (1964). There, the physician or psychologist administers a test in a strictly standardized procedure, and the subject, in consequence, feels himself to be in a test situation. For a physician, this might sometimes force rather unnatural behaviour which could seriously disturb the atmosphere associated with trust and confidence in the normal physician–patient relationship. We found that the more the test

Figure 1

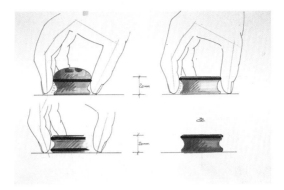

Figure 2

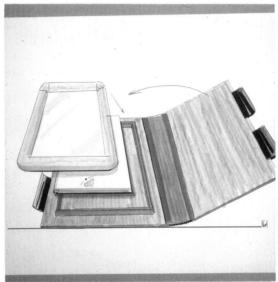

Figure 5

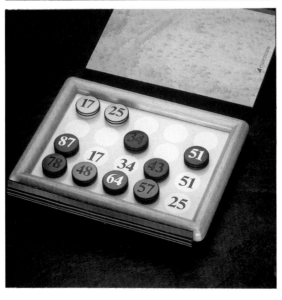

Illustrations to Chapter 9

Figure 8

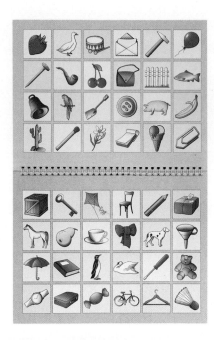

Figure 3

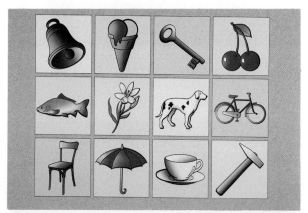

Figure 4

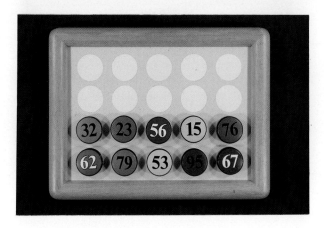

material and the reinforcing instructions created a challenging game-type situation requiring cognitive effort without the neutral or aloof character of a typical psychological test situation, the more it was accepted by our patients and, as already mentioned, the reliability and validity of the test results were higher. The test instructions should, of course, explain the aims and relevance of the test procedure – for example, that objective data for the evaluation of the patient's complaints or expected treatment effects are to be obtained.

Within the scope of the SKT project, we have reached some of the mentioned aims and, to a certain extent, solved some of the problems concerning the use of the test in clinical practice. One important finding in all our studies concerning the SKT project is that for a psychometric test to be practicable and routinely administered, adaptation of the test materials and procedures is required; the specific situation of the patients, the diagnosis and severity of the disease or, in general, the setting and the expected results are to be taken into consideration.

The SKT Project

In order to show our approach, I would like to briefly describe the SKT material and test procedure. We are aware that we have not reached, nor can we expect to reach, a final solution to the problems concerning the measurement of cognitive disturbances caused by diseases like dementia with the SKT. However, the huge amount of empirical data obtained in clinical studies encourages us to once again point out the advantages of the basic assumptions and of the deviations from 'classical' psychological test procedures underlying the SKT. The constant improvement and adaptation of the test materials and test procedure for routine clinical application and of course the documentation of its sensitivity to treatment effects in international clinical studies are probably the main causes of its success as a psychometric test within the field of dementia. With the aim of further improving its practicability, we asked a designer to carry out some ergonomic studies which brought about recommendations for changes in the test material as shown in Figures 1 (suggestions for the ergonomic improvement of magnetic blocks – see colour plate) and 2 (the new version of the SKT, encased in wood – see colour plate). This test version will be available in 1992, after we have finished our confirmatory studies concerning reliability and validity. The test procedure of the new form is identical to that of the available SKT. It is our aim that both forms should be interchangeable with regard to the norm values, in order that the results from studies in which the available form has been used can be compared with results obtained using the new form. The considerable amount of time and effort required for the adaptation is the reason for the delay in issuing the new form.

The tableau for the first subtest (Figure 3, see colour plate) shows 12 objects (Form A) which the patient is asked to name as quickly as possible and then to try to keep in mind. The time needed to perform this task in seconds is the raw score for Subtest I. The tableau is turned over immediately after the last object has been named. Subtest I serves as a basis for the following memory tests as well as for a measurement of the ability to name objects.

In Subtest II the patient is then asked to recall the named objects. The number of objects correctly recalled within 60 s gives the raw score for Subtest II, which serves as a measure of immediate recall. The test results are recorded on a registration form.

After the registration of the number of correctly recalled objects, the tableau which was shown at the beginning is presented to the patient again for a short learning phase which gives him or her another chance to commit the 12 objects to memory.

The patient then has to read a set of randomly chosen numbers (Figure 4 – position of magnetic blocks for Subtest III – see colour plate) as quickly as possible. The number of seconds which this takes is the raw score of Subtest III. After that, the patient is asked to arrange the numbers into rank order (Subtest IV) (Figure 5, see colour plate). Then he or she has to put them back into the original order. Again, the number of seconds taken is equal to the raw score for Subtest V.

For Subtest VI, the patient has to count symbols; in Form A, for example, the patient is asked to count squares (Figure 6).

In Subtest VII, the patient is asked to read letters; in Form A, the tableau shows the capital letters A and B (Figure 7). This subtest is part of a group of well-known cognitive interference tests which were described by Cattell in 1946 and Cattell and Tiner in 1949 which measure cognitive rigidity. The patient is asked to name the letter 'A' when he or she reads 'B', and to call it 'B' when actually there is an 'A' to be read. This serves

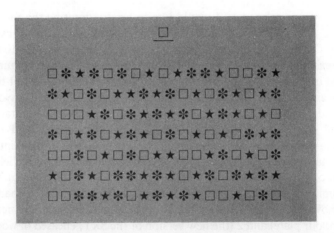

Figure 6.

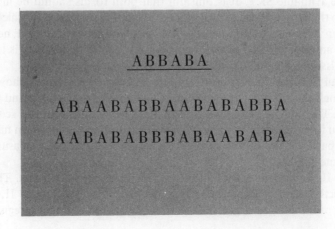

Figure 7.

to assess cognitive flexibility and aspects of concentration which are very sensitive even to mild disturbances due to brain diseases like dementia.

The patient is then asked to recall the objects once again. The number of correct items named within 60 s is the raw score for Subtest VIII, which measures an aspect of memory performance: delayed recall after distractions.

The last subtest serves to assess recognition, a rather stable, perhaps the most steady, memory function. Forty-eight objects which include the 12 objects shown on the first tableau are presented (Figure 8, see colour plate). The number of correctly identified objects equals the raw score of Subtest IX.

In general, the patients have exactly 60 s to pass the memory tests; for each of the other tests, 60 s are the maximum. That means, if a patient needs only 10 s to pass a subtest, he will immediately proceed with the next one. Generally, the SKT takes 10 to 15 min, including giving instructions and transforming the raw scores into norm values. The latter is performed by referring to the norm value tables which are available for three different intelligence and four different age groups.

The summarized score of the nine subtests serves to estimate the severity of disturbance in terms of clinically orientated descriptions of the magnitude of organic brain disease or dementia. For example, a total score ranging from 9 to 13 points indicates a mild organic brain syndrome which is associated with the clinical descriptions of, for example, Lauter (1980), stage 2 and 3 of the Global Deterioration Scale (GDS) (Reisberg, 1983), less than 24 points in the Mini-Mental State Examination (MMSE) (Folstein *et al.*, 1975) or more global descriptions of mild stages of dementia which we found in DSM-III-R or ICD 9-CM.

Using the parallel forms of the SKT (five parallel forms called A to E are available), the course of the disease can be documented as shown in Figure 9. This is only a comfortable way of presenting the SKT results and records the clinical course or

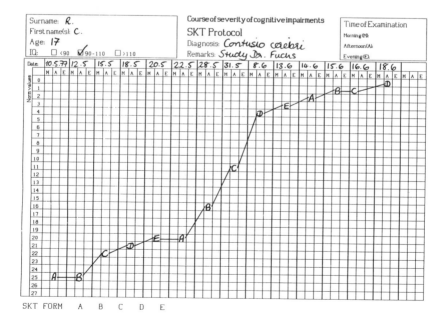

Figure 9.

therapeutic effects using data obtained with the SKT. At the moment, we are collecting data for the purpose of international validation from clinical trials in the UK, the USA and the Netherlands. Studies in France, Italy and Belgium will hopefully also be terminated soon. We are currently involved in setting up a data pool. The collected data should allow those using the SKT to estimate, for example, the outcome of a particular therapy by referring to study results obtained with the SKT in trials of similar patient groups and types of drugs. References to the available version of the SKT can be found in a summarized form in Erzigkeit (1989a) and, of course, in the latest (4th) edition of the SKT manual (Erzigkeit, 1989b).

Acknowledgement

I would like to thank Miss Catherine Sheppard for her aid in translating this contribution into English.

References

Arnold, K. R. (1983) *Untersuchungen zu Aspekten der Normierung, Reliabilität und Validität eines Testsystems zur Erfassung von Aufmerksamkeits- und Gedächtnisstörungen.* Dissertation, Friedrich Alexander University, Erlangen-Nürnberg.

Arnold, K. and Heerklotz, B. (1980) Bewertung von Depressions- und Befindlichkeits-Skalen bei alkoholischen Durchgangs-Syndromen. *Neurol. Psychiat.*, **6**, 217–20.

Cattell, R. B. and Tiner, L. (1949) The varieties of structural rigidity. *J. Pers.*, **17**.

Cattell, R. B. (1946) The riddle of perseveration I and II. *J. Pers.*, **14**, 229–67.

Erzigkeit, H. (1977) *Manual zum SKT. Formen A–E – vorläufiges Manual.* Munich: Vless, Vaterstetten.

Erzigheit, H. (1986) Manual zum SKT. 2. Neu bearbeitete Auflage. Ebersberg: Vlass-Verlag.

Erzigkeit, H. (1989a) The SKT – a short cognitive performance test as an instrument for the assessment of clinical efficacy of cognition enhancers. In: Bergener, M. and Reisberg, B. (eds) *Diagnosis and Treatment of Senile Dementia*, pp. 164–74. Springer.

Erzigkeit, H. (1989b) *Manual zum SKT.* Weinheim: Beltz Test GmbH.

Folstein, M. F., Folstein, S. E. and McHugh, P.R. (1975) 'Mini-Mental State'. A practical method for grading the cognitive state of patients for the clinician. *J. Psychiatr. Res.*, **12**, 189.

Fuchs, H. H. (1979) *Validierungsuntersuchungen zum SKT.* Dissertation, Friedrich Alexander University, Erlangen-Nürnberg.

Kirkilonis, T. (1978) *Empirische Untersuchung über die Anwendbarkeit psychopathometrischer Verfahren in der ärztlichen Allgemeinpraxis.* Dissertation, School of Medicine, Friedrich Alexander University, Erlangen-Nürnberg.

Lauter, H. (1980) Demenzen. In: Peters, U. H. (ed.) *Die Psychologie des 20 Jahrhunderts.* Vol. X. Zurück: Kindler.

Lehrl, S. and Erzigkeit, H. (1977) Psychopathometrische Verfahren bei der Prüfung von Psychopharmaka. Zur Frage der Rentabilitätserhöhung. *Pharmacospsychiatry*, **12**, 25–37.

Michel, L. (1964) Allgemeine Grundlagen psychometrischer Tests. In: Heiss, R. (ed.) *Handbuch der Psychologie*, Vol. 6, pp. 19–70. Göttingen: Hogrefe.

Reisberg, B. (ed.) (1983) *Alzheimer's Disease. The Standard Reference*, pp. 173–87. New York: The Free Press.

Witkowski, R. J. (1983) *Rückfallalkoholismus. Eine medizinsoziologische Analyse.* Wiesbaden: Akademische Verlagsgesellschaft.

10

Appropriate Psychometric Testing of Cognitive Enhancers in Human Pharmacological Studies with Healthy Volunteers

Helmut Ott

Department of Pharmacopsychology, Schering AG, Berlin, Germany

Introduction

Presently, one of the most challenging tasks in human pharmacology with healthy volunteers is to identify cognitive enhancing properties pharmacodynamically in new chemical entities (NCEs) designed for anti-dementia indications. Up to now, no standard drug among the nootropics has been accepted. Therefore, a researcher may find himself in the situation of looking for the effects of 'weak' partial agonists, 'weak' antagonists or 'weak' inverse partial agonists, if he works with beta-carbolines, a new class of benzodiazepine receptor ligands. Since these compounds are said to be 'weak' in action, one may ask what should be measured when there is nothing to measure (pharmacodynamically).

The question is: what obstacles are involved in identifying enhancing qualities of an NCE in human pharmacological trials with healthy subjects? Some important general problems are obvious:

1. The first and most significant task during phase I studies is to identify the proper dose range between the least effective and maximally tolerated dose, based on the adequate bioavailability and pharmacokinetics of the NCE.
2. To identify even small and subtle cognitive enhancing properties of a new drug, one needs very sensitive test models such as pharmaco-electroencephalography (EEG), visual analogue scales or memory tests. With such tests, ceiling and floor effects have to be kept in mind.

    Ceiling effects arise due to the test construction, e.g. subjects behave qualitatively better or more quickly than expected with a particular test, or are due to the fact

---

Dementia: Molecules, Methods and Measures. Edited by I. Hindmarch, H. Hippius and G. K. Wilcock
© 1991 John Wiley & Sons Ltd

that human volunteers function at an optimal level with respect to physical, physiological and psychological mechanisms. From numerous studies conducted over the past
20 years, we know that the sedative and other detrimental effects of most candidates for
hypnotics, neuroleptics, anti-depressants and other psychotropic drug classes can be
relatively easily determined (Spiegel, 1988; Wittenborn, 1987; Hindmarch, 1984). In
contrast, it will not be easy to enhance 'normal' functions with a supposed cognitive
enhancing NCE under these normal conditions. One solution to this problem may
be to decrease physical and psychological functions artificially by means such as stress,
fatigue, sedative compounds, etc., and to antagonize these lowered states by the NCE.

The *floor effects* of a certain test, e.g. digit-symbol substitution test (DSST), may
ensue from a misunderstanding of the task as a whole, or because even the simplest
items are too difficult. However, these do not occur primarily in healthy volunteers,
but in demented patients who are the target population of psychological testing during
clinical trials in phases II and III of the drug development.

The appropriately designed tests for human pharmacology should, in our opinion,
also be used with demented patients, not only those with mild to moderate dementia,
but also in severe cases. However, most of our test procedures exhibit drastic floor
effects in this poorly functioning population.

3. Many problems, including the floor and ceiling effects, arise if we want to use the
   same models and test concepts in animal pharmacology. Only a few models have
   been accepted which allow a transfer of results from animal research to human
   pharmacological and clinical work: for example, EEG, vigilance tasks, some memory
   tests and some psychomotor tasks (Flicker, 1988).
4. The irreversibility of and the progressive decrease in the intellectual functioning in
   Alzheimer patients causes other problems for the comparability of human pharmacological results to clinical results. In patients, we expect deceleration or even cessation
   of the progressive course of the disease, whereas, in healthy human volunteers, we
   would like to see reversibility of the induced changes. The latter will receive the drug
   only for short periods, whereas patients will be subjected to long-lasting or even life-
   long treatment. Additionally, one has to consider treatment response latencies, and to
   address the question as to whether they are the same in healthy volunteers as in patients.

With these basic questions in mind, we will suggest how some of these problems may
be solved.

A review of the literature on dementia, anti-dementia drugs and testing methods could
include hundreds of articles on these subjects. Therefore, our task will not be to organize
all these partly conflicting results in a detailed framework, but merely to point out that
'all roads lead to Rome'. A lot of working groups have different approaches to cope
with the difficulties in anti-dementia drug research in human pharmacology. Our working
group's experience may contribute to the matter, and may even be a voice in the concert
of pharmacological research in cognitive enhancers. From this practical point of view,
our test procedures, study results and established guidelines may be acknowledged and
evaluated as an example of a scientific approach to the intensively pursued goal, i.e.
to identify cognitive enhancing properties in healthy human volunteers.

Some Ideas for Phase I Trials with Putative Cognitive Enhancing Drugs

To cope with the above mentioned difficulties, our human pharmacological unit tries
to make the observations in the first application of a new compound as precise as possible.
Some of our main ideas are given below.

Dose Titration

The first step in human pharmacopsychology is to identify the proper dose after single and multiple application. This is based on knowledge from animal pharmacology and toxicology, but primarily on human pharmacokinetics, which should show sufficient bioavailability, proper absorption, and peak and elimination characteristics. Acceptable standard deviations of the pharmacokinetics and sufficient stability data on the compound must be obtained before any clinical development can take place.

Dosage may be increased up to the limit of the maximally tolerated dose or to the limit set by animal toxicological data, where it may often be helpful to the study to conduct increasing tolerability investigations, in order to estimate kinetically or behaviourally relevant dosage limits. During the testing of the maximal tolerable dose, we may stress that all 'clinical symptoms and side effects' in healthy volunteers really follow the same pharmacodynamic course as all other more or less sensitive neuropsychological or physiological test parameters, but the observations and ratings by medically trained observers, in most cases, will be cruder than standardized laboratory test systems.

Observer Ratings of the Medicated Subjects

Standard observer ratings, like adverse reaction reports, will be performed at critical time points and critical phases according to a detailed time schedule by the medically trained staff, who are continuously present.

Self-ratings

The subjects will be trained or requested to be aware of changes in their own physical and mental states, and to note these experiences in diaries, subjective notices, visual analogue scales, scales for mood and well-being, neurophysiological symptom lists, etc.

Anchor Test

The DSST is used as an anchor test in most of our human pharmacological studies. This complex psychomotor and mental test gives information about the reliability of the supposed drug effect in the different independent trials.

Clinical EEG

In the very first applications of the NCE, a concomitant clinical EEG will be needed for the detection of convulsive episodes and other electrophysiologically detectable changes. This measure of caution points to the danger that all cognitive enhancers may have excitational potency. The clinical EEG may also be used as an inclusion or exclusion criterion.

Videotaping

Videotaping of the subject's behaviour in and out of bed is used for post hoc detection of small changes in behaviour. The videotaping may only be done in critical phases of adverse drug reactions, or systematically by time sampling of certain expected or unexpected behavioural changes.

Design

Basically, the study will be randomized, double-blind and placebo controlled, preferably with independent groups of subjects for each dose level. The number and choice of subjects per group (e.g. three verum / one placebo, seven verum / three placebo, six verum / six placebo or 18 verum / 18 placebo) are dependent on the goal of the specific study, and the level of certainty with which a relevant difference should be detected and statistically confirmed by means of a specific method. There will be no so-called 'pre-pilot trials' to get the 'first medical impressions' of the supposed NCE qualities. In the case of emergencies, the code is only broken by non-participating, medically trained persons.

Data Inspection and Evaluation

After the end of the study, quick and exhaustive inspection and evaluation of all data for every dose level will be made before the next dose step is realized. This ensures that no information is lost, and reduces the danger that false alarms occur which stop the next dose-finding step.

Aged Subjects

In agreement with several guidelines for research on healthy volunteers, older healthy subjects will be included as early as possible during the first trials of the developmental phase I. In this early stage, only male subjects should participate. However, aged women with no child-bearing potential should also be included as early as possible, in order to identify sex-related differences of the NCE (Hawkins, 1988; Freeman, 1978; Ingram and Ingram, 1989; Commission of the European Communities, 1990; Bethge *et al.*, 1989).

Psychometric and Neurophysiological Testing

Guided by special hypotheses, appropriate psychometric and neurophysiological testing in phase II may take place. In particular, performance enhancement, vigilance-inducing properties, antagonism or interactions will be studied not only during phase I, but also during phases II and III, especially for the so-called labelling profile to be claimed for drug registration purposes.

These crucial ideas, among others, ensure optimal control and dose recommendation, including safety aspects for the phase II patient trials. In particular, the dose range between the least effective and the maximal tolerable dose of the NCE will be helpful for the first clinical dose-finding studies in patients.

Selection Criteria for Psychometric Testing

After having reviewed the basic questions in the human pharmacological study of cognitive enhancers, we will now focus on adequate criteria for selecting appropriate psychometric and neurophysiological test procedures according to the DSM-III-R syndromes of dementia (APA, 1987).

The DSM-III-R manual defines dementia in essence as 'impairment in short- and long-term memory, associated with impairment in abstract thinking, impaired judgement, other disturbances of higher cortical function, or personality change . . . the disturbance is severe enough to interfere significantly with work or usual social activities or relation-ships with others' (APA, 1987, p. 103). Current research on nootropic drugs concentrates on two central organically associated mental disorders, namely senile dementia of the Alzheimer type (SDAT) and multi-infarct dementia (MID). An attempt was made to design appropriate tests according to the established diagnostic criteria of SDAT and MID, especially the detrimental neuropsychological and physiological functions, for use in human pharmacological studies with healthy volunteers as well as in clinical studies with patients. The results are shown in Table 1.

In the two left-hand columns, the clinical target syndromes (A–F) of SDAT and MID are represented; the column showing MID also includes focal neurological signs (G) as well as cerebrovascular disease (H), which are not demonstrable in SDAT. The clinical courses of the two types of dementia are different: SDAT has a progressive course, whereas MID has a 'stepwise deteriorating course with "patchy" distribution of deficits early in the course' (APA, 1987, p. 123). In the next column, the most important neuropsychophysiological dysfunctions are listed. The headings correspond to points A–F, and the subheadings 1–4 refer to the corresponding points in the DSM-III-R manual (APA, 1987, p. 107). In the next column, there are examples of how these test concepts were made operational, once as a manual test and once as a computerized version. The last column shows the operation of the corresponding test concepts in patients.

As can be clearly seen in Table 1, testing methods exist for all higher cortical functions – even vigilance measurement – and a large proportion of these can also be applied with the aid of computers. For the patient population with SDAT and MID, some test concepts are lacking; one may be content with neurological examinations, case histories and medical examinations. Obviously, there are no clinical factors to be investigated in healthy volunteers, whereas in patients, comprehensive medical, neurological and physical examinations are necessary. As mentioned above, the substance-related effects will be reversible in healthy volunteers, but in patients, an attempt is made to stop or counteract the progressive process.

In the final column of Table 1, indications of computerized testing methods have been intentionally excluded, since this subject is to be dealt with in more detail below.

Automated testing in psychology began in 1967. At first, progress was slow, but it has since developed more and more into a strong trend, and has begun to replace manual methods (Cull and Trimble, 1987). The great advantage of the computerized presentation of psychological test tasks is that objectivity and reliability are clearly improved in comparison with manual versions, and that the validity aspects and, especially, the pharmacosensitivity can thus be more precisely investigated and the validity coefficients increased. The relationships between the theoretical testing criteria objectivity, reliability and validity (Lienert, 1969), as well as pharmacosensitivity, are shown in Figure 1. The following aspects of computerization are further benefits for establishing methodological reliability whose importance should not be underestimated:

1. Precise registration of reaction times.
2. Quantitative test evaluations, including plausibility checks and individual comparisons to the standards (directly on site and immediately after test application).
3. Results which can be represented in tabular and graphic form.
4. Transference of the automated data for biometric processing.

Thus it is only natural that automated methods are given preference in the search for appropriate tests for the characterization of nootropic drugs.

Table 1. Examples of human pharmacological tests with respect to the DSM-III-R criteria for dementia. In the two left-hand columns, '+' indicates that an impaired neuropsychophysiological function is associated with SDAT or MID according to DSM-III-R criteria. The next column lists the neuropsychophysiological functions, which are classified here from A to H according to the DSM-III-R criteria as proposed by the American Psychiatric Association. In the three columns to the right, these neuropsychophysiological functions are operationalized by examples of tests or concepts. A distinction is made between test applications in healthy volunteers and patients; '+' indicates that a computerized version is available for testing in volunteers

Clinical target syndrome: (impairment of)		Neuropsychophysiological function/course	Operationalization by test concepts/tests (examples)		
SDAT	MID		Volunteers Manual	Volunteers Computerized	Patients
+	+	**A** Memory	Word lists (free recall)	–	Visuospatial memory
			Recognition	+	Everyday memory battery
			Delayed pattern retention	+	Case history
		B At least one of the following:			
+	+	(1) Abstract thinking (or)	Raven, logical reasoning	+	BCRS*
			Pauli performance	+	MMSE†
			Arithmetic		
+	+	(2) Judgment for everyday activities (or)			IADL‡
					PSMS§
+	+	(3) Other higher cortical functions/ information processing (or)			
		Language-aphasia	Verbal fluency (free association)	–	Aphasia examination
			Colour naming	–	
			Nuremberg Geriatric Inventory	–	
		Psychomotor skills (apraxia, visuomotor coordination)	Tapping, pegboard	+	Apraxia examination
			Tracking, reaction time	+	

	Feature	Test	
+	Perception, cognition-agnosia, preservation	Agnosia examination	+
		Digit-symbol, rapid information processing	
		Colour word, Stroop,	−
		Trail making	−
	Construction abilities, concept formation	Object sorting	+
		Block design	−
+	(4) Personality, mood, aggression	Visual anaologue scales	+
		Adjective check list	+
		Mood scale	+
+	C Interferes with work and social activities (driving)		−
		Driving simulator	+
		On-the-road-test	+
+	D Not occurring during delirium (vigilance, attention)	EEG	+
		Macworth clock	+
		Case history	
		RDRS-2¶	
−	E Organic factors		
−	G Focal neurological signs	Medical examination	
+	H Cerebrovascular disease	Neurological examination	
		Physical examination	
+	F Course of dementia	Reversibility	
progressive			
+ stepwise deteriorating with patchy distribution		Deceleration or stopping of progression	

Note: *Brief Cognitive Rating Scale (Reisberg and Ferris, 1988)
† Mini-Mental State Examination (Cockrell and Folstein, 1988)
‡ Instrumental Activities of Daily Living Scale (Lawton and Brody, 1988)
§ Physical Self Maintenance Scale (Lawton and Brody, 1980)
¶ Rapid Disability Rating Scale-2 (Linn,1988)

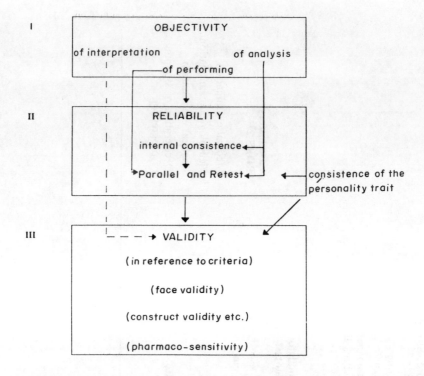

Figure 1. Modified theoretical criteria of test construction according to Lienert (1969). This figure shows the relationships between objectivity, reliability and validity. If a test is objective in performance and analysis (i.e. parametrization), then the internal consistency of the test is high, and parallel and retest values will also be high. This especially holds true when the measured personality trait or other psychological function is constant. Validity refers to the ability of the method to accurately reflect that construct for which it was intended. This can be achieved via different mathematical procedures. For example, if the test in question correlates highly to an external criterion, this is known as 'criterion validity'. If a test is sensitive enough to distinguish between the effects of placebo and certain standard medications, or even between different dosages of the same compound, it is called 'pharmacosensitive'

Experience with clinical neuropsychological testing methods for demented patients is not yet very comprehensive. Two recent examples are described in greater detail below.

In a large series of manually conducted standard tests with two groups of aged patients (one group of SDAT patients, one group with Parkinson's syndrome), Huber *et al.* (1989) were able to demonstrate that these groups of patients performed more poorly than the control groups in all scores. Furthermore, the SDAT group's scores were equivalent to or poorer than those of the Parkinson group, except in the factors 'verbal fluency' and Raven's matrices. In a similar large-scale, non-computerized battery of tests, another group of authors (Storandt and Hill, 1989) clearly differentiated between 'mild' and 'questionable' dementia, with a distinct tendency toward better performance in the matched control group.

In a review article by Flicker (1988), 64 tests were evaluated in order to establish whether they are *age-sensitive* or *sensitive for the investigation of dementia syndromes*. Only 61% of the tests proved to be age-sensitive, whereas, not unexpectedly, nearly all (92%) of the tests indicated demential degeneration, since the degree of age-related cognitive disturbances is usually not as great as for disturbances caused by dementia. He also investigated the neuropsychological tests for floor and ceiling effects, and showed that 69% had floor effects and 17% had mixed effects. Only 8% reached a sufficient degree of difficulty so that both demented and healthy individuals could be subjected to the same test. Among these tests were finger tapping, reaction time, digit span and telephone dialing. Flicker reached the conclusion that the vast majority of the tests have too narrow a range of difficulty, i.e. they were designed in such a way that they are either too easy or too difficult for dementia research. Even the so-called 'simplified' test variants are not comparable to the original, so that dementia and non-dementia age groups cannot be directly assigned to the same scale.

The fulfilment of theoretical test criteria seems to be a nearly insurmountable task. Flicker's survey of 64 neuropsychological tests revealed that in 25% of the tests, no parallel forms for reproduction of the test results are available, or data on reliability are missing. In 39% of the tests, there is no information regarding construct validity, in 58% no information on face validity, and in 75–78% of the tests there are no indications of the pharmacosensitivity in association with scopolamine or cognitive enhancers. Tests suitable for interspecies comparisons are, at 13%, likewise rather scantily represented in this list. Although 50% of these tests are widely distributed, the proportion of computerized tests in this review (28%) leaves much to be desired. Tests for the diagnosis of linguistic functions and long-term memory of remote events (months or years past) have been either overlooked or neglected in dementia research.

Because of this rather discouraging state of affairs, it appears advisable to have a closer look at recent developments in computer-supported test systems.

Computer-supported Test Batteries

Table 2 shows six examples of test batteries, most of which were designed with computer support. It can be seen in this table that nearly all authors addressed the DSM-III-R criteria for dementia, i.e. 'memory', 'psychomotor skills' and 'vigilance'. Tests for 'judgment of everyday activities', 'constructional abilities' and 'social activities' are for the most part lacking, probably due to the fact that these data are elicited by questionnaires such as the Instrumental Activities of Daily Living (Lawton and Brody, 1988). Most of these test batteries include at least some allowance for information on objectivity, reliability and validity. Only two batteries are completely automated and do not require manual operation by the test administrator. Three of the test batteries use the touchscreen as a modern technical development, so that the answers/reactions are entered immediately by screen contact, and not via keyboards or other key fields. The latter are most often out of view of the stimulus display, so that in these testing methods the subject needs a certain amount of practice for quick answering coordination. All six test batteries are suitable for patients, and five are suitable for healthy volunteers.

The specific subtests which are used in the individual test batteries are not dealt with in greater detail here; the reader is referred to the individual papers detailed at the end of this chapter. According to the information available to us, there do not appear to be any subtests common to all the test batteries. The individual subtests in the batteries vary greatly both in concept as well as in execution and parameters. They are comparable only on the abstract level of general neuropsychological functions, such as 'memory' or 'vigilance', etc.

Standardization of a Computer-supported Psychoexperimental Test Battery

An example for the construction and control methods of a computerized test battery in accordance with established theoretical criteria (Lienert, 1969) can be seen in the study

Table 2. Examples of human pharmacological test batteries with respect to the DSM-III-R criteria for dementia. The far left column lists the neuropsychophysiological functions, which are classified here from A to D according to the DSM-III-R criteria as proposed by the American Psychiatric Association; '+' indicates that the corresponding neuropsychophysiological functions are addressed in the six test batteries under comparison. Brackets indicate ambivalence regarding whether these functions are represented in the test batteries. The term 'standardization' refers to fulfilment of the test criteria outlined in Figure 1. Again, brackets indicate ambivalence. The term 'mode' indicates whether the tests are applied manually, with the aid of computers, or even with a touchscreen

Neuropsychophysiological functions	Corkin et al., 1986 (Neuropsychological Battery)	Larrabee and Crook, 1988 (Computerized Everyday Memory Battery)	Ferries, et al., 1988 (NYU Comp. TB f. Assessment Cognition)[1]	Morris, et al., 1987 CANTAB[2]	Hindmarch et al., 1984 Subhan, 1984	Ott et al., 1989 (Computer Supported Psychoexperimental Test Battery)
A *Memory:*						
Immediate, late	+	+	+		+	+
'Spatial', learning				+		
B1 *Abstract thinking:*						
Concept formation, planning			+	+		+
B2 *Judgment* for everyday activities						

B3 *Higher cortical functions:*					
Language	+	(+)			+
Psychomotor skills, psychomotor speed (practice)	+	+	+	+	+
Visuomotor coordination, balance	+				+
Perception, cognition				+	+
Constructional abilities (concept formation)					
B4 *Personality:*					
Mood, aggression				+	+
C *Interference with work and social activities:*					
Driving (simulation)	+	+	+		+
D *Vigilance, attention*	+	+	+	(+)	+
Standardization: objectivity (O), reliability (R), validity (V)	(O)(R)(V)	OR(V)	OR	OR(V)	O(V)R
Mode: manual (M), computerized (C), touchscreen (T)	M	MCT	CT	CM	CM
Appropriate for: patient (Pt), volunteers (Vol)	Pt	Pt	Pt Vol	Vol Pt	Vol Pt

[1] New York University computerized test battery for assessing cognition in aging and dementia.
[2] Cambridge Neuropsychological Test Automated Battery.

by Ott *et al.* (1989). In these investigations, the authors applied a computer-supported psychoexperimental test battery to 36 male volunteers in a clinical phase I study. This battery comprised the following tests:

1. *Tapping.* In the tapping test, the subject is instructed to tap with a metal pin as quickly as possible in the middle of a metal plate. This test is used to measure simple psychomotor activity, reactive inhibition and fatigue.
2. *Pegboard.* The pegboard test consists of the transference of metal pins into holes from one side of the panel to the other, making possible the measurement of gross motor function, accuracy of arm aiming and dexterity.
3. *Video tracking.* This exercise involves manoeuvring the tracking signal with a joystick to follow the target signal as closely as possible. This test measures visuomotor coordination.
4. *Pauli memory performance test.* Here the subject is to add or subtract memorized digits to allow the measurement of continuous attention, perseverance and effort.
5. *Multiple reaction time test.* In this test, the subject reacts as quickly as possible by finger pressure (allowing the measurement of simple visual reaction time) in comparing one symbol with a second symbol which appears a few seconds after disappearance of the first (to test delayed retention/delayed matching).
6. *Visual analogue scales.* Here the subject enters his or her mood state on a 100 mm scale between two poles described by contrasting adjectives, thus indicating stress, exhaustion, fitness, etc.

In order to establish the highest possible degree of objectivity, a stringent standardization procedure of testing was established prior to application; all 36 test subjects were given identical tasks under identical conditions. The computer-supported test battery was administered on three subsequent study days with three measurements separated by an interval of 2 h between each test run. A fourth study day with the same measurement points in the morning, noon and afternoon took place after a seven-day interval.

The learning curves of the individual subjects as well as of the whole group were plotted. To compare the different reliability values between learning onset (resulting in low coefficients) and the stable learning plateau (resulting in high coefficients), the retest reliability coefficients were established between days 1 and 4 and days 3 and 4 (Figure 2).

Based on the resulting high reliability coefficients, the duration of some tests could even be shortened, e.g. the tapping test from 1 min to 0.5 min, the Pauli memory performance test from 10 min to 5 min, etc. To ensure construct validity, 18 parameters were selected and subjected to a factor analysis with Varimax rotation. Only six factors were permitted. Approximately 75% ($\pm$ 3%) of the variance was explained. Four acceptable factors were found and were classified as:

1. Mood ('Befindlichkeit').
2. Cognition (mental abilities, mental processes).
3. Motor performance (gross and fine movements, purely psychomotor performance).
4. Visuomotor coordination.

Using such a computer-supported test battery, it is possible to investigate pharmacological influence on a certain psychological function with regard to its learning plateau or concerning the acquisition of a specific function. In addition, the pharmacokinetic courses of CNS compounds can be pharmacodynamically portrayed in a sensitive manner.

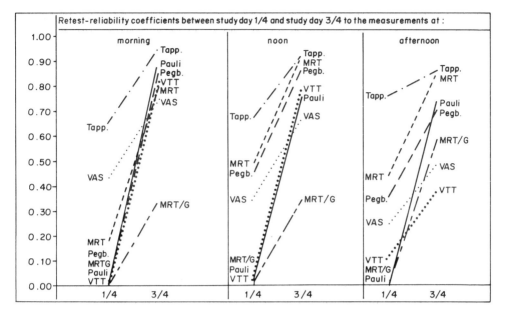

Figure 2. Retest reliability coefficients in a computer-supported test battery. This figure shows a comparison of the different reliability coefficients (*r*) between learning onset (low *r*) and the stable learning plateau (high *r*) resulting from the correlations between days 1 and 4 (1/4) and days 3 and 4 (3/4) at morning, noon and afternoon sessions. The coefficients for 3/4 range between $r = 0.35$ (MRT/G) and $r = 0.92$ (Tapp.). Tapp. = tapping test; Pauli = Pauli memory performance test; Pegb. = pegboard test; VTT = video tracking test; MRT = multiple reaction time test; VAS = visual analogue scales; MRT/G = MRT with memory

Pharmacosensitivity of Tests and Computer-supported Test Batteries after Administration of Stimulants and Cognitive Enhancers

The performance-enhancing effects of 'psychostimulants', 'psychoenergizers', 'nootropics' or, as most recently described, 'cognitive enhancers' (Pepeu, 1989) have been the subject of investigation for a long period of time. Wittenborn (1988) evaluated 15 tests, all having a certain association with 'memory load', according to whether benzodiazepines or non-benzodiazepines had any significant effects on performance. As expected, no cases of performance-enhancing effects were seen in 109 studies after administration of different benzodiazepines; performance-decreasing effects, however, were seen in 90 clinical tests (i.e. 83%). Among the non-benzodiazepines, especially caffeine, nicotine and alcohol, which were administered in 71 experiments, performance was significantly enhanced in 12 cases (i.e. 17%); however, the opposite was true in 27 (38%) of the experiments. The pharmacosensitive tests included 'verbal recall', 'paired association', 'number recall', 'number in sequence', 'DSST', 'symbol copying test' and 'picture recognition'. Based on these observations in healthy volunteers, Wittenborn concluded that the stimulating and memory-enhancing effects of stimulants can certainly be measured psychometrically, meaning that these testing concepts are pharmacosensitive for so-called cognitive enhancers and psychostimulants.

In a study by the present authors (Ott *et al.*, 1980) using electromechanical equipment which was the precursor of that used in the standardized, computer-supported test battery discussed above (Ott *et al.*, 1989), it was demonstrated that 20 mg dextroamphetamine sulphate and 30 mg methylphenidate had a significant performance-enhancing effect versus placebo on tapping, aiming, pegboard and the Pauli performance test with and without memory.

To a certain extent, the often quoted and promising computer-supported method known as 'critical flicker fusion' (CFF) (Hindmarch, 1988) appears to be a suitable index for decreased performance in association with sedatives (Hindmarch, 1988, p. 79), but in an extended study of 32 subjects it did not differentiate between methylphenidate and placebo (Ott and Christea, 1982). This is probably less a result of the psychostimulant than of the method applied, which deserves fundamental criticism both in terms of technique and of neurophysiology (Ott and Kranda, 1982).

After 1968, clinical investigations and the introduction of Hydergin (co-dergocrine mesylate; Hydergine), a dihydrogenated ergot alkaloid, gave rise to an extremely strong impulse toward a pharmacological treatment of senile dementia, cerebrovascular disease and other associated age-related mental diseases. In a review of 26 clinical studies, McDonald (1979) noted that with Hydergin versus placebo or other reference substance, the effects were measured only by clinical rating scales in interview situations, but not by objective tests such as single or disjunctive reaction time measurement or by apparative memory tests.

On the other hand, however, the use of so-called objective measuring instruments does not guarantee success in promoting a given substance gerontopharmacologically as performance enhancing, as could be shown by the results of our investigation of ergot alkaloids. Extensive experiments with healthy volunteers as well as some patients in a home for the aged, using apparative psychological test methods, rating scales (McDonald and Rohloff, 1983), and EEG readings, revealed no relevant changes after single-dose administration or application over several weeks. The question arose as to whether this lack of change was due to the substance, the dosage and duration of treatment or the inadequate sensitivity of the measurement instruments. This is precisely the point at which the greatest problem in current gerontopharmacology and dementia therapy can be seen, i.e. that no pharmacological standard of therapy has yet been established by which the sensitivity of the measuring instruments could be gauged. With the demand for pharmacosensitive, computer-supported methods of measurement, one may by no means omit rating scales, and electrophysiological and neurophysiological methods in a study, because psychophysiological functions vary greatly, particularly with advanced age – perhaps due to the very long-term individualization – and are nearly impossible to correlate (Aufdembrinke *et al.*, 1988).

Beta-carbolines

In succession to the benzodiazepine derivatives, which function as so-called *full agonists* with the effects of anxiolysis, sedation and sleep, muscle relaxation, anti-convulsion and amnesia (pharmacological examples are diazepam and lormetazepam), the discovery was made of benzodiazepine receptor ligands such as flumazenil, which possess antagonistic properties. The search for further ligands broadened the spectrum to include so-called *partial inverse agonists* which, like full inverse agonists, can induce anxiety, stimulation, elevated muscle tone, convulsions and enhanced memory functions (Dorow *et al.*, 1987b). With these discoveries, the new pharmacological principle of bidirectional effects on the behavioural level was born (Stephens and Jensen, 1987). Thus in the SDAT area of benzodiazepine receptor ligand research, therapists currently place their hopes in the partial inverse antagonists. If the effects of stimulation, vigilance raising and enhancement of memory performance can be separated from the other, undesirable characteristics of the inverse antagonists, then the progression of the above mentioned symptoms of Alzheimer's disease and MID could be stopped, or at least retarded.

Full antagonists might also show a comparable effect, according to the hypothesis of Sarter *et al.* (1988). This hypothesis states that the cholinergic transmission of the remaining acetylcholine neurons becomes synergistically amplified when benzodiazepine receptor ligands on the acetylcholine gamma-aminobutyric acid (GABA) complex are blocked via a benzodiazepine antagonist. This 'disinhibition' increases acetylcholine release and enhances choline uptake. Since it has already been reported that choline plays an important role in normal memory functions, and that Alzheimer patients possess this enzyme in reduced amounts, it therefore seems reasonable that even a slight increase in choline transmission might have a beneficial effect in the memory processes in patients with Alzheimer's disease.

Subsequent to isolated pharmacological animal tests to establish the profile of these NCEs e.g. enhancement of vigilance and memory function, the results of initial human pharmacological application of weak inverse agonists show that there may be a chance to realize the above described pharmacological concept. The compound ZK 93426 is one of the possible candidates. After intravenous administration of 0.04 mg in several double-blind, placebo-controlled studies, performance enhancement was seen in the following tests: logical reasoning and picture difference task, visual memory and word list, especially in long-term retrieval, and visual analogue scales referring to feelings of drive (Duka *et al.*, 1988). Additionally enhanced wakefulness was obvious in multiple sleep latency tests (Dorow *et al.*, 1987a). So far, ZK 93426, as a weak partial agonist, has proven to exert small but significant intrinsic activities at different pharmacodynamic levels.

The Scopolamine Model as an Age-deficit Paradigm (Dementia Model)

As mentioned above, the cholinergic hypothesis is of central importance for the degenerative age-related diseases SDAT and MID (Ferris *et al.*, 1983; Brinkmann *et al.*, 1982); it therefore appears logical to establish an artificial age-deficit paradigm (Drachmann and Leavitt, 1974; Bartus *et al.*, 1982). Scopolamine is a relatively well-tolerated anticholinergic substance that influences mainly the memory (Drachmann and Leavitt, 1974; Bartus *et al.*, 1981) and also vigilance in EEG, especially pharmaco-EEG (Itil and Fink, 1966; Fink, 1969). It is expected that cognitive enhancers can be detected by partial or total antagonization of the scopolamine-suppressant behavioural effects (Sannita *et al.*, 1987).

In our investigations using the scopolamine model (Ott *et al.*, 1990), the beta-carboline candidate ZK 93426 partially counteracted the scopolamine effects in the DSST and pharmaco-EEG (Ott, 1990, unpublished data).

Future Perspectives

Appropriate psychometric testing of putatively cognitive enhancing drugs in human pharmacological phase I trials is possible. Many tests have been proven to be sensitive to age, dementia, scopolamine and cognitive enhancers. In the near future, more and more tests will be computerized and standardized according to theoretical test criteria, e.g. objectivity, reliability and validity, as well as pharmaco-sensitivity. Floor and ceiling effects will be minimized by reconstruction of the tests. Computer testing programs will be more easily exchangeable between research groups, based on the worldwide increase in common industry standards in computer technology. Compounds with 'cognitive enhancing' properties, e.g. beta-carbolines, will be available and, hopefully, some of them will be accepted as standards. There is a great need for worldwide consensus conferences to establish standards for testing anti-dementia drugs in animal, human pharmacological and clinical research in order to shorten the time necessary to develop effective nootropics for therapeutic application (Amaducci *et al.*, 1989).

Age and dementia-related deficit models such as the scopolamine model may be extremely useful to detect and confirm the antagonistic and cognitive enhancing properties of NCEs. Stress models such as long-term performance tests (e.g. reaction time tests) and natural deficit models such as the investigation of subvigilant older subjects or sleep deprivation paradigms are possibly useful, but there is little evidence for their effectiveness as research tools in the area of cognitive enhancers.

Labelling trials, including examination of the interaction of the NCE with alcohol (Willumeit *et al.*, 1984; Ott *et al.*, 1990) and with different long-term medication regimens, increase the willingness of the registration authorities to accept the new substance, and contribute to the clarification of the mechanisms involved in different effects, including side effects.

Acknowledgements

The author wishes to thank Dr B. Aufdembrinke, Dr T. Duka, Dr F. Dahlke, Dr R. Dorow, Dr K. Fichte, Mr A. Rohloff and Dr B. Voet for assistance and advice, and Mr B. Young for help preparing the text. Thanks are also due to Miss B. Grossmann for bibliographic support, and to Mrs U. Hippler for graphics and J. Lohmann for photography.

References

Amaducci, L., Angst, J., Bech, P., Benkert, O., Bruinvels, J., Engel, R. R., Gottfries, C. G., Hippius, H., Levy, R., Lingjaerde, O., López-Ibor, J. J. Jr, Orgogozo, J. M., Pull C., Saletu, B., Stoll, K. D. and Woggon, B. (1989) Consensus Conference on the Methodology of Clinical Trials of 'Nootropics', Munich, June 1989. Report of the Consensus Committee.

American Psychiatric Association (1987) *Diagnostic and Statistical Manual of Mental Disorders – DSM-III-R*. Washington, D.C.: American Psychiatric Association.

Aufdembrinke, B., Ott, H. and Rohloff, A. (1988) Measures of memory and information processing in elderly volunteers. In: Hindmarch, I. and Ott, H. (eds) *Benzodiazepine Receptor Ligands, Memory and Information Processing* (Psychopharmacology Series 6), pp. 48–64. Berlin, Heidelberg: Springer Verlag.

Bartus, R. T., Dean, R. L., Sherman, K., Firedman, E. and Beer, B. (1981) Profound effects of combining choline and piracetam on memory enhancement and cholinergic functions in aged rats. *Neurobiol. Aging*, **2**, 105–11.

Bartus, R. T. *et al.* (1982) The cholinergic hypothesis of geriatric memory dysfunction. *Science*, **217**, 408–17.

Bethge, H., Czechanowski, B., Gundert-Remy, U., Hasford, J., Kleinsorge, H., Kreutz, G., Letzel, H., Mueller, A. A., Selbmann, H. K. and Weber, E. (1989) Empfehlungen zur Ermittlung, Dokumentation, Erfassung und Bewertung unerwünschter Ereignisse im Rahmen der klinischen Prüfung von Arzneimitteln. *Arzneim.-Forsch./Drug Res.*, **39**, 10.

Brinkmann, S. D., Pomara, N., Goodnick, P. J., Barnett, N. and Domino, E. F. (1982) A dose-ranging study of lecithin in the treatment of primary degenerative dementia (Alzheimer's disease). *J. Clin. Psychopharmacol.*, **2**, 181–5.

Cockrell, J. R. and Folstein, M.F. (1988) Mini-mental state examination (MMSE). *Psychopharmacol. Bull.*, **24**(4), 689–95.

Commission of the European Communities (1990) Good clinical practice for trials on medicinal products in the european community. Provisional address: rue de la loi 200, B-1049 Brussels.

Corkin, S., Growdon, J. H., Sullivan, E. V., Nissen, M. J. and Huff, F. J. (1986) Assessing treatment effects: a neuropsychological battery. In: Poon, L. W. (ed.) *Clinical Memory Assessment of Older Adults*, pp. 156–167. Washington, D. C.: American Psychological Association.

Cull, C. A. and Trimble, M. R. (1987) Automated testing and psychopharmacology. In: Hindmarch, I. and Stonier, P. D. (eds) *Human Psychopharmacology – Measures and Methods*, pp. 113–54. Chichester: John Wiley and Sons.

Dorow, R., Duka, T., Höller, L. and Sauerbrey, N. (1987a) Clinical perspectives of beta-carbolines from first studies in humans. *Brain Res. Bull.*, 3, 319–26.

Dorow, R., Duka, T., Sauerbrey, N. and Höller, L. (1987b) β-Carbolines: new insights into the clinical pharmacology of benzodiazepine receptor ligands. In: Dahl, S., Gram, F., Paul, S. M. and Potter, W. Z. (eds) *Clinical Pharmacology in Psychiatry*, pp. 37–51. Berlin, Heidelberg: Springer Verlag.

Drachman, D. and Leavitt, J. (1974) Human memory and the cholinergic system. *Arch. Neurol.*, 30, 113–21.

Duka, T., Edelmann, V., Schütt, B. and Dorow, R. (1988) β-Carbolines as tools in memory research: human data with the β-carboline ZK 93426. In: Hindmarch, I. and Ott, H. (eds) *Benzodiazepine Receptor Ligands, Memory and Information Processing* (Psychopharmacology Series 6), pp. 246–60. Berlin, Heidelberg: Springer Verlag.

Ferris, S. H. and Crook, T. (1983) Cognitive assessment in mild to moderately severe dementia. In: Crook, T., Ferris, S. and Bartus, R. (eds) *Assessment in Geriatric Psychopharmacology*, pp. 178–86. Mark Powley Associates.

Ferris, S. H., Flicker, C. and Reisberg, B. (1988) NYU computerized test battery for assessing cognition in aging and dementia. *Psychopharmacol. Bull.*, 24(4), 699–702.

Fink, M. (1969) EEG and human psychopharmacology. *Annu. Rev. Pharmacol. Toxicol.*, 9, 241–58.

Flicker, C. (1988) Neuropsychological evaluation of treatment effects in the elderly: a critique of tests in current use. *Psychopharmacol. Bull.*, 24(4), 535–56.

Freeman, M. M. (1978) General considerations for the clinical evaluation of drugs. Washington, D. C.: Order No. FDA 77-3040. US Department of Health, Education and Welfare.

Hawkins, B. S. (1988) Perusing the literature. *Controlled Clin. Trials*, 9, 152–62.

Hindmarch, I. (1984) Psychological performance models as indicators of the effects of hypnotic drugs on sleep. In: Hindmarch, I., Ott, H. and Roth, T. (eds) *Sleep, Benzodiazepines and Performance/Psychopharmacology Supplementum 1*, pp. 58–68. Berlin, Heidelberg, New York, Tokyo: Springer Verlag.

Hindmarch, I. (1988) Information processing, critical flicker fusion threshold and benzodiazepines: results and speculations. In: Hindmarch, I. and Ott, H. (eds) *Benzodiazepine Receptor Ligands, Memory and Information Processing* (Psychopharmacology Series 6), pp. 79–89. Berlin, Heidelberg: Springer Verlag.

Huber, S. J., Shuttleworth, E. C. and Freidenberg, D. L. (1989) Neuropsychological differences between the dementias of Alzheimer's and Parkinson's diseases. *Arch. Neurol.*, 46, 1287–91.

Ingram, D. and Ingram, V. (1981) *An Introduction to Human Volunteer Studies*. Manchester: Clinical Pharmacology Unit, University Hospital of South Manchester.

Itil, T. M. and Fink, M. (1966) Anticholinergic drug-induced delirium (experimental modification, quantitative EEG and behavioral correlations). *J. Nerv. Ment. Dis.*, 143, 492–507.

Larrabee, G. J. and Crook, T. (1988) A computerized every day memory battery for assessing treatment effects. *Psychopharmacol. Bull.*, 24(4), 695–97.

Lawton, B. and Brody, E. M. (1988) Instrumental activities of daily living (IADL) scale: original observer-rated version. *Psychopharmacol. Bull,* 24(4), 785–9.

Lienert, G. A. (1969) *Testaufbau und Testanalyse*. Weinheim: Beltz Verlag.

Linn, M. W. (1988) Rapid disability rating scale-2 (RDRS-2). *Psychopharmacol. Bull.*, 24(4), 799–801.

McDonald, R. J. (1979) Hydergine: a review of 26 clinical studies. *Pharmacopsychiatr. Neuropsychopharmakol.*, 12(6), 407–22.

McDonald, R. and Rohloff, A. (1983) Effects of lisuride on psychomotor functions and recall memory in elderly healthy volunteers. In: Calne, D. B. *et al.* (eds) *Lisuride and other Dopamine Agonists*, pp. 515–28. New York: Raven Press.

Morris, R. G., Evenden, J. L., Sahakian, B. J. and Robbins, T. W. (1987) Computer-aided assessment of dementia: comparative studies of neuropsychological deficits in Alzheimer-type dementia and Parkinson's disease. *Cogn. Neurochem.*, 21–36.

Ott, H. and Kranda, K. (1982) *Flicker Techniques in Psychopharmacology*. Weinheim, Basel: Beltz Verlag.

Ott, H., Fichte, K. and Herrmann, W. M. (1980) Beitrag zur humanpharmakologischen Klassifizierung von Psychopharmaka: Das psychologische Leistungsprofil. *Arzneimittelforschung*, 1198.

Ott, H., Cristea, R. and Fichte, K. (1982) The evaluation of drug effects on CFF by three different methods. In: Ott, H. and Kranda, K. (eds) *Flicker Techniques in Psychopharmacology*, pp. 65-76. Weinheim, Basel: Beltz Verlag.

Ott, H., Seitz, O., Voet, B. and Bösel, R. (1989) Standardization of a computer supported psychoexperimental test-battery covering the psychological functions psychomotor performance, cognition, visuo-motor coordination, and mood: objectivity, reliability, and validity. Abstracts of the IV World Conference on Clinical Pharmacology and Therapeutics. *Europ. J. Clin. Pharmacol.*, **36**.

Ott, H., Rohloff, A., Seitz, O. and Voet, B. (1990) Acute CNS-depressive effects of scopolamine 0.5 mg s.c. on EEG, psychomotor performance, cognitive functions and mood in healthy volunteers. *Poster, 10th Congress of the European Sleep Research Society*, 20-25 May, Strasbourg.

Pepeu, G. (1989) Cognitive enhancing agents – introduction. *Prog. Neuropsychopharmacol. Biol. Psychiatry*, **13**, 45-6.

Reisberg, B. and Ferris, S. H. (1988) Brief cognitive rating scale (BCRS). *Psychopharmacol. Bull.*, **24**(4), 629-36.

Sannita, W. G., Maggi, L. and Rosadini, G. (1987) Effects of scopolamine (0.25-0.75 mg i.m.) on the quantitative EEG and the neuropsychological status of healthy volunteers. *Neuropsychobiology*, **17**, 199-205.

Sarter, M., Schneider, H. H. and Stephens, D. N. (1988) Treatment strategies for senile dementia: antagonist beta-carbolines. *Trends Neurosci.*, **1**, 13-17.

Spiegel, R. (1988) *Einführung in die Psychopharmakologie*. Bern, Stuttgart, Toronto: Hans Huber.

Stephens, D. N. and Jensen, L. H. (eds) (1987) Bidirectional effects of β-carbolines in behavioral pharmacology. *Brain Res. Bull.*

Storandt, M. and Hill, R. (1989) Very mild dementia of the Alzheimer type, II. psychometric test performance. *Arch. Neurol.*, **46**, 383-6.

Subhan, Z. (1984) The effects of benzodiazepines on short-term memory and information processing. In: Hindmarch, I., Ott, H. and Roth, T. (eds) *Sleep, Benzodiazepines and Performance/Psychopharmacology Supplementum 1*, pp. 173-181. Berlin, Heidelberg, New York, Tokyo: Springer Verlag.

Willumeit, H. P., Ott, H. and Neubert, W. (1984) Simulated car driving as a useful technique for the determination of residual effects and alcohol interaction after short- and long-acting benzodiazepines. In: Hindmarch, I., Ott, H. and Roth, T. (eds) *Sleep Benzodiazepines and Performance*, pp. 133-51. Springer Verlag.

Wittenborn, J. R. (1987) Psychomotor tests in psychopharmacology. In: Hindmarch, I. and Stonier, P. D. (eds) *Human Psychopharmacology – Measures and Methods*, pp. 69-78. Chichester: John Wiley and Sons.

Wittenborn, J. R. (1988) Assessment of the effects of drugs on memory. In: Hindmarch, I. and Ott, H. (eds) *Benzodiazepine Receptor Ligands, Memory and Information Processing* (Psychopharmacology Series 6), pp. 67-78. Berlin, Heidelberg: Springer Verlag.

11

Clinical Assessment Instruments and Neuropsychological Tests

*L. Israel, †DJ. Kozarevic and ‡J. M. Orgogozo

*Internal Medicine and Gerontology Department, Grenoble
University Hospital, France,
†Research Department, University Clinical Centre, Belgrade,
Yugoslavia, and ‡Neurology Department, Raymond Pellegrin Hospital,
Bordeaux, France

Introduction

Since the recognition of Alzheimer's disease as an important public health problem, the measurement of pathological cognitive changes in the elderly has become an area of increasing interest. The past two decades have seen a proliferation of tests, rating scales and mental status questionnaires designed for the screening, diagnosis and long-term monitoring of demented patients. Such instruments may be of interest to both clinicians and researchers.

Facing a dementia syndrome, the clinician is frequently concerned with problems of differential diagnosis. In daily practice he has in particular to distinguish dementia from depression or other psychiatric impairments. He should also attempt to define the type of dementia and assess the severity of the disease, evaluate related or dependent behavioural disorders and assess the level of dependency of his patient. In addition he has to estimate the possible evolution, i.e. the prognosis of the disease. Proper instruments, such as rating scales and neuropsychological tests, could help to achieve these requirements in a more efficient way. These tools also allow researchers to study and follow groups of patients on a common comparative basis. By doing so, normative data, which are essential for multicentric studies, are provided.

Rating scales are very useful in standardizing the clinical examination of demented patients through oriented observation. Although they may not appear so to a clinician concerned with a single case, they are essential when it is necessary to compare groups

Dementia: Molecules, Methods and Measures. Edited by I. Hindmarch, H. Hippius and G. K. Wilcock
© 1991 John Wiley & Sons Ltd

of patients, with regard to their similarities and differences at single or different points in time. Such standardized assessments permit investigators to make more homogeneous judgments. Furthermore, when the severity of the dementia syndrome reaches a certain threshold, when tests are no longer applicable because of a floor effect or an incapacity of the patient to collaborate, rating scales remain the only way to quantify objectively the deficiences.

The purpose of this chapter is to present and discuss a selection of commonly used rating scales, neuropsychological tests and questionnaires designed to measure specific features of the dementia syndrome.

Neuropsychological tests and rating scales are two forms of psychometric investigation techniques, and sometimes the difference between them is unclear. The well-known author Wechsler (1981) uses the term scale instead of test for the content of his battery, while others such as Roth *et al.* (1986) use the term test (IMC tests) for designing a questionnaire. Tests are standardized tasks proposed to a patient, who has to actively fulfil them and whose reactions and responses are scored. Application of tests therefore assumes the patient's participation. On the contrary, rating scales are based exclusively on the judgment of the rater, who scores the capacity or behaviour of the patient in various domains, either through direct observation or through the description of relatives or caregivers (informants).

Clinical Instruments: Global Assessments and Rating Scales

Global assessment generally refers either to an overall rating of the patient's clinical condition, or to a composite score derived by summing individual scores from different items or instruments. One of the main overall rating instruments used for global assessment is the Clinical Global Impression (CGI). This integrative measurement is based on an interview with the patient by an observer, who rates his global impression on a 7-point scale.

This type of global assessment is not specific to dementia, and it is often used as an integrated indicator of efficacy and tolerance of drug treatments. Although global ratings are sometimes extremely useful, they appear insufficient by themselves to demonstrate an improvement. For instance, a withdrawn, apathetic patient might be stimulated and activated by a compound (e.g. alcohol), which may make that patient look better while in fact it deteriorates his cognitive abilities. Therefore a global assessment should not be used alone: an additional objective measure is needed to demonstrate concomitant changes in cognitive functions and memory.

A more comprehensive and discriminating approach is to apply rating scales that measure several domains, i.e. cognitive impairments, memory, behaviour, etc. Scales are much more specific than empirical description of symptomatology, but they are still subjective. An exhaustive presentation of such scales can be found in a number of manuals and textbooks (Crook *et al.*, 1983; Guelfi, 1986; Israel *et al.*, 1984; MacDowell and Newell, 1987; Van Riezen and Segal, 1988).

Rating scales are exclusively based on subjective observer judgment (observer dependent bias), while neuropsychological tests are an objective way of measuring different types of behaviour, performance and cognitive abilities of the patient. However, the test situation and the implicit influence of the examiner may also significantly distort the results of the tests (situation dependent bias).

Theoretical Considerations of Rating Scales

Several rating scales were developed to assess the dementia syndrome (Israel *et al.*, 1986). They differ in their *technical aspects*, in their *content* and in the level of qualifications required by the *rater*.

Technical aspects. Scaling is a set of procedures used to assign numerical weights to individual items meant to reflect the severity of behavioural or cognitive impairments. From a technical point of view the following different types can be distinguished: nominal, ordinal, interval and ratio scales.

In nominal scales, numbers are assigned arbitrarily with no implication of an order in the category. Such scales may only be used for a classification; no statistical analysis can be carried out.

In ordinal scales, the classification implies a distinct numerical order within the categories. However, there is no assumption concerning the relative distance between the different values assigned to each category; non-parametric statistical methods such as a rank order correlation can be used.

In interval scales, individual values are also ordered along a vector, but a numerical difference in one region of the scale is assumed to be equivalent to the same numerical difference in another region of the scale. In consequence, addition and subtraction are permissible (but not multiplication or division). Statistical analysis such as the Pearson correlation factor analysis or discriminate analysis can be used with such scales.

Only in ratio scales are all types of statistical operation allowed.

Scales used to assess dementia syndrome are generally ordinal scales or sometimes nominal, but interval or ratio scales have almost never been used.

In addition, each variable is explored using items, and each item is scored using a scaling system which is usually different for each rating scale. This scoring can either be dichotomic (yes–no, present–absent), i.e. conditional, or can include some degrees (generally from 3 to 7). In this case a digit is used to indicate the possible scoring, but intervals between the digits are not equivalent so that these digits have no cardinal value but are codes that could just as well be indicated by ordered letters such as a, b, c, d.

Content. Many variables, such as behaviour, cognition, attention, memory, mood, affectivity and sociability, can be assessed. Some scales are unidimensional, assessing only one aspect, while others are more comprehensive and multidimensional, assessing several signs, symptoms or different functions. In addition, scales might be specific to dementia syndrome or non-specific; in the first case they are designed to assess several features of the dementia syndrome, and in the second case they describe status or behavioural characteristics which are relevant both to demented and non-demented persons.

The few recently developed scales designed specifically to assess Alzheimer's disease include the Dementia Rating Scale (Hughes *et al.*, 1982), the Global Deterioration Scale (GDS) (Reisberg *et al.*, 1982), the Mattis Dementia Scale (Mattis, 1976), the Alzheimer's Disease Assessment Scale (ADAS) (Mohs *et al.*, 1983) and the Extended Scale for Dementia (Lau *et al.*, 1988).

Table 1. Rating scales

Title	References	Country	Population	Rater	Number of items and grades	Time required	Training
Stockton Geriatric Rating Scale	Meer and Baker, 1966	USA	Inpatients	Medical staff, nurse	33 items; 3 grades	10 min	No
Dementia Scale	Blessed et al., 1968	UK	Whole population	Physician, psychologist, nurse's aide	11 items; 4 grades	35–40 min	Light
Instrumental Activities of Daily Living Scale	Lawton and Brody, 1969	USA	Whole population	Physician, psychologist, medical staff	14 items; 3–5 grades	30 min	Light
D. Test	Ferm, 1974	Finland	Outpatients	Physician, psychologist, nurse's staff	13 items; 6 grades	30 min	Light
Sandoz Clinical Assessment-Geriatric (SCAG)	Salzman, 1983 Shader et al., 1974 Georges et al., 1977	USA	Outpatients	Physician, psychologist, nurse	19 items; 7 grades	20 min	Mild
Ischaemia Score	Hachinski et al., 1975	Canada	Whole population	Physician	9 or 13 items; yes–no	5 min	Intensive
Performance Test of Activities of Daily Living	Kuriansky and Gurland, 1976	USA	Whole population	Physician, psychologist, nurse	16 items; 3 grades	20 min	Minimum
Check List Differentiating Pseudo-dementia from Dementia	Wells, 1979	USA	Inpatients	Physician	22 items	15 min	Neurological experience
Edinburgh Psychogeriatric Dependency Rating Scale	Wilkinson and Graham-White, 1980	UK	Whole population	Nurse	36 items; different grades from 2 to 6	5 min	Light

Scale	Reference	Country	Population	Rater	Structure	Time	Training
Clifton Assessment Procedures for Elderly (CAPE)	Pattie and Gilleard, 1981	UK	Whole population	Physician, psychologist, nurse's aide	Variable	15–25 min	Light
Rapid Disability Rating Scale	Linn and Linn, 1982	USA	Whole population	Nurse, informant, relatives	18 items; 4 grades	5 min	Light
GBS Scale	Gottfries et al., 1982	Sweden	Whole population	Physician, psychologist, nurse	26 items; 7 grades; 4 subscales	30 min	Light
Behavioural Mood Disturbance and Stress Scale	Greene et al., 1982	UK	Outpatients	Relatives	31 items; 5 grades	15–20 min	No
Rating Scale for Diagnosis of Alzheimer's and Pick's Disease	Gustafson and Nilsson, 1982	Sweden	Whole population	Physician	12 and 19 clinical signs; global score	5 min	Neurological experience
Clinical Dementia Rating Scale (CDR)	Berg et al., 1982 Hughes et al., 1982	USA	Whole population	Neurologist, psychiatrist, psychologist	6 items, 5 levels each	10 min	Brief
Global Deterioration Rating Scale (GDS)	Reisberg et al., 1982	USA	Whole population	Physician, psychologist	7 levels	15 min	Clinical experience
Functional Dementia Scale	Moore et al., 1983	USA	Whole population	Caregiver	20 items; 3 subscales	10 min	Light
Comprehensive Psychiatric Rating Scale (CPRS)	Bucht and Adolfsson, 1983	Sweden	Whole population	Psychiatrist, psychologist, physician	33 items; 7 grades	10 min	
Brief Cognitive Rating Scale (BCRS)	Reisberg et al., 1983a,b	USA	Whole population	Psychiatrist, psychologist	10 axes, 7 levels each	80 min	Necessary
Geriatric Evaluation by Relatives (GERRI)	Schwartz, 1983	USA	Whole population	Informant, relatives	49 items; 5 grades	15 min	No
Dementia Behaviour Scale	Haycox, 1984	USA	Inpatients	Medical staff, nurse etc.	8 categories; 7 levels	10 min	Light

(continued)

Table 1. (*continued*)

Title	References	Country	Population	Rater	Number of items and grades	Time required	Training
Alzheimer's Disease Assessment Scale (ADAS)	Rosen *et al.*, 1984	USA	Whole population	Physician, psychologist	21 items; 5 levels	10 min	In neuro-psychology
Clinical Rating Scale for Symptoms of Psychosis in Alzheimer's Disease (SPAD)	Reisberg and Ferris, 1985	USA	Whole population	Psychiatrist, psychologist	9 items; 3 levels	5 min	Necessary
FAST	Reisberg *et al.*, 1986	USA	Whole population	Psychiatrist, psychologist	16 items; 7 grades	5 min	Psychiatric experience
CAMDEX	Roth *et al.*, 1987	UK	Whole population	Physician, psychologist	Interview (psychologist necessary)		Psychiatric experience
New Hierarchic Dementia Scale	Cole and Dastoor, 1987	Canada	Whole population	Physician, psychologist, nurse's aide	20 subscales; 5–10 items per scale	30 min	Necessary
Cornell Scale for Depression in Dementia	Alexopoulos *et al.*, 1988	USA	Whole population	Physician, psychologist, nurse's staff	19 items; 3 grades	80 min	Necessary
Nurse's Observation Scale for Geriatric Patients (NOSGER)	Brunner and Spiegel, 1990, Spiegel *et al.*, 1991	Switzerland	Whole population	Nurse's staff, informant, relatives	30 items; 5 grades	30 min	Light

Raters. Evaluation of treatment responses generally covers several areas, assessed by different raters.

1. Symptomatic manifestations rated by the physician, based on signs and symptoms.
2. The cognitive functioning rated either through scales or mental status questionnaires (physician, nurse, psychologist).
3. The patient's performance on various tasks, as determined by neuropsychological tests, rated by the physician or by a psychologist.
4. Social adjustment and activities of daily living (ADL) rated by relatives, nurses, caregivers, social workers or lay persons, for example with the often used Katz index of ADL (Katz *et al.*, 1962) or the more complex instrumental activities of daily living (IADL) (Lawton and Brody, 1969; Loewenstein *et al.*, 1989).
5. The patient's reported experience based on self assessment (interview, questionnaire or rating scale) when such an evaluation is still possible.

For clinical assessment, raters might belong to different fields: medical doctors, psychologists, nurses or even non-professionals such as relatives, friends or social workers. The data gathered are collected either during the clinical examination or through permanent observation during a certain period by a caregiver responsible for the patient.

Classification and Review of Rating Scales

Rating scales are different from one another and could be classified according to a variety of criteria (Poitrenaud, 1984, 1987) (specific versus non-specific, depending on the rater, depending on the variable, etc.). We have chosen to review them according to their use, for two main reasons. Firstly, the selection of any scale is mainly determined by what goal its properties are able to fulfil. Secondly, when speaking about use we presume the prior demonstration of validity and reliability, as well as the existence of previous studies establishing its usefulness and interest. By doing so we attempt to incorporate the *goals* of the users, the *purpose* of the scale and the *aim* of measurement (Figure 1).

Tools developed for diagnostic purposes are not always identical to instruments designed for assessing severity or measuring changes. In the first and second case, one has to identify a condition and/or its intensity through signs and symptoms. A single measurement is needed based on cross-sectional studies. In the third case, changes in different chronological stages must be measured. Several assessments at different intervals are required and longitudinal studies are necessary. This is why we have distinguished scales which enable: (1) A contribution to *diagnosis*, (2) assessment of *severity*, and (3) measurement of *changes* (Table 2).

The *diagnostic* scales can be divided into:

a. Scales which differentiate patients with cognitive impairment, but who are not necessarily considered as demented, from those without impairment (Reisberg, 1986).
b. Scales which establish the presence of dementia, but without specificity to aetiology. If the aetiology could be specified, these scales are indicated by the sign (a) in the table.
c. Scales which facilitate the differential diagnosis between dementia and other psychiatric disorders (Gottlieb *et al.*, 1988; Johansen *et al.*, 1985). Such scales which differentiate between the two most frequent forms of dementia, i.e. 'degenerative' (senile dementia of the Alzheimer's type) and 'vascular', even if this differentiation

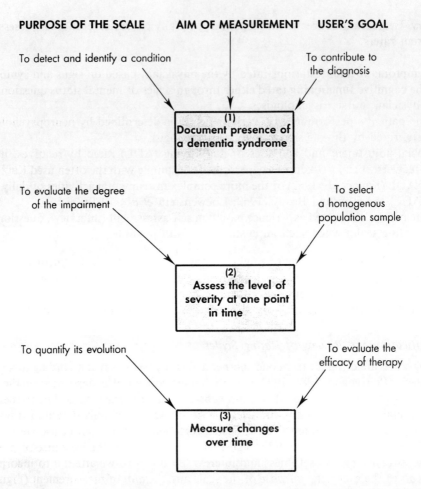

Figure 1. Rationale for the classification of rating scales according to their main objective

can only be reliably done at autopsy. Among the scales used for this purpose, some use only clinical items, rated by a neurologist (Hachinski *et al.*, 1975; Olafson *et al.*, 1989), and some also use the results of laboratory tests such as the computerized tomography (Loeb and Gandolfo, 1983).

The scales designed to assess *severity* may be distinguished by two subcategories:

1. Scales which specifically assess cognitive impairment in order to separate mild from severe cases (Storandt *et al.*, 1984).
2. Scales which are not specific to the dementia syndrome but indicate a level of dependency (Israel and Waintraub, 1986).

Scales which are measuring *changes* differ from those measuring severity by the fact that longitudinal studies contribute to the establishment of their validity (Katzman *et al.*, 1988; Lolk *et al.*, 1988; Stern *et al.*, 1987). This type of scale may be used for assessing drug effects.

It is interesting to observe that it is only since 1982 that instruments have been

Table 2. Classification of rating scales according to the use

Use 1	Use 2	Use 3	Reference	Specificity	Validation studies
	✓		Meer and Baker, 1966*	NS	v3, v4, r1, r2
c			Blessed et al., 1968	S	v4, r1, r2
	✓		Lawton and Brody, 1969*	NS	v3, v4, r1, r2
	✓		Ferm, 1974*	S	v4, v5, r1, r2, r3
	✓	✓	Shader et al., 1974*	NS	v2, r1, r4, s1, s2
c			Hachinski et al., 1975	S (a)	v3, v4
a, b	✓		Kuriansky and Gurland, 1976*	NS	v1, v2, v3, r1
c			Wells, 1979	S	v3, v4, v5, r2
c	✓	✓	Pattie and Gilleard, 1981*	NS	v2, v3, r2
	✓		Linn and Linn, 1982*	NS	v2, v3, v4, v5, r1, r2, s2
b	✓	✓	Gottfries et al., 1982*	S	r1
	✓		Greene et al., 1982	S	v2, r2
c			Gustafson and Nilsson, 1982	S (a)	v4, r3
	✓		Hughes et al., 1982	S	v3, v5, r1
	✓		Reisberg et al., 1982	S	v3, v4, r1
	✓		Moore et al., 1983	S	v2, v3, r1, r2, r3
	✓	✓	Bucht and Adolfsson, 1983	S	v2, r1, r3, r4
	✓		Cole et al., 1983	S	v3, r1, r2
a,b	✓		Reisberg et al., 1983a,b	S	v3, v4
	✓	✓	Schwartz, 1983	S	v3, r1, r3, s1
	✓		Haycox, 1984	S	v3, v4, r1, r2
	✓	✓	Rosen et al.,1984	S	v3, v4, r1, r2
b, c			Reisberg and Ferris, 1985	S	v4
b, c	✓		Reisberg et al., 1986	S	v3
a, b, c			Roth et al., 1987*	S	v3, r1
c	✓	✓	Alexopoulos et al., 1988	S	v3, r1, r3, s1
	✓	✓	Spiegel et al., 1991	S	v2, v3, v4, r1, r2, s1, s2

Note: Use 1 = contributes to the differential diagnosis between (a) patients cognitively impaired from those who are not; (b) demented from non-demented patients; and (c) dementia and other psychiatric disorders.
Use 2 = assesses severity.
Use 3 = measures changes.
  * = multidimensional.
  NS = non-specific but used for demented patients;
    S = specifically designed for demented patients; (a) = determines aetiology.
Validity: v1 = content; v2 = construct; v3 = concurrent; v4 = external; v5 = predictive.
Reliability: r1 = inter-rater; r2 = test-retest; r3 = internal consistency; r4 = cross-validation.
Sensitivity: s1 = inter-individual; s2 = intra-individual.

specifically designed for demented patients. Before 1982 tools used to assess the severity of the dementia syndrome were either tests (Table 3) or mental status questionnaires, both serving general purposes. In the latter case, the answers to different questions were expressed through a global rating. A group of questionnaires is listed in Table 4. The main advantage of such clinical assessments was that no special training was required for the rater. Threshold values indicated whether cognition was significantly impaired or not. Nevertheless, such scores had a low *specificity*, depending very closely on the cultural level. In this sense questionnaires could neither contribute to a diagnosis nor assess changes. Nevertheless, if mental status questionnaires are not as sensitive to changes as neuropsychological tests, they still might differentiate efficiently normals from pathological patients, and thus be used for the inclusion of patients in studies in order to select a homogeneous population.

Table 3. Tests

Title	Reference	Country	Form	Population	Rater	No. of items	Time required	Training	Applications
Three Dimensional Praxis Test	Benton, 1962	USA	Non-verbal test	Whole population	Psychologist	3 subtests	16 min	Learning the diagnosis	Clinical practice
Set Test	Isaacs and Akhtar, 1972	UK	Psychometric test	Whole population	Psychologist, physician care staff	4 subtests	5 min	Minimum	Clinical practice, screening of dementia
Visual Retention Test	Benton, 1974	USA	Psychometric test	Whole population	Psychologist	10 items	5 min	Intensive	Clinical practice, diagnosis, research
Mini-Mental State Examination	Folstein et al., 1975	USA	Psychometric test	Whole population	Physician, psychologist, nurse's aide	11 subtests	10 min	Light	Clinical practice, screening of functional disorders, diagnosis, prognosis
Stimulus Recognition Test	Brink et al., 1979	USA	Psychometric test	Whole population	Psychologist	10 items	12 min	To get familiar with the technique	Clinical practice, diagnosis, research
Extended Scale for Dementia	Hersch, 1979	Canada	Psychometric test	Whole population	Psychologist	23 subtests	60 min	Light	Clinical practice, research, drug trials, diagnosis
Kendrick Battery for Detection of Dementia	Kendrick et al., 1979	UK	Psychometric test	Whole population	Physician, psychologist, nurse's aide, social worker	2 subtests	15 min	½ day regular repeating	Clinical practice, diagnosis, drug trials, research, screening for dementia
Bilan d'évaluation du Syndrome Démentiel	Israel et al., 1979	France	Questionnaire tests	Whole population	Psychologist, physician, occupational therapist	Clinical approach	25 min	Necessary	Clinical practice, care planning

Source: Israel et al. (1984).

Table 4. Questionnaires

Title	Reference	Country	Population	Rater	No. of items	Time required	Training	Applications
Mental Test Score	Hodkinson, 1972	UK	Inpatients	Psychologist, physician, nurse's aide	10 questions	3 min	No	Clinical, screening
Dementia Screening Scale	Hasegawa, 1974	Japan	Whole population	Physician, psychologist	11 questions	15 min	No	Diagnosis, research, epidemiological studies
Abbreviated Mental Test	Qureshi and Hodkinson, 1974	UK	Inpatients	Physician, psychologist, nurse's aide	10 items	3 min	No	Clinical practice, diagnosis
Short Portable Mental Status Questionnaire	Pfeiffer, 1975	USA	Whole population	Physician, psychologist, nurse's aide, social worker	10 questions	2 min	No	Functional diagnosis, prognosis, drug trials, surveys
Geriatric Mental State Schedule	Copeland et al., 1976	UK	Whole population	Physician, psychologist, nurse, social worker	600 items	30–40 min	Intensive	Research, diagnosis, epidemiological studies prognosis
Philadelphia Mental Status Questionnaire	Fishback, 1977	USA	Whole population	Physician, nurse, nurse's aide	35 items	10 min	No	Clinical diagnosis, organicity
Cognitive Capacity Screening	Jacobs et al., 1977	USA	Whole population	Physician, psychologist, professionals	30 items	5 min	To get familiar with the technique	Clinical functional diagnosis
Confusion Assessment Schedule	Slater and Lipman, 1977	UK	Whole population	Non-qualified	21 items	10 min	No	Clinical functional diagnosis
Modified Tooting Bec Questionnaire	Denham and Jeffreys, 1978	UK	Inpatients	Psychologist, physician, nurse's aide	16 items	3 min	No	Clinical prognosis, care planning
Orientation Scale for Geriatric Patients	Berg and Svensson, 1980	Sweden	Inpatients	Physician, psychologist, nurse's aide, social worker	10 questions	5 min	No	Clinical, diagnosis, research, drug trials, prognosis

Neuropsychological Tests

Neuropsychological tests occupy an important role in clinical assessment because they are more objective than interview methods, and more sensitive to changes in a pathological condition than conventional psychometry. In general they can be used with demented patients as well as with those with mild cognitive impairments.

While the clinical approach is exclusively qualitative, the neuropsychological approach refers simultaneously to tests and to clinical judgment. In this sense this approach differs also from traditional psychometry in which results are based and expressed exclusively on quantitative performance scores.

Unfortunately, they are not appropriate for all patients with dementia, and some severely demented patients cannot perform even the simplest recognition tasks.

Historically there have been two main neuropsychological traditions: European and American. In Europe, the Soviet tradition was developed by A. R. Luria (1980), who was the first to stress the importance of observation of the patient's behaviour when performing different tasks. Since 1960 The School of Geneva under the influence of J. de Ajuriaguerra also developed a neuropsychological approach (Bel-Air School). The American tradition is represented by H. Reitan (1979), who emphasized the use of a standardized test battery designed to reflect the full range of mental impairments associated with brain lesions. The evaluation of cognitive dysfunctions is made on the basis of comparisons with a normal reference group.

Conditions Required

Such tests require certain conditions in their design. They need to be simple, especially if demented patients are to be examined, and sensitive enough to assess changes. One must be careful to avoid floor or ceiling effects. They also require certain validity conditions, particularly face validity and inter-rater reliability. The best neuropsychological tests are those which fulfil the following requirements (Henderson and Huppert, 1984):

1. The test should be culture-free, or at least appropriate for different languages and cultures. If not, norms for each country are required.
2. It should correlate well with universally accepted criteria, and relate closely to the behavioural problems for which a trial treatment has been undertaken.
3. Several – at least four or five – parallel forms should be available, in order to avoid a training effect when repeating the test.

To achieve a better interpretation of the differential rates of decline observed, another requirement for measuring changes appears extremely important: standards for different rates of decline in different functions, and a clear identification of the component of a function should be *previously* available.

Applications

Neuropsychological tests currently used to assess drug effects on cognitive functions in the elderly were reviewed by Lezak in 1983, Grant and Adams in 1986 and more recently by Flicker in 1988. For each of the tests reviewed, indications are given concerning sensitivity to the cognitive loss associated with ageing and with dementia, as well as construct, content and face validity, broad difficulty range, duration, repeatability, widespread use and ease of computerization, sensitivity to pharmacological agents and comparison with the animal models.

One of the most comprehensive and most used instruments available at present is the ADAS designed by Rosen *et al.* (1984). The ADAS was developed to assess the major cognitive, behavioural and affective dysfunctions characteristic of Alzheimer's disease (Schwarb *et al.*, 1988). None of the other scales already mentioned, except the Brief Cognitive Rating Scale (BCRS) which correlates well with psychometric batteries (Lolk *et al.*, 1988), rates these three primary areas. Selection of the original 40 items was based on clinical observations of memory dysfunction, disorientation, behavioural and affective disturbances and on experimental investigations of various components of language, memory and praxis. The final form of the scale comprises 21 items with significant inter-rater reliability (ranging from 0.659 to 1) and significant test–retest reliability of 1-month interval between test sessions, ranging from 0.514 to 1 for patients with Alzheimer's disease. The cognitive subscale, composed of items evaluating memory, language and praxis functions, had an inter-rater reliability of 0.989 and a test–retest reliability of 0.915 (excluding the two memory tests). The non-cognitive behaviour subscale, whose items evaluate components of depression, concentration, cooperation, psychotic disturbances and motor activity, had an inter-rater reliability of 0.947 and a test–retest reliability of 0.588. For the total score, inter-rater reliability was 0.986 and test–retest reliability was 0.838.

Concurrent validity of the ADAS was demonstrated by the significant correlations among the subscales and total scores with scores on the Memory Information Test (Blessed *et al.*, 1968), for which r ranged from -0.419 to 0.775 and the Dementia Rating Scale, with r ranging from 0.455 to 0.642. Scores on these two instruments correlated significantly with measures of the histopathological changes characteristic of Alzheimer's disease. Construct validity was evidenced by the significant correlations between the two subscales ($r = 0.588$) and between the total score and cognitive ($r = 0.824$) and non-cognitive subscales ($r = 0.666$).

The total ADAS scale therefore indicates impairments in several combined areas, and the scale appears significantly sensitive to overall decline, possibly more than the Blessed Scale (Blessed *et al.*, 1968), Katzman's (Katzman *et al.*, 1983) or the Mini-Mental State Examination (MMSE) (Folstein *et al.*, 1975).

A Neuropsychological Test Battery was proposed by the CERAD (Consortium to Establish a Registry for Alzheimer's Disease) (Morris *et al.*, 1988). It includes seven frequently used measures of memory, language, praxis:

1. Verbal fluency (Isaacs and Akthar, 1972).
2. Modified Boston Memory Test (Kaplan *et al.*, 1978).
3. MMSE (Folstein *et al.*, 1975).
4. Word list memory.
5. Constructional praxis (Rosen *et al.*, 1981).
6. Word list recall.
7. Word list recognition.

Table 5. Qualitative assessment of severity of dementia syndrome through functional levels of organization (Geneva School)

SPEECH	PRAXIS				GNOSIS			
	I Constructive	II Ideomotor	III Ideation	IV Dressing	I Visual	II Auditory	III Somatognosis	IV Stereognosis
1) Inability to find the right word	Onset of constructual graphic apraxia in the form of impaired ability to reproduce perspective (draws cube but base is missing)	Preserved	Preserved	Preserved	Difficulties in recognizing pictures of objects – at first if they are incomplete, blurred or superimposed Poppelreuter	Preserved	Digital auto-topoagnosia (when the examiner touches the finger of one hand the patient locates this in the other hand)	Preserved
2) Paraphrasias	Loss of perspective in graphic praxic constructural reproduction	Difficulties in copying complicated hand gestures	Preserved	Preserved	More severe difficulties	Preserved	Constant digital auto-topoagnosia	Preserved

3) Substitution of words	Drawing cubes in two faces, then in one face	Difficulties in copying conventional symbolic gestures (military salute, crossing himself, etc.)	Preserved	Difficulties with dressing Trouble with putting on pieces of clothing on proper parts of body	Unable to identify drawing of objects, but correct identification of objects is still possible	Preserved	Difficulties in somatognosis	Bilateral stereognosis. Difficulties in recognizing objects by feeling with fingers
4) Distorted words – Mistakes made in forming individual words	Jumbling of parts of the model in drawing 'Closing in'	Ideomotor apraxia	Praxis difficulties in ideation: with object, without object, imitating when shown how How one handles an iron, a coffee mill. If unable to demonstrate, he has to do it with right object	Puts on clothes in an incorrect order	Is able to classify colours	Preserved	Body auto-topoagnosia	Loss of normal reactions to pain
				Undressing impossible	Unable to classify		Inability to localize pain	

Reproduced with permission of the authors.

Whether such batteries will be sensitive enough to measure changes induced by an experimental treatment remains to be determined, even if most if not all of these subtests have been included in one or another drug trial in the past (Orgogozo and Israel, 1990.

Longitudinal Studies

A few studies of the changes on neuropsychological tests and scales in patients with dementia can serve as illustrative examples of how to estimate the potential sensitivity of these instruments. Barclay *et al.* (1985) compared the 5-year outcome of 199 patients with Alzheimer's disease, 69 with vascular dementia and 43 with so-called 'mixed' dementia (with clinical features of both primary and vascular dementia). Measurements using the MMSE (Folstein *et al.*, 1975), Haycox Scale (Haycox, 1984) and BDRS (Brief Dementia Rating Scale) (Blessed *et al.*, 1968), among other things, showed with all these instruments a consistent decline over time, with no significant differences between the groups. This may mean either that there is truly no difference in cognitive and behavioural outcome between the three diagnostic categories, or that the instruments are not sensitive enough to show a difference, since there was a significant difference in mortality, a reliable indicator of a worse outcome (Go *et al.*, 1978), in the vascular dementia group.

Stern *et al.* (1987) followed 65 patients with probable Alzheimer's disease for at least 6 months, with an extended version of the MMSE as the cognitive end-point, and the BDRS (non-cognitive part of the Blessed Scale) as the functional end-point. They found that cognitive deterioration was slightly more rapid than functional decline, which again might be a real fact, but might just as well be a consequence of a relative lack of sensitivity of the BDRS to changes in functional status. It should also be kept in mind that daily activities are often routinized in elderly people, and that assistance from the family and caregivers often distorts the measurement of the real capacities of the patient.

Katzman *et al.* (1988) reviewed four longitudinal studies with the Blessed IMC (Information, Memory, Concentration) test (Blessed *et al.*, 1968) in senile dementia. The mean annual rate of increase in the IMC scores was 4.4 errors (on a maximum possible of 33) per year, independently of education and of age, but was quite variable among individuals, with a ceiling effect for those most impaired. It was concluded, rightly in our opinion, that this measured rate of worsening (+ 4.4 per year) and its variance (SD ± 3.6, SEM ± 0.3) can be used as a basis for designing drug trials in Alzheimer's disease.

Lolk *et al.* (1988) did a short-term study in 57 patients with mild to moderate dementia of the primary or vascular type using the Sandoz Clinical Assessment-Geriatric Scale (SCAG) (Shader *et al.*, 1974) and the BCRS (Reisberg *et al.*, 1983a). Changes were assessed by comparing the differences between the end and the beginning of the follow-up. They found a slight increase in the SCAG scores, possibly due to a training effect, and a stability of the BCRS over time, the latter being well correlated in individual cases with a battery of psychometric tests, which was not the case with the SCAG. From these results the authors question the validity of the SCAG as an outcome measure of drug effects in trials on demented patients.

Berg *et al.* (1988) followed 43 patients with senile dementia of the Alzheimer type, in comparison to 58 age-matched controls, over 5 years. Among a series of outcome measures, the Clinical Dementia Rating Scale (CDR) (Hughes *et al.*, 1982) was found to be the most sensitive to deterioration of cognitive function in the demented patients, while the controls were stable with all the instruments. The conclusion was that the different measures are complementary, but that the two components of the Blessed Scale (Blessed *et al.*, 1968) (cognitive and non-cognitive) are less sensitive to change than the CDR, the 'sum of boxes' taken from this scale being possibly the best measure of deterioration in demented patients.

Lastly, Forette *et al.* (1989) correlated changes in the MMSE (Folstein *et al.*, 1975) and the factors of the SCAG (Shader *et al.*, 1974) in 55 patients with senile dementia of the Alzheimer type followed-up for 1 year. The mean decline in MMSE was 3.3 (from 16.7 ± 3.7 to 13.3 ± 7.4), while only two factors of the SCAG changed significantly: factor II (cognitive functioning) and factor III (apathy), by $+2.7$ and $+3.0$, respectively. So even if the MMSE was not designed to measure changes in cognitive function, it seems at least as good as the known sensitive factors of the SCAG to measure changes over time in demented patients. Whether this will also be true for measuring drug effects remains to be demonstrated in clinical trials.

Discussion

When summarizing the main problems linked with clinical assessment instruments and neuropsychological tests, we have to underline the great variability of the instruments reviewed, as well as the differences arising from examining demented patients compared with normals or patients with psychiatric disorders (Gottlieb *et al.*, 1988).

Variability

In particular we have noticed the variety of purposes, the diversity of scoring systems, the heterogeneity of population samples, the multiplicity of variables and the diversity of raters. In fact there is no 'ready to wear' instrument which could fulfil all purposes. Besides, at this point in time, there is no consensus that any single instrument can be considered to be adequately sensitive to mild degrees of impairment in various age groups across a broad range of cultures and educational levels. The two main reasons for this appear to be firstly the discrepancies in the current theoretical understanding of pathological decline in the elderly and, secondly, some methodological inadequacies of instrument design, in particular the content of the material used is sometimes too abstract and unrelated to the concrete situation of daily life.

Considering the first point, the debate continues as to whether dementia can be considered as a separate disease entity, distinct from an accelerated normal ageing process. In 1985, Berg summarized the argument against the conceptualization of dementia as an accentuated form of normal ageing, while in the field of neuro-psychometry many authors demonstrated evidence of decline in cognitive functions in the demented which is not observed in normal ageing. The existence of fundamental quantitative as well as qualitative differences is almost generally accepted, but the threshold of what can be called 'Age-associated impairment' is still uncertain.

At the moment there is also little agreement about the criteria for improvement, which probably vary depending on whether the treatment is intended to satisfy the patient, the family, the physician or the society. Nevertheless, a treatment efficacy may be proven on different assessment levels, and trends should be in the same direction for different raters using different tools. This is a necessary but not a sufficient condition. Effects should also be evidenced on parameters that are important for the patient and provide him with a true therapeutic benefit (clinically relevant versus irrelevant effects).

Considering the patients, who are the most important and the central target point of any trial, we must stress that they are essentially characterized by a tremendous variability. The variability from one patient to another can often conceal the effect of the treatment. Care should therefore be taken to detect responsive subjects in order to investigate their fluctuations and to analyse their particular features and characteristics. It is in this sense that neuropsychological tests need to be used in conjunction with clinical assessment, and this is why the use of the ADAS appears adequate, although further studies are needed.

A difference in response to drugs could be observed not only between different pathological conditions but also among different subjects belonging to the same category and sometimes only because of the interaction of age and cultural level.

A distinction should be made especially between healthy subjects with age-associated cognitive impairment and patients with the pathological conditions of dementia. To mix them up in a same drug trial makes analysis very confusing, and even destructive to the conclusions. Changes may not always be measured through the same instrument for patients with mild cognitive impairments and those with dementia who are at the extreme of a normal distribution of variables. A standardized clinical assessment could be applied to these different samples of the population, and this is another reason for which the ADAS scale is interesting as it may be appropriate to both mild and moderately demented as well as normal aged subjects.

Selection of Instruments

The selection of an instrument must never be an automatic routine (Israel and Waintraub, 1983). It should in fact be the last step of a preliminary thorough thinking in order to define the most adequate outcome criteria. *Evaluation is not an end-point in itself, but only a way of reaching a definite target*. In consequence, the selection of instruments should be done according to the main purpose of the research.

For instance, if one wants to facilitate diagnosis for screening cases, the choice of an adequate instrument will depend on preliminary studies establishing significant differences between groups of demented and non-demented patients. *In no case could a scale replace a diagnosis*. It can only facilitate the probability to establish it, and one must not forget that the validity of a scale had to be established first by considering the diagnosis as a reference.

The majority of scales aim to assess behavioural abnormalities which are the consequence of the dementia syndrome, and provide no information on aetiology, except the specially designed scales such as the Hachinski *et al.* (1975), Portera-Sanchez *et al.* (1982) and Gustafson (1982, 1985) scales. If the purpose of the user is only to select a group of homogeneous patients, he must choose an instrument assessing the severity of the condition (CDR, GDS or BCRS) or setting a minimal threshold like the MMSE (Bleecker *et al.*, 1988).

While there is no theoretical objection to choosing the same instrument for selecting patients and measuring changes, in practice it is better to use different tools. In fact, the most sensitive scales for selecting patients are not the most sensitive to drug-induced changes, because diagnostic tools, for which intra-class stability is predominant, are not good tools for measuring changes (Berg *et al.*, 1988).

Clinical Relevance and Use as Outcome Criteria

We should bear in mind that psychometric tools only measure differences, and are *neither necessarily valid as outcome criteria nor correspond to clinically relevant changes*.

Considering the aims of a trial, do we have in mind to improve a condition, to maintain it or to slow down its deterioration? Perhaps a combination of these different targets at different levels of assessment will be the best choice, but how to choose? The answer to these questions is important in order to determine an agreement for some specific outcome criteria in relation to the purpose of the trial and to the therapeutic benefit expected. For instance, if a person is progressively losing her autonomy because of cognitive impairment or other associated factors, intervention methods, and in particular drug therapy, may reinforce and develop compensatory mechanisms which tend to maintain the balance by increasing substitution strategies and resistance to stress. So when the purpose is to maintain a function, the outcome measures should focus on coping and compensatory mechanisms, and not only on impairments. But if the purpose of a drug is to enhance one or several specific cognitive functions such as attention, perception or memory, the outcome measures should focus on these specific activities.

Thus, the first step in developing treatment for cognitive impairments should be a clear definition of the specific clinical entities for which therapy is to be undertaken. Do we intend to restore or improve impaired functions or to enhance preserved ones? In fact, we are actually dealing with fundamental but still not well-defined criteria of clinically relevant changes. And in spite of this, we have to define some precise measurement of objective changes. It is quite a challenge.

Here a dilemma has to be faced. A change in a condition can be studied only if we are able to identify it reliably. However, we do not know in advance which features will be distinctive or specific. More longitudinal studies are needed for that. In consequence the criteria chosen are only tentative at this stage (Henderson and Huppert, 1984). We should be quite clear about this. At the present empirical stage, it is our interpretation of the observed effects of a treatment which allows us to refine our knowledge of dementing disorders, and not the contrary. This is why we believe it is premature to claim that an instrument is sufficiently sensitive to measure changes indicating improvement, as long as recognized criteria have not been established first. In this sense, before deciding on the value of an instrument, it is necessary to first define the relevant clinical criteria for improvement or deterioration, and only then attempt to establish the necessary norms which will serve as a reference for the assessors.

References

Alexopoulos, G. S., Abraham, R. C., Young, R. C. *et al.* (1988) Cornell scale for depression in dementia. *Biol. Psychiatry*, **23**, 271–84.

Barclay, L. L., Zemcov, A., Blass, J. P. and Sansone, J. (1985) Survival in Alzheimer's disease and vascular dementia. *Neurology*, **35**, 834–40.

Bel-Air School (1984) Schedules of Bel-Air. In: Israel, L. *et al.* (eds) *Source Book of Geriatric Assessment*, p. 339. Basel: Karger.

Benton, A. L. and Fogel, M. L. (1962) Three Dimensional Praxis Test: A clinical test. *Arch. Neurol.*, **7**, 347–54.

Benton, A. L. (1974) *Revised Visual Retention Test: Clinical and Experimental Application*, 4th edn. New York: The Psychological Corporation.

Berg, L. (1985) Does Alzheimer's disease represent an exaggeration of normal aging? *Arch. Neurol.*, **42**, 737–9.

Berg, S. and Svensson, T. (1980) An orientation scale for geriatric patients. *Age Ageing*, **9**, 215–9.

Berg, L., Hughes, C. P., Coben, L. A. *et al.* (1982) Mild senile dementia of Alzheimer type: research diagnostic criteria, recruitment, and description of a study population. *J. Neurol. Neurosurg. Psychiatry*, **45**, 962–8.

Berg, L., Miller, J. P., Storandt, M., Duchek, J., Morris, J. C., Rubin, E. H., Burke, W. J. and Coben, L. A. (1988) Mild senile dementia of the Alzheimer type: 2. Longitudinal assessment. *Ann. Neurol.*, **23**, 477–84.

Bergin, A. E. and Lambert, M. J. (1978) The evaluation of therapeutic outcomes. In: Garfield, S. L. and Baergin, A. E. (eds) *Handbook of Psychotherapy and Behavior Changes: An Empirical Analysis*, 2nd edn. New York: Wiley.

Bleecker, M. L., Bolla-Wilson, K., Kawas, C. and Agnew, J. (1988) Age-specific norms for the Mini-Mental State Exam. *Neurology*, **38**, 1565–8.

Blessed, G., Tomlinson, B. E. and Roth, M. (1968) The association between quantitative measures of dementia and senile change in the cerebral grey matter of elderly subjects. *Br. J. Psychiatry*, **114**, 797–811.

Brink, T. L. *et al.* (1979) Senile confusion: assessment with a new stimulus recognition test. *J. Am. Geriatr. Soc.*, **27**(3), 126–9.

Brunner, C. and Spiegel, R. (1990) Eine Validierungsstudie mit der NOSGER (Nurses' Observation Scale for Geriatric Patients), einem neuen Beurtellungsinstrument für die Psychogeriatrie. *Z. Klin. Psychol.*, **19**, 211–19.

Bucht, G. and Adolfsson, R. (1983) The comprehensive psychopathological rating scale in patients with dementia of Alzheimer type and multi-infarct dementia. *Acta Psychiatr. Scand.*, **68**(4), 263–70.

Cole, M. G. and Dastoor, D. (1987) A new hierarchic approach to the measurement of dementia. *Psychosomatics*, **28**(6), 298–304.

Cole, M. G., Dastoor, D. P. and Koszycki, D. (1983) The hierarchic dementia scale. *J. Clin. Exp. Gerontol.*, **5**(3), 219–34.

Copeland, J. R. M. *et al.* (1976) A semi-structured clinical interview for the assessment of diagnosis and mental state in the elderly: the geriatric mental state schedule. *Psychol. Med.*, **6**, 439–59.

Crook, T., Ferris, S. and Bartus, R. (1983) *Assessment in Geriatric Psychopharmacology*. New Canaan, Connecticut: Mark Powley Associates.

Denham, M. J. and Jeffreys, P. M. (1978) Routine mental testing in the elderly. *Medicine*, **1**, 1.

Ferm, L. (1974) Behavioural activities in demented geriatric patients: study based on evaluations made by nursing staff members and on patients' scores on a simple psychometric test. *Gerontol. Clin.*, **16**, 185–94.

Fishback, D. B. (1977) Mental status questionnaire for organic brain syndrome with a new visual counting test. *J. Am. Geriatr. Soc.*, **25**(4), 167–70.

Flicker, C. (1988) Neuropsychological evaluation of treatment effects in the elderly: a critique of tests in current use. *Psychopharmacol. Bull.*, **24**(4), 535–56.

Folstein, M. E., Folstein, S. E. and McHugh, P. R. (1975) Mini-Mental State: a practical method for grading the cognitive state of patients for the clinician. *J. Psychiatr. Res.*, **12**, 189–98.

Forette, F., Henry, J. F., Orgogozo, J. M., Dartigues, J. F., Pere, J. J., Hugonot, L., Israel, L., Loria, Y., Goulley, F., Lallemand, A. and Boller, F. (1989) Reliability of clinical criteria for the diagnosis of dementia. A longitudinal multicenter study. *Arch. Neurol.*, **46**, 646–8.

Georges, D., Lallemand, A., Coustenoble, J. *et al.* (1977) Validation par l'analyse factorielle d'une échelle d'évaluation clinique des troubles de la sénescence cérébrale. Application à l'essai thérapeutique. *Thérapie*, **32**, 173–80.

Go, R. C. P., Todorov, A. B., Elston, R. C. and Constantidinis, J. (1978) The malignancy of dementia. *Ann. Neurol.*, **3**, 559–61.

Gottfries, C. G., Brane, G. and Steen, G. (1982) A new rating scale for dementia syndromes. *Gerontology*, **28**(2, suppl.), 20–31.

Gottlieb, G. L., Gur, R. E. and Gur, R. C. (1988) Reliability of psychiatric scales in patients with dementia of the Alzheimer type. *Am. J. Psychiatry* **145**, 857–60.

Grant, I. and Adams, K. M. (1986) *Neuropsychological Assessment of Neuropsychiatric Disorders*. New York: Oxford University Press.

Greene, J. G., Smith, R., Gardiner, M., *et al.* (1982) Measuring behavioural disturbance of elderly demented patients in the community and its effects on relatives: a factor analytic study. *Age Ageing*, **11**, 121–6.

Guelfi, J. D. (1986) Echelles d'évaluation des états démentiels. In: *Les Thérapeutiques de la Démence*, pp. 149–59. Paris: Maloine.

Gustafson, L. (1985) Differential diagnosis with special reference to treatable dementia and pseudodementia conditions. *Dan. Med. Bull.*, **32**(1, suppl.), 55–60.

Gustafson, L. and Nilsson, L. (1982) Differential diagnosis of presenile dementia on clinical grounds. *Acta Psychiatr. Scand.*, **65**, 194–209.

Hachinski, V. C., Iliff, L. D., Zilhka, E. *et al.* (1975) Cerebral blood flow in dementia. *Arch. Neurol.*, **32**, 632–7.

Hasegawa, K. (1974) *Validity and Reliability of Rating Scales for Psychogeriatric Assessment. The Study on Hasegawa's Dementia Scale.* Kawasaki: St Marianna University, Department of Psychiatry.

Haycox, J. A. (1984) A simple, reliable clinical behavioral scale for assessing demented patients. *J. Clin. Psychiatry*, **45**, 23–4.

Henderson, A. S. and Huppert, F. A. (1984) The problem of mild dementia. *Psychol. Med.*, **14**, 5–11.

Hersch, E. L. (1979) Development and application of the extended scale for dementia. *J. Am. Geriatr. Soc.*, **27**(8), 348–54.

Hodkinson, H. M. (1972) Evaluation of a mental test score for assessment of mental impairment in the elderly. *Age Ageing*, **1**, 233–8.

Hughes, C. P., Berg, L., Danziger, W. *et al.* (1982) A new clinical scale for the staging of dementia. *Br. J. Psychiatry*, **140**, 566–72.

Isaacs, B. and Akhtar, A. J. (1972) The set test: a rapid test of mental function in old people. *Age Ageing*, **1**, 222–6.

Israel, L. and Waintraub, L. (1983) Méthodes d'évaluations psychométriques en gériatrie. Le choix d'un instrument et ses critères de fiabilité. *Presse Méd.*, **12**(48), 3124–8.

Israel, L. and Waintraub, L. (1986) Autonomie ou capacité fonctionnelle? Revue critique de quelques échelles actuellement utilisées en gériatrie pour l'évaluation des activités de la vie quotidienne. *Psychol. Medicale*, **18**(14), 2225–31.

Israel, L. *et al.* (1979) Bilans d'évaluation des effets d'une rééducation psychomotrice sur des sujets atteints de démence. *Encéphale*, **V**, 269–84.

Israel, L., Kozarevic, D. and Sartorius, N. (1984) *Source Book of Geriatric Assessment*, Vols 1 and 2. Basel: Karger.

Israel, L., Waintraub, L. and Fillenbaum, G. G. (1986) Assessing the dementia(s) in clinical practice and population surveys: review of the literature since 1965. In: Bès, A. *et al.* (eds) *Senile Dementias: Early Detection*, pp. 592–603. London: John Libbey Eurotext.

Jacobs, J. W. *et al.* (1977) Screening for organic mental syndrome in the medically ill. *Ann. Intern. Med.*, **86**, 40–6.

Johansen, A. M., Gustafson, L. and Risberg, J. (1985) Psychological evaluation in dementia and depression. *Dan. Med. Bull.*, **32**(1, suppl.), 60–2.

Kaplan, N. E., Goodglass, H. and Weintraub, S. (1978) The Boston Naming Test. Boston: VA Medical Center.

Katz, S., Moskowitz, A. B., Jackson, B. A. *et al.* (1962) Studies of illness in the aged, the index of ADL: a standardized measure of biological and psychological function. JAMA, **185**, 914–9.

Katzman, R., Brown, T., Fuld, P. A., Peck, A., Schechter, R. and Schimmel, H. (1983) Validation of a short orientation-memory-concentration test of cognitive impairment. *Am. J. Psychiatry*, **140**(6), 734–9.

Katzman, R., Brown, T., Thal, L. J., Fuld, P. A., Aronson, M., Butters, N., Klauber, M. R., Wiederholt, W., Pay, M., Renbing, X., Ooi, W. I., Hofstetter, R. and Terry, R. D. (1988) Comparison of rate of annual change of mental status score in four independent studies of patients with Alzheimer's disease. *Ann. Neurol.*, **24**, 453–4.

Kendrick, D. C. *et al.* (1979) The revised Kendrick battery: clinical studies. *Br. J. Soc. Clin. Psychol.*, **18**, 329–40.

Kuriansky, J. and Gurland, B. (1976) The performance test of activities of daily living. *Int. J. Aging Hum. Dev.*, **7**(4), 343–52.

Lau, C., Wands, K., Merskey, H., Boniferro, M., Carriere, L., Fox, H. and Hachinski, V. (1988) Sensitivity and specificity of the extended scale for dementia. *Arch. Neurol.*, **45**, 849–53.

Lawton, M. P. and Brody, E. M. (1969) Assessment of older people: self maintaining and instrumental activities of daily living. *Gerontologist*, **9**, 179–86.

Lezak, M. D. (1983) *Neuropsychological Assessment*, 2nd edn. New York: Oxford University Press.

Linn, M. W. and Linn, B. S. (1982) The rapid disability scale-2. *J. Am. Geriatr. Soc.*, **30**(6), 378–82.

Loeb, C. and Gandolfo, C. (1983) Diagnostic evaluation of degenerative and vascular dementia. *Stroke*, **14**, 399–401.

Loewenstein, D. A. *et al.* (1989) A new scale for the assessment of functional status in Alzheimer's disease and related disorders. *J. Gerontol.*, **44**, P114–21.

Lolk, A., Nielsen, H. and Kragh-Sorensen, P. (1988) Procedures in evaluating dementia – a study of conjoint application of two rating scales (SCAG and BCRS) and psychometric tests. *Acta Psychiatr. Scand.*, **78**, 592–8.

Luria, A. R. (1980) *Higher Cortical Functions in Man*. New York: Basic Books.

MacDowell, I. and Newell, C. (1987) *Measuring Health. A Guide to Rating Scales and Questionnaires*. New York: Oxford University Press.

Mattis, S. (1976) Mental status examination for organic mental syndrome in the elderly patient. In: Bellak, L. and Karasu, T. B. (eds) *Geriatric Psychiatry. A Handbook for Psychiatrists and Primary Care Physicians*, pp. 79–121. New York: Grune and Stratton.

Meer, B. and Baker, J. A. (1966) The Stockton geriatric rating scale. *J. Gerontol.*, **21**, 392–403.

Mohs, R. C., Rosen, W. G. and Davis, K. L. (1983) The Alzheimer's disease assessment scale: an instrument for assessing treatment efficacy. *Psychopharmacol. Bull.*, **19**(3), 448–50.

Moore, J. T., Bobula, J. A., Short, T. B. *et al.* (1983) A functional dementia scale. *J. Fam. Pract.* **16**(3), 449–503.

Morris, J. C., Mohs, R. C., Rogers, H., Fillenbaum, G. and Heyman, A. (1988) Consortium to establish a registry for Alzheimer's disease (CERAD) clinical and neuropsychological assessment of Alzheimer's disease. *Psychopharmacol. Bull.*, **24**(4), 641–52.

Olafsson, K., Korner, A., Bille, A., Jensen, H. V., Thiesen, S. and Andersen, J. (1989) The GBS scale in multi-infarct dementia and senile dementia of Alzheimer type. *Acta Psychiatr. Scand.*, **79**, 94–7.

Orgogozo, J. M. and Israel, L. L. (1990) New aspects of the treatment of dementia. In: Orgogozo, J. M. and Gottfries, C. G. (eds) *Progress in Dementia Research*, pp. 111–36. Carnsworth: Parthenon Publishing Group.

Pattie, A. M. and Gilleard, C. J. (1981) *Manual of the Clifton Assessment Procedures (CAPE)*. Kent: Hodder and Stoughton.

Pfeiffer, E. (1975) A short portable mental status questionnaire for the assessment of organic brain deficit in elderly patients. *J. Am. Geriatr. Soc.*, **23**(10), 433–41.

Pichot, P., Girard, B. and Dreyfus, J. C. (1970) L'échelle d'appréciation gériatrique de Stockton (SGRS). Etude de la version française. *Rev. Psychol. Appl.*, **20**, 245–58.

Poitrenaud, J. (1984) Place de la psychométrie dans l'exploration des syndromes démentiels. In: *Fondation Nationale de Gérontologie. Maladie de type Alzheimer et autres démences séniles: actes du colloques des 30 et 31 Janvier 1984, Paris*, 144–52.

Poitrenaud, J. (1987) L'évaluation neuropsychologique des déficits cognitifs dans les états démentiels du sujet âgé. *Rev. Geriatr.*, **12**(6), 245–57.

Portera-Sanchez, A., Del Ser, T., Bermejo, F. and Arrondo, J. M. (1982) Clinical diagnosis of senile dementia of Alzheimer type and vascular dementia. In: Terry, R. D., Bolis, C. L. and Toffano, G. (eds) *Neural Aging and its Implications in Human Neurological Pathology*, pp. 169–88. New York: Raven Press.

Qureshi, K. N. and Hodkinson, H. M. (1974) Evaluation of a ten-question mental test in the institutionalized elderly. *Age Ageing*, **3**, 152–7.

Reisberg, B. (1986) Dementia: a systematic approach to identifying reversible causes. *Geriatrics*, **41**(4), 30–46.

Reisberg, B. and Ferris, S. H. (1985) A clinical rating scale for symptoms of psychosis in Alzheimer's disease. *Psychopharmacol. Bull.*, **21**, 101–4.

Reisberg, B., Ferris, S. H., De Leon, M. J. *et al.* (1982) The global deterioration scale (GDS): an instrument for the assessment of primary degenerative dementia (PDD). *Am. J. Psychiatry*, **139**, 1136–9.

Reisberg, B., London, E., Ferris, S. H. *et al.* (1983a) The brief cognitive rating scale: language, motoric and mood concomitants in primary degenerative dementia. *Psychopharmacol. Bull.*, **19**(4), 703–8.

Reisberg, B., Schneck, M. K., Ferris, S. H. *et al.* (1983b) The brief cognitive rating scale (BCRS): findings in primary degenerative dementia (PDD). *Psychopharmacol. Bull.*, **19**, 47–50.

Reisberg, B., Ferris, S. H. and De Leon, M. J. (1986) Senile dementia of the Alzheimer type: diagnostic and differential diagnostic features with special reference to functional assessment staging. In: Traber, J. and Gispen, W. H. (eds) *Senile Dementia of the Alzheimer Type*. Berlin, Heidelberg: Springer Verlag.

Reitan, R. M. (1979) *Halstead-Reitan Neuropsychological Test Battery*, pp. 18–37. Tucson AZ: University of Arizona, Neuropsychological Laboratory.

Rosen, G. W. (1981) *Rosen Drawing Test*. Bronx, NY: VA Medical Center.

Rosen, G. W., Terry, R. D., Fuld, D. A., Katzman, R. and Peck, A. (1980) Pathological verification of ischemic score in differentiation of dementia. *Ann. Neurol.*, **7**, 486–8.

Rosen, G. W., Mohs, R. C. and Davis, K. L. (1984) A new rating scale for Alzheimer's disease. *Am. J. Psychiatry*, **141**(11), 1356–64.

Roth, M., Thym, E., Mountjoy, C. Q. *et al.* (1986) Camdex: a standardized instrument for the diagnosis of mental disorder in the elderly with special reference to the early detection of dementia. *Br. J. Psychiatry*, **149**, 698–709.

Salzman, C. (1983) The Sandoz clinical assessment geriatric scale. In: Crook, T., Ferris, S. and Bartus, R. (eds) *Assessment in Geriatric Psychopharmacology*. New Canaan, Connecticut: Mark Powley Associates.

Schwarb, S., Koberle, S. and Speigel, R. (1988) The Alzheimer's disease assessment scale (ADAS): an instrument for early diagnosis of dementia? *Int. J. Geriatr. Psychiatr.*, **3**, 45–53.

Schwartz, G. (1983) Development and validation of the Geriatric Evaluation by Relatives Rating Instrument (GERRI). *Psychol. Rep.*, **53**, 479–88.

Shader, R.I., Harmatz, J. S. and Salzman, C. (1974) A new scale for clinical assessment in geriatric populations: Sandoz Clinical Assessment-Geriatric (SCAG). *J. Am. Geriatr. Soc.*, **22**, 107–13.

Slater, R. and Lipman, A. (1977) Staff assessments of confusion and situation of confused residents in homes for old people. *Gerontologist*, **6**, 523–30.

Spiegel, R., Brunner, C., Phil, L., Ermini, D., Monsch, A., Notter, M., Puxty, J. and Tremmel, L. (1991) A new Behavioral Assessment Scale for Geriatric Out- and In-Patients: the NOSGER (Nurses' Observation Scale for Geriatric Patients). *J. Am. Geriat Soc.*, **39**, 339–47.

Stern, Y., Mayeux, R., Sano, M., Hauser, W. A. and Bush, T. (1987) Predictors of disease course in patients with probable Alzheimer's disease. *Neurology*, **37**, 1649–53.

Storandt, M. *et al.* (1984) Psychometric differentiation in mild senile dementia of Alzheimer type. *Arch. Neurol.*, **41**, 497–9.

Van Riezen, H. and Segal, M. (1988) *Comparative Evaluation of Rating Scales for Clinical Psychopharmacology*. Amsterdam: Elsevier.

Wechsler, D. (1981) *Wechsler Adult Intelligence Scale – Revised*. New York: Psychological Corporation.

Wells, C. E. (1979) Pseudodementia. *Am. J. Psychiatry*, **136**(7), 895–900.

Wilkinson, I. M. and Graham-White, J. (1980) Psychogeriatric dependency rating scales (PGDRS). A method of assessment for use by nurses. *Br. J. Psychiatry*, **137**, 558–65.

12

EEG Brain Mapping in Dementia and Gerontopsychopharmacology

B. Saletu

Department of Psychiatry, University of Vienna, Austria

Introduction

Biological measures have gained increasing importance in the clinical diagnosis and treatment of dementia, particularly as far as imaging techniques are concerned. While structural techniques, including computerized tomography (CT), magnetic resonance imaging (MRI) and sonographic measures, play a role in predominantly diagnostic assessments of dementias, functional measures, such as xenon measurement of cerebral blood flow (XeCBF), SPECT (single photon emission computed tomography), positron emission tomography (PET), electroencephalography (EEG) and EP (evoked potential) brain mapping, and magnetic resonance spectroscopy, may be utilized not only in diagnostic but also in therapeutic assessments. Out of the various imaging methods, EEG and EP brain mapping seem to be highly suitable ones as they are readily available, inexpensive, high time-resolution methods for objective and quantitative evaluations of the neurophysiological basis of dementia and its treatment (Itil *et al.*, 1985; Herrmann and Schärer, 1986; Saletu, 1989; Saletu *et al.*,1987a,c, 1988, 1989a,b). The aim of this chapter is to present recent findings on the utilization of EEG mapping in the diagnosis and differential diagnosis of dementia, to describe the relationship between CT, EEG, clinical and psychometric measures and to show its relevance in psychopharmacological trials.

Methods

Data on the diagnostic aspects and interrelationships between different measures were obtained in 111 demented hospitalized patients (77 females, 34 males) aged between 58 and 98 (mean 82) years and diagnosed according to DSM-III criteria. The patients

Dementia: Molecules, Methods and Measures. Edited by I. Hindmarch, H. Hippius and G. K. Wilcock
© 1991 John Wiley & Sons Ltd

had been off all psychopharmaceutical agents for at least 14 days and were subdiagnosed as either senile dementia of the Alzheimer-type (SDAT) or multi-infarct dementia (MID) according to the Hachinski score (<4 = SDAT; >7 = MID) and CT, resulting in 54 SDAT and 57 MID patients. The groups did not differ in regard to sex, age, or Sandoz Clinical Assessment-Geriatric (SCAG) score (70 ± 6 vs. 70 ± 8). EEG recordings and clinical and psychometric evaluations were carried out before and 8 weeks after treatment. CT measures included 10 cerebrospinal fluid (CSF) space variables as well as 17 cortical density measures underneath the EEG electrodes ($1.7\,mm^3$ cubes, measured in Hounsfield units). Clinical investigations were carried out by means of SCAG score/factors, and the psychometric tests included the digit-symbol substitution test (DSST), the trail making test and the digit span test. Three-minute vigilance controlled EEGs (V-EEG) were recorded by means of Nihon-Kohden 4317F and 4321F polygraphs (time constant: 0.3 s; high frequency response: 35 Hz; frequency range: 0.5–35 Hz; amplification: approximately 1–20 000; maximal noise level: $2\,\mu V$ peak to peak). Seventeen leads were digitized on-line by a Hewlett Packard Vectra system with a sampling frequency of 102.4 Hz, resulting in a frequency resolution of 0.2 Hz. Topographic brain mapping was carried out based on a method described in detail elsewhere (Duffy *et al.*, 1981; Anderer *et al.*, 1987, 1989a,b; Saletu *et al.*, 1987a) by means of Hewlett Packard Vectra computers.

Pharmaco-EEG studies with the aim of classifying nootropics and determining their cerebral bioavailability were carried out in double-blind, placebo-controlled trials in groups of 10–15 normal healthy elderly volunteers above the age of 60 (Saletu, 1981, 1987, 1989; Saletu *et al.*, 1987a,b, 1989a, 1990). The subjects received randomized single oral doses of the experimental compound, placebo and eventually a reference compound at weekly intervals. Evaluations were carried out at the 0, 2, 4, 6 and 8 h after oral drug administration.

Long-term investigations with nootropics were carried out in patients as described above (Saletu *et al.*, 1983, 1985, 1987c, 1988).

Results

EEG maps of SDAT and MID Patients Compared with Controls

SDAT patients demonstrated increased delta/theta activity over both frontopolar (Fp), frontotemporal (FT), occipitotemporal (OT), parietal (P) and occipital (O) regions, as well as over the left temporal (T) and central (C) regions (Figure 1)*. An alpha attenuation was observed over both Fp regions, and a beta decrease over both P and left OT, C and vertex areas. The dominant frequency was slowed over the left O, C and FT and right P, OT and F regions. The centroid of the total activity was slowed down over the whole posterior region with a maximum over the parietal area and over both Fp and the left FT regions. Concerning absolute power we observed a significant increase in total power over both T as well as right Fp regions. Likewise, there was an increase in absolute delta power over both Fp, FT, P and OT, the left O as well as right T and

---

*Please note that the figures to this chapter can be found in a separate plate section, together with their descriptive legends.

Illustrations to Chapter 12

Figure 1. Differences between SDAT patients and controls and between MID patients and controls in EEG brain maps (V-EEG, AV, $n = 2 \times 24$). Statistical probability maps depicting inter-group differences in relative power of 1.3–7.5 Hz, 7.5–13 Hz and 13–35 Hz activity, the dominant frequency of the alpha activity and the centroid of the total activity (1.3–35 Hz) are shown in the two columns on the left, and absolute power differences are shown in the two columns on the right. Orange, red and purple colours represent significant ($P < 0.01$, $P < 0.001$ and $P < 0.0001$, respectively) increases, while green, light blue and dark blue indicate significant ($P < 0.01$, $P < 0.001$ and $P < 0.0001$, respectively) decreases compared with controls. SDAT patients demonstrate increased delta/theta activity, decreased beta activity and a slowed dominant frequency and centroid mostly over the parietal regions compared with controls. MID patients demonstrate an augmented delta/theta activity over the whole brain, and attenuated beta activity and a slowed dominant frequency and centroid, indicating a decrease in vigilance. Differences in absolute power are only seen in low frequency bands (1.3–7.5 Hz) and total power

Figure 2. Topographic brain maps of relative power in the 3.5–7.5 Hz EEG activity obtained in a typical SDAT and MID patient. While the SDAT patient (Hachinski score: 2; SCAG score: 57) demonstrates a diffuse slight increase in theta activity (left brain map), the MID patient (Hachinski score: 12; SCAG score: 77) shows a marked augmentation of theta activity over the left hemisphere and right frontopolarly which is due to multiple infarcts in brain regions supplied by the left anterior, middle and posterior cerebral artery and right anterior cerebral artery (right brain map). There is a small maximum–minimum difference in the SDAT patients as opposed to a large one in the MID patient. Moreover, there is a small left–right asymmetry in the SDAT patient, but a marked one in the MID patient

Figure 3. Brain maps of correlations between a CT measure (greatest distance between anterior horns) and 36 EEG variables in dementia ($n = 91$). Each of the 36 maps show the topographic display of correlation coefficients between the CT measure and a specific EEG variable. The upper part of the figure shows correlation maps regarding 13 absolute power variables, the middle part regarding 12 relative power variables, and the lower part regarding 11 centroid and dominant frequency measures. The eight-colour key represents positive (hot/red colours) and negative (cold/blue colours) correlation coefficients; significance levels are shown in the lower right corner. The larger the distance between the anterior horns the more delta/theta activity can be seen over the frontopolar regions

Figure 4. Brain maps of correlations between a CT measure (width of the third ventricle) and 36 EEG variables in dementia ($n = 91$). For technical description of maps and colour key, see legend of Figure 3. The wider the third ventricle, the more delta/theta and slow alpha power and the less beta activity and the slower the centroid of the total activity

Figure 5. Brain maps of correlations between a CT measure (cortical density in Hounsfield units) and 36 EEG variables in dementia ($n = 91$). For technical descriptions of maps and colour key, see legend of Figure 3. The less the cortical density in the CT, the higher the delta and theta activity in the EEG, which is specifically seen in regard to absolute power over both temporal, frontotemporal and temporo-occipital areas, with a left-sided accentuation

Figure 6. Brain maps of correlations between psychopathology (total SCAG score) and 36 EEG variables in dementia ($n = 91$). For technical descriptions of maps and colour key, see legend of Figure 3. The more delta/theta activity, the less alpha and beta activity and the slower the centroid of the total activity, the higher the SCAG score (which reflects psychopathology)

Figure 7. Brain maps of relations between cognitive disorders (rated by SCAG) and 36 EEG variables in dementia ($n = 91$). For technical descriptions of maps and colour key, see legend of Figure 3. The more pronounced the theta activity, mostly over the left hemisphere, the more pronounced the cognitive disorder

Figure 8. Brain maps of correlations between affective disorders (rated by SCAG) and 36 EEG variables in dementia ($n = 91$). For technical description of maps and colour key, see legend of Figure 3. The higher the delta/theta activity, the less the beta activity and the slower the centroid, mostly over the posterior regions with a right-sided accentuation, the worse the affect

Figure 9. Brain maps of correlations between psychometric performance (trail making test) and 36 EEG variables in dementia ($n = 91$). For technical description of maps and colour key, see legend of Figure 3. The higher the delta/theta activity, the less the alpha activity and the slower the centroid, the worse the performance in the trail making test

Figure 10. Brain maps of correlations between mnestic performance (digit span test) and 36 EEG variables in dementia ($n = 91$). For technical description of maps and colour key, see legend of Figure 3. The higher the delta/theta activity, the lower the alpha activity and the slower the centroid of the total activity, the worse the memory

Figure 11. Pharmaco-EEG maps of differences between 600 mg pyritinol and placebo 1 h after oral drug administration in three absolute power variables (left column), three relative power variables (middle column) and in total power, the centroid and centroid deviation (right column). Each statistical probability map represents the results of a statistical comparison by t-test of drug-induced to placebo-induced changes. The eight-colour scale shows differences between drug-induced and placebo-induced changes (based on t values expressed in P values): dark blue = decrease at $P < 0.01$; light blue = decrease at $P < 0.05$; dark green = decrease at $P < 0.10$; light green = trend toward decrease; light yellow = trend toward increase; dark yellow = increase at $P < 0.10$; red = increase at $P < 0.05$; lilac = increase at $P < 0.01$. Pyritinol 600 mg induces in regard to absolute power a trend toward a decrease in 1.3–7.5 Hz and a significant increase in alpha and beta power, and in regard to relative power a significant decrease in delta/theta and increase in alpha activity. Further, it augments total power and accelerates the centroid. The findings indicate an improvement in the vigilance of the aged subjects ($n = 12$)

Figure 12. Statistical probability maps of changes in relative power of 13–16 Hz beta activity in aged subjects 2, 4, 6 and 8 h after 30 mg, 60 mg nicergoline and 5 mg co-dergocrine mesylate (CDM) compared with placebo ($n = 12$). While 30 mg nicergoline produces a significant increase in slow beta activity after 4 and 6 h, 60 mg nicergoline produces such changes as early as in 2 h with a peak effect at 4 h; 5 mg CDM also produces a beta augmentation with a maximum at 4 h

Figure 13. Topographic brain maps of the absolute power in the delta activity of a therapy-responsive (left side) and therapy-resistant (right side) MID patient before and 8 weeks after therapy (20 mg nicergoline/day). The topogram of absolute power in delta activity (1.3–3.5 Hz) before treatment is shown in the upper image, that after treatment in the lower one. Nose is shown to the right, left ear to the top and right ear to the bottom of the image. Blue colours represent low delta activity (20, 30 and 40 pW), red colours indicate high pathological delta power (70, 80, 90 and 100 pW). Pretreatment, delta power is high over the sites of the infarcts (left hemisphere, red colours). After treatment, the infarct still can be seen, but the surrounding brain tissue improved markedly in its function (indicated by blue colours). In contrast, the therapy-resistant patient (right side) shows an increase in slow activity

Figure 14. Pharmaco-EEG maps of differences between xanthinol nicotinate- and placebo-treated SDAT patients (left side) and MID patients (right side). Statistical probability maps concerning the relative power of the combined delta/theta, alpha 1, alpha 2, combined beta activity as well as the relative power of the dominant frequency are demonstrated, depicting differences between the drug- and placebo-induced changes in terms of P values (red colours = increase; blue colours = decrease). In SDAT patients 8 weeks of treatment with 3 g xanthinol nicotinate per day ($n = 19$) results, compared with placebo ($n = 21$), in an increase in slow alpha, decrease in fast alpha, increase in occipital and decrease in vertex beta activity and in an augmentation of relative power of the dominant frequency over various brain regions. In MID patients 8 weeks therapy with 3 g xanthinol nicotinate ($n = 26$) induces, compared with placebo ($n = 23$), an attenuation of delta/theta and augmentation of beta activity over the FT and T regions as well as a decrease in relative power of the dominant frequency and slow alpha activities over the left C and P regions

Figure 15. Differences between xanthinol nicotinate- and placebo-induced changes in SDAT ($n = 19/21$) (upper map) and MID ($n = 26/23$) (lower map) based on multivariate T^2 obtained from a multivariate test in repeated measures ANOVA. Analysis is three way: by group (drug or placebo), by week (0 or 8) and by frequency (delta/theta, alpha 1, alpha 2 or beta) for each electrode. Significant ($T^2 > 2.57$, $P < 0.05$) drug effects can be observed over the frontal region in SDAT patients and in fronto temporal regions in MID patients

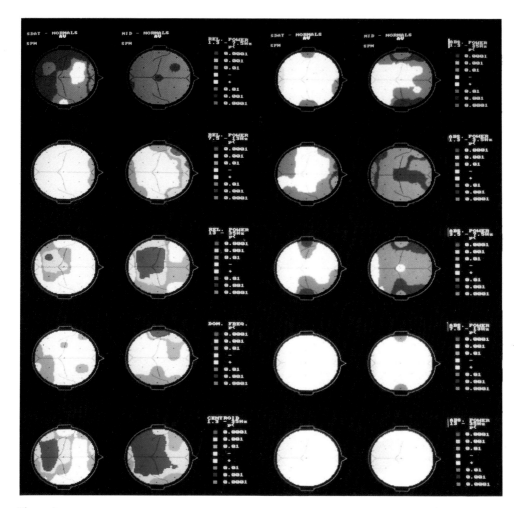

Figure 1

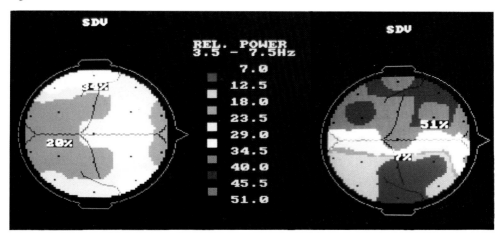

Figure 2

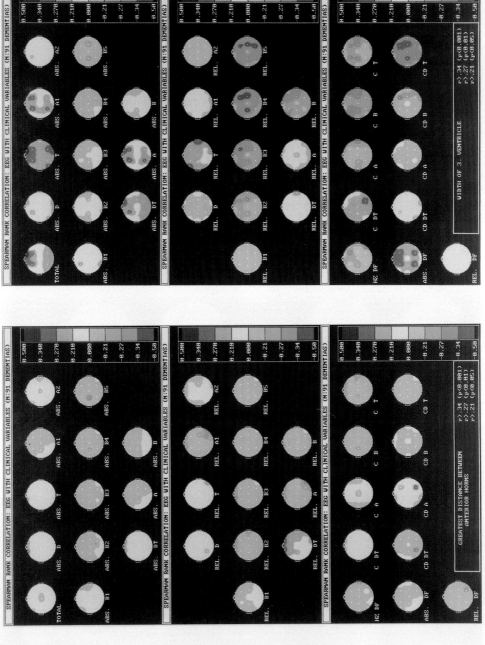

Figure 4

Figure 3

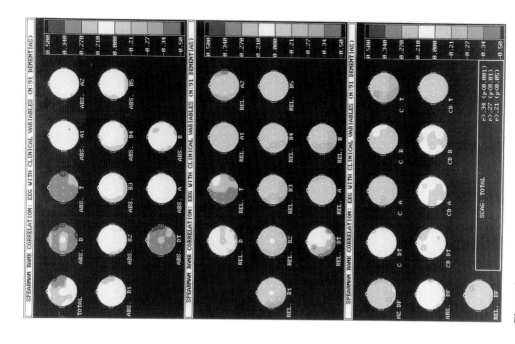

Figure 5

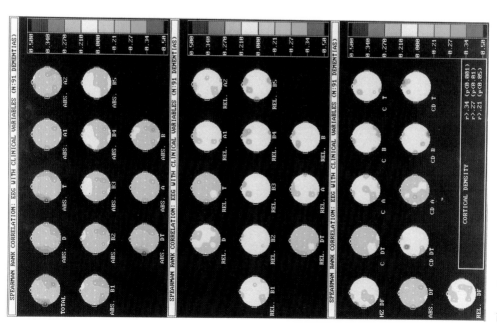

Figure 6

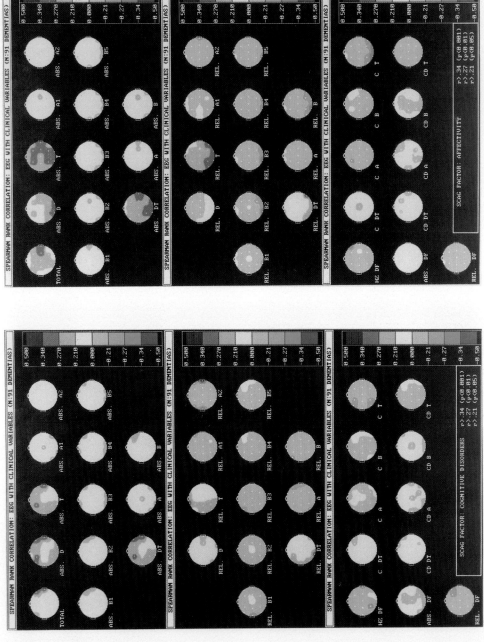

Figure 7

Figure 8

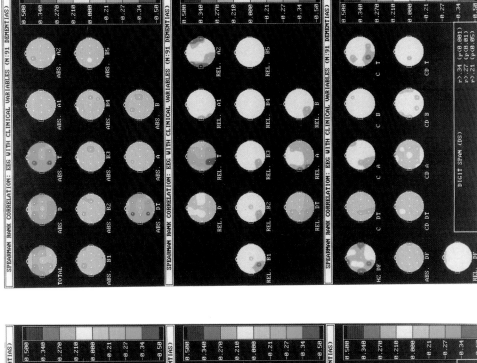

Figure 9

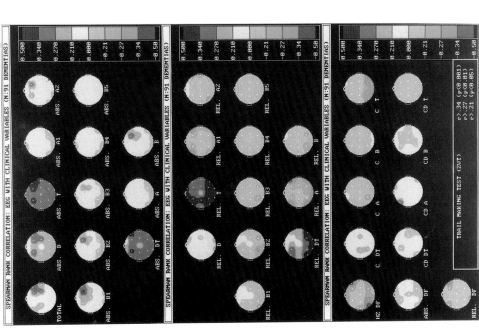

Figure 10

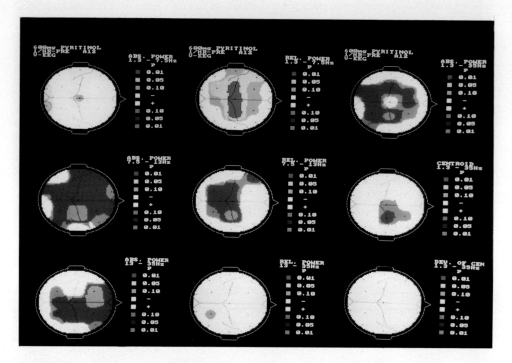

Figure 11

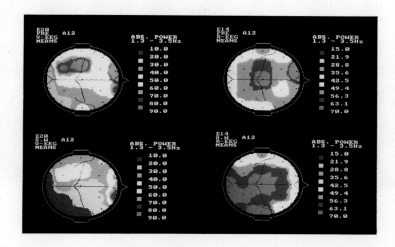

Figure 13

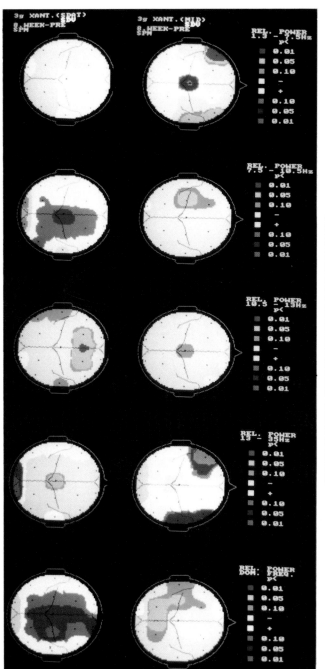

Figure 14

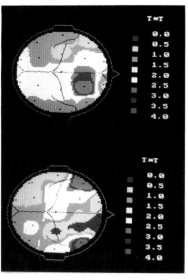

Figure 15

TOPOGRAPHIC BRAIN MAPS (SPM) OF CHANGES IN RELATIVE POWER OF 13 - 16 Hz
BETA ACTIVITY OF ELDERLIES 2,4,6,and 8 HOURS AFTER 30mg and 60mg NICERGOLINE
AND 5mg CO-DERGOCRINE MESYLATE (CDM) AS COMPARED WITH PLACEBO (N:12)

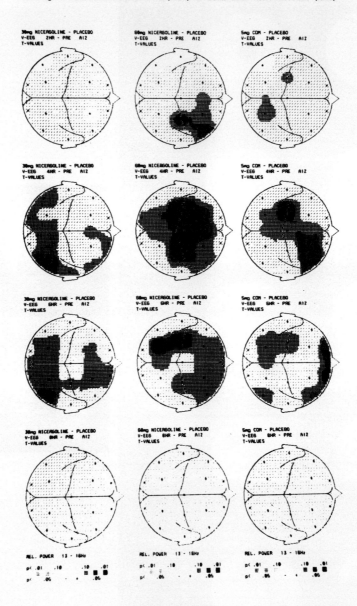

Figure 12

Table 1. EEG power spectra data (means and standard deviations) in SDAT and MID patients and controls (V-EEG, O_r-AV)

Variable	SDAT (n = 24)		MID (n = 24)		Controls (n = 24)	
Absolute power (pW)						
Total power (1.3–35 Hz)	79.1	(63.6)	121.6	(126.2)	89.8	(107.0)
Delta (1.3–3.5 Hz)	13.0	(15.0)	15.4	(13.5)	5.3	(4.4)
Theta (3.5–7.5 Hz)	17.3	(16.8)	34.7	(47.4)	12.7	(25.2)
Delta/theta (1.3–7.5 Hz)	30.4	(29.2)	50.1	(58.9)	18.0	(29.2)
Alpha (7.5–13 Hz)	38.7	(41.6)	57.3	(74.9)	56.3	(77.9)
Beta (13–35 Hz)	10.0	(12.0)	14.3	(8.3)	15.4	(18.4)
Relative power (%)						
Delta (1.3–3.5 Hz)	16.5	(11.2)	15.6	(8.6)	7.9	(4.7)
Theta (3.5–7.5 Hz)	20.9	(12.5)	24.1	(14.5)	12.4	(9.9)
Delta/theta (1.3–7.5 Hz)	37.4	(19.6)	39.7	(19.7)	20.3	(12.5)
Alpha (7.5–13 Hz)	47.3	(18.3)	43.7	(17.2)	58.7	(16.2)
Beta (13–35 Hz)	15.3	(10.0)	16.6	(10.2)	20.9	(12.2)
Centroid (total) (Hz)	9.1	(2.0)	9.2	(2.0)	10.7	(1.7)

O_r-AV = right occipital–common average reference lead.

C regions. Theta power was increased significantly over both T and C and the right FT and Fp regions. There were no significant differences in absolute alpha and beta power. Table 1 depicts the differences in the raw values of EEG power spectra (means and standard deviations) between SDAT and controls and also between SDAT and MID patients. As can be seen, delta activity is augmented in SDAT patients by two standard deviations of the normal control values.

Comparison of MID patients with normals demonstrated a highly significantly augmented relative power in the delta/theta bands all over the brain (Figure 1). The relative power of the alpha activity was decreased in the peripheral regions such as the Fp, FT, T, OT and O areas. The relative power of the beta activity was attenuated almost everywhere. The dominant frequency was slowed over both T, FT and OT regions, but this change was more pronounced over the left than the right hemisphere. On the other hand, the centroid slowing was seen almost over the entire brain, with a slight accentuation over the left hemisphere. Total power was slightly augmented over both T, FT and FP as well as left OT and right C regions. Delta power was markedly and ubiquitously augmented. Theta power also appeared augmented over the whole brain of MID patients except the O and the vertex areas. Absolute alpha power was augmented bitemporarily. There were no differences between MID patients and controls in absolute beta power.

Comparing 54 SDAT patients with 57 MID patients, the latter showed less beta activity and a slower centroid than the former, specifically over both frontal regions. A better discrimination between the two subtypes of dementia was obtained utilizing two new measures: the difference between the maximum and minimum value of a certain EEG variable in the map, and interhemispheric asymmetries (Saletu *et al.*, 1988). In regard to the first measure it became obvious that EEG alterations in the SDAT appear to be diffuse, whereas in MID patients there are marked differences between the various brain areas (Figure 2). Based on these minimum–maximum differences the groups could be discriminated at the $P = 0.007$ level, with 63.1% of the cases correctly classified based on stepwise discriminant function analysis of the differences between the maximum and the minimum power values in nine relative power variables. Based on power asymmetry differences, the two subgroups could be discriminated at the $P = 0.014$ level.

Correlations between CT and EEG Measures

Utilizing Spearman rank correlation between 11 CT measures and 36 EEG variables, we obtained so-called correlation maps showing the relationships between one CT variable (e.g. width of the third ventricle or the greatest distance between the lateral ventricles at the level of the cella media) and 36 EEG variables (Figures 3–5). The greater the distance between the lateral ventricles (indicating brain atrophy), the more delta/theta activity was seen and the less the alpha and beta power over various brain regions. Furthermore, the more atrophy, the slower the centroid of the total activity over the anterior brain regions, but specifically over both FT areas. While the width of the third ventricle as well as the distance between the choroid plexuses was highly significantly and widely correlated with EEG measures (Figure 4), there were only small and topographically limited correlations between the greatest distance between the anterior horns and EEG measures (Figure 3). The larger the distance between the anterior horns, the higher the relative power in the delta/theta activity over both Fp regions, the less alpha activity and the slower the centroid (Figure 3). Cortical density was correlated negatively with absolute delta/theta power, mostly over the T, FT and OT regions with a left-sided accentuation; the more pronounced the cortical atrophy, the more the delta/theta activity (Figure 5).

Correlations between EEG Measures and Psychopathology

Correlation maps between EEG measures and the overall psychopathology as measured by means of the SCAG score demonstrated that the more pronounced the delta/theta activity and the less the beta activity and the slower the centroid, specifically over the left TO and P regions, the worse the psychopathology as rated by the SCAG score (Figure 6). In regard to the SCAG factors, cognitive disorders were, for instance, correlated positively to theta power values over the left hemisphere (Figure 7), whereas affective disorders were correlated positively with more right-sided absolute theta power (Figure 8). Some SCAG factors such as interpersonal relations showed only few correlations to EEG measures. Impairment of self care was correlated negatively with alpha activity, mostly over both FT, T and OT areas, with a right-sided accentuation.

Correlations between EEG and Psychometric Measures

Highest correlations were obtained between EEG and psychometric measures, such as the DSST, trail making test and digit span test (Figures 9 and 10). The higher the delta/theta activity and the slower the centroid of the total power spectrum, the less digits were substituted by symbols (Figure 9). Moreover, the higher the delta/theta activity, the less the alpha and beta activity and the slower the centroid of the total power spectrum, the worse the performance in the trail making test and in the digit span test. Interestingly, it seemed that in the digit span test there was a left-sided accentuation of the findings (Figure 10).

Pharmaco-EEG Mapping in Gerontopsychopharmacology

Anti-hypoxidotics/nootropics produce significant changes in the quantitatively analysed EEG of normal elderly subjects characterized by a decrease in slow activity and an increase in alpha and/or beta activity (Saletu, 1981, 1987, 1989; Saletu and Grünberger, 1985; Saletu *et al.*, 1987a, 1990). These changes are opposite to the alterations in brain function found during normal and pathological ageing and are indicative of improvement in vigilance. Figure 11 depicts pharmaco-EEG maps 1 h after oral administration of 600 mg pyritinol compared with placebo. While delta power shows a trend towards a decrease, a significant increase is observed in regard to alpha and beta power. Relative delta/theta power decreases significantly over the vertex region, centrally, left frontotemporally and parietally, while alpha activity increases. Total power increases, as does the centroid and the absolute power of the dominant frequency. Drugs inducing such changes include representatives of different drug classes such as co-dergocrine mesylate, nicergoline, vincamine, vinconate, SL 76188, tinofedrine, suloctidil, piracetam, etiracetam, aniracetam, tenilsetam, buflomedil, CRL 40028, CRL 40476, piridoxilate, Actovegin, hexobendine, pyritinol and Duxil (an almitrine/raubasine combination). Moreover, we found that these neurophysiological alterations were associated with behavioural changes such as improvement in complex reaction, psychomotor activity, reaction time, mood, affectivity, attention variability and tapping, and an increase in critical flicker fusion (CFF) (Saletu and Grünberger, 1985). This association was not only found in acute studies, but also after chronic administration of antihypoxidotics in the elderly, which supports the idea that improvement of vigilance is linked to improvement in adaptive behaviour in man.

Pharmaco-EEG mapping may also be utilized to explore dose-efficacy and time-efficacy relationships (Figure 12) as well as the bioequipotency of different galenic formulations of nootropics (Saletu *et al.*, 1987a, 1989b, 1990).

EEG Mapping in Therapeutic Monitoring of Demented Patients

Topographic brain mapping of the EEG during nootropic treatment of demented patients may be utilized to monitor the therapeutic efficacy of drugs inasmuch as vigilance improvement may objectively and quantitatively be shown (Saletu *et al.*, 1987c, 1988). Patients who show vigilance improvement have a better therapeutic outcome than those who do not show the typical decrease in slow and increase in alpha and/or alpha-adjacent beta activity (Figure 13). The type of vigilance improving effect of a nootropic, as well as the target area of its action, may differ in degenerative and vascular dementia. As can be seen in Figure 14, SDAT patients exhibit as the most prominent change an increase in relative alpha 1 power, mostly over the vertex region, after 8 weeks of treatment with 3 g xanthinol nicotinate daily, while vascular dementia cases exhibit a decrease in delta/theta and an increase in beta activity as the most prominent change. This is of interest as the Clinical Global Impression (CGI), SCAG, DSST, trail making test and digit span test performance improved in both subgroups of dementia to a similar extent when compared with placebo (Table 2). However, if one analyses EEG drug effects by MANOVA considering time (weeks 0 and 8), groups (drug and placebo) and relative power variables (delta/theta, alpha 1 and 2, and beta), the action of the drug in SDAT patients is seen mostly over the frontal region, while in MID patients it is seen mostly over both frontotemporal regions (significant Hotelling's T^2 values >2.57, $P<0.05$) (Figure 15).

Table 2. Clinical changes in SDAT and MID patients after 8 weeks' therapy with 3 g xanthinol nicotinate and placebo

		SDAT (n = 52)					MID (n = 56)						
		Xanthinol nicotinate (n = 26)		Placebo (n = 26)		Diff. SX-SP U-test	Xanthinol nicotinate (n = 28)		Placebo (n = 28)		Diff. MX-MP U-test	Other Diff. U-test
		Pre	8 weeks	Pre	8 weeks		Pre	8 weeks	Pre	8 weeks		
CGI:	MD	6.00	4.00*	6.00	6.00	†	6.00	4.00*	6.00	6.00	†	SP vs. MX† SX vs. MP†
	x̄	5.38	4.23	5.46	5.38		5.43	4.39	5.39	5.50		
	SD	0.75	1.27	0.81	0.85		1.03	1.26	1.10	1.35		
SCAG:	MD	69.0	63.5*	71.5	71.0	†	70.5	63.0*	71.0	70.0	†	SP vs. MX† SX vs. MP†
	x̄	69.7	64.5	70.7	69.5		69.6	64.1	69.5	69.1		
	SD	5.5	6.5	6.3	6.8		7.4	8.3	7.9	8.8		
Digit symbol substitution test:	MD	11.5	16.5*	9.5	12.0*	†	11.5	17.0*	11.0	13.0*	†	SP vs. MX† SX vs. MP†
	x̄	12.2	16.9	10.8	12.9		11.3	17.3	11.9	13.6		
	SD	4.6	5.8	4.7	6.7		3.8	5.4	6.3	6.8		
Trail making test:	MD	91.5	82.8*	117.8	108.3*	n.s.	102.3	93.3*	98.0	93.3*	n.s.	n.s.
	x̄	99.8	93.4	117.1	111.4		110.9	104.3	113.9	106.9		
	SD	47.6	47.0	33.3	35.2		42.8	43.4	51.1	39.5		
Digit span test:	MD	7.0	8.0*	6.0	6.5	†	7.0	8.0*	7.0	6.0	†	SP vs. MX† SX vs. MP†
	x̄	6.8	7.7	6.7	6.7		6.9	7.6	6.8	6.6		
	SD	1.0	1.2	1.2	1.3		1.4	1.1	1.6	1.5		

Note: *$P < 0.01$ (Mann–Whitney U-test); †$P < 0.01$ (Wilcoxon); n.s. = not significant.
Diff. = difference; SX = SDAT/xanthinol nicotinate; SP = SDAT/placebo; MX = MID/xanthinol nicotinate; MP = MID/placebo.

Discussion

Both SDAT and MID patients show highly significant differences in their brain maps compared with normal healthy aged subjects. While the former demonstrate neurophysiological aberrations, such as an increase in delta/theta activity, a decrease in beta activity, and a slowing of the dominant frequency and the centroid of the total activity, specifically in the parietal and temporal regions and described also as the most abnormal ones by neuropathologists, neurochemists and neuroimagers (Najlerahim and Bowen, 1988; Risberg, 1981; Duara *et al.*, 1986; Haxby *et al.*, 1986; Tamininga *et al.*, 1987; Frackowiak *et al.*, 1981; Friedland *et al.*, 1983, 1985; Bustany *et al.*, 1983; Creasey *et al.*, 1986; Pettergrew *et al.*, 1987), MID (multi-infarct dementia) patients exhibited a marked increase in slow activity compared with controls over the whole brain, which may be due to the fact that infarcted brain regions and their penumbras produce generally more pronounced EEG abnormalities than degenerated ones and that – as they are located in different regions of individual patients – they may add up in the mean SPM (statistical probability map) of the total patient group. Our findings of a slowed centroid of the total activity over the parietal regions are of interest in the light of the PET findings of Frackowiak *et al.* (1981) that MID patients showed most pronounced defects in the parietal regions.

That EEG slowing, reflecting a decrease in vigilance in the sense of Head (1923) and Bente (1977), is correlated to radiological, psychopathological and psychometric data was demonstrated by means of correlation maps based on Spearman rank correlations. The greater the anterior horn distance, lateral ventricle distance and Evan's index, as well as the less the cortical density, the more delta, theta and the less alpha and beta activity in the EEG maps. Moreover, the higher the delta/theta and the less alpha – and beta – activity, the higher the SCAG scores and the worse the psychometric performance.

The best discrimination between the two main subgroups of dementia were obtained utilizing maximum–minimum differences in relative power as well as power asymmetry. By means of discriminant analysis of maximum–minimum differences in nine relative power variables obtained in 17 channels, both dementia groups could be differentiated at the level of $P = 0.006$. By means of the latter, 63.1% of the cases were correctly classified. Asymmetry was also regarded as the most typical cerebral blood flow characteristic of MID patients evaluated by means of the Xenon-133 inhalation method (Risberg, 1981). Utilizing PET, Benson *et al.* (1983) and Kuhl *et al.* (1985) described scattered metabolic defects in the brains of MID patients.

In gerontopsychopharmacology, EEG mapping may be utilized in order to classify nootropic compounds as well as to determine their bioavailability in their target organ – the human brain. Nootropics induce EEG alterations characterized by a decrease in delta/theta activity and an increase in alpha and/or beta activity (Saletu, 1981, 1987, 1989; Saletu *et al.*, 1987a, 1989a, 1990). These alterations are the opposite of age-related changes and are indicative of vigilance improving properties. EEG mapping may be also utilized in monitoring therapeutic progress in patients. As was described previously (Saletu *et al.*, 1987c), patients showing vigilance improvement had a better therapeutic response than those who did not show neurophysiological changes indicative of improvement in vigilance in the pharmaco-EEG maps. Finally, EEG maps may give valuable information about the mode of action of nootropic agents. While in our xanthinol nicotinate study (Saletu *et al.*, 1988) both verum-treated groups showed electrophysiological signs of an improvement in vigilance in their brain maps, they exhibited differences in regard to the topography of these effects. While SDAT patients exhibited significant differences from placebo over the frontal regions, MID patients showed the maximum changes over the frontotemporal areas. This is of interest as in the course of an Alzheimer dementia parietal and temporal areas are first afflicted and only at a later stage of the disease frontal areas follow. Thus, the drug may have a chance to work in regions where neurons are still surviving.

Summary

EEG brain mapping is a readily available, inexpensive, high-time-resolution method for the objective and quantitative evaluation of the neurophysiological basis of dementia. In 111 mildly to moderately demented patients diagnosed according to DSM-III of both the degenerative (SDAT) and vascular (MID) type we investigated not only differences between SDAT, MID patients and normal controls, but also explored the relationships between CT scans, EEG maps, clinical rating and psychometric tests. CT measures included 10 CSF space variables as well as 17 cortical density measures; clinical investigations consisted of the SCAG score/factors, DSST the trail making test and the digit span forward test. SDAT patients showed in brain maps slightly to moderately more slow and less alpha and beta activity as well as a slowing of the dominant frequency and the centroid than normal controls, which was most prominent in the parietal and temporal regions. MID patients exhibited markedly augmented delta/theta and attenuated alpha and beta activity and a slowing of the dominant frequency and centroid ubiquitously. These neurophysiological findings suggest a deterioration in vigilance. Differences between SDAT and MID patients were found mostly in measures of differences between maximum and minimum power and right/left differences in the maps. Brain maps of correlation coefficients between CT and EEG variables demonstrated that the wider the CSF spaces and the less the cortical density, the more delta/theta and the less alpha and beta activity in the EEG. Moreover, the higher the delta/theta and the less the alpha and beta activity, the higher the SCAG scores and the worse the psychometric performance. From the pharmacological point of view, pharmaco-EEG mapping may be utilized to classify nootropic drugs and to determine cerebral bioavailability based on dose- and time-efficacy relationships. Moreover, the method can be applied in therapeutic monitoring: therapy-responsive patients show typical vigilance improvement in their brain maps, while therapy-resistant ones do not. Finally, different types and topographical distributions can shed some light on the mode of action of nootropic drugs in dementias of different aetiologies.

References

Anderer, P., Saletu, B., Kinsperger, K. and Semlitsch, H. (1987) Topographic brain mapping of EEG in psychopharmacology – Part I. Methodological aspects. *Methods Find. Exp. Clin. Pharmacol.*, **9**(6), 371–84.

Anderer, P., Semlitsch, H. V. and Saletu, B. (1989a) Ein Korrekturverfahren zur Reduktion okularer Artefakte in der EEG- und ERP- Tomographie. In: Saletu, B. (ed.) *Biologische Psychiatrie*, pp. 82–5. Stuttgart, New York: Thieme.

Anderer, P., Semlitsch, H. V., Saletu, B. and Filz, L. (1989b) Die Strategie der Artefaktbehandlung im 'Brain-Electrical-Signal-Topography' (BEST) – System. In: Saletu, B. (ed.) *Biologische Psychiatrie*, pp. 86–9. Stuttgart, New York: Thieme.

Bartels, P. H. and Subach, J. A. (1976) Automated interpretation of complex scenes. In: Preston, E. and Onoe, M. (eds) *Digital Processing of Biomedical Imagery*, pp. 101–14. New York: Academic Press.

Benson, D. F., Kuhl, D. E., Randall, A., Hawkins, A., Phelps, M. E., Cummings, J. L. and Tsai, S. Y. (1983) The fluorodeoxyglucose F scan in Alzheimer's disease and multi-infarct dementia. *Arch. Neurol.*, **40**, 711–14.

Bente, D. (1977) Vigilanz: Psychophysiologische Aspekte. *Verh. Dtsch. Ges. Inn. Med.*, **83**, 945–52.

Bustany, P., Henry, J. F., Sousalline, F. and Comar, D. (1983) Brain protein synthesis in normal and demented patients – a study by positron emission tomography with C-L-methionine. In: Magistretti, P. L. (ed.) *Functional Radionucleotides in Aging of the Brain*, pp. 319–26. New York: Raven Press.

Creasey, H., Schwartz, M., Frederickson, H., Haxby, J. H. and Rapoport, S. I.(1986) Tomography in dementia of the Alzheimer type. *Neurology*, **36**, 1563–8.

Duara, R., Grady, C., Haxby, J., Sundaram, M., Cutter, N. R., Heston, L., Moore, A., Schlageter, N., Larson, S. and Rapoport, S. I. (1986) Positron emission tomography in Alzheimer's disease. *Neurology*, **36**, 879–87.

Duffy, F. H., Bartels, P. H. and Burchfield, J. L. (1981) Significance probability mapping: an aid in the topographic analysis of brain electrical activity. *Electroencephalogr. Clin. Neurophysiol.*, **51**, 455–62.

Frackowiak, R. S. J., Pozzilli, C., Legg, N. J., du Poulay, G. H., Marshall, J., Lenzi, G. L. and Jones, T. (1981) Regional cerebral oxygen supply and utilization in dementia. A clinical and physiological study with oxygen 15 and positron tomography. *Brain*, **104**, 753–78.

Friedland, R. P., Budinger, T. F., Ganz, E., Yano, Y., Mathis, C. A., Koss, B., Ober, B. A., Heusmann, R. H. and Derenzo, S. E. (1983) Regional cerebral metabolic alterations in dementia of the Alzheimer type. Positron emission tomography with (F) fluorodeoxyglucose. *J. Comput. Assist. Tomogr.*, **7**, 590–698.

Friedland, R. P., Brun, A. and Budinger, R. F. (1985) Pathological and positron emission tomography correlations in Alzheimer's disease. *Lancet*, **i**, 228.

Haxby, V., Grady, C. L., Duara, R., Schlageter, N., Berg, G. and Rapoport, S. I. (1986) Neocortical metabolic abnormalities precede non-memory cognitive defects in early Alzheimer type dementia. *Archiv. Neurol.*, **43**, 882–5.

Head, H. (1923) The conception of nervous and mental energy. II. Vigilance: A physiological state of the nervous system. *Br. J. Psychol.*, **14**, 125–47.

Herrmann, W. M. and Schärer, E. (1986) Das Pharmako-EEG und seine Bedeutung für die klinische Pharmakologie. In: Kümmerle, D. S., Hinterhuber, G. and Spitzy, K. U. (eds) *Klinische Pharmakologie*, pp. 1–71. Landsberg: Ecomed.

Itil, T. M., Shapiro, D. M., Eralp, E. L., Akmann, A., Itil, K. Z. and Garbizu, C. (1985) A new brain function diagnostic unit, including the dynamic brain mapping of computer analyzed EEG, evoked potentials and sleep (a new hardware/software system and its application in psychiatry and psychopharmacology). *New Trends Exp. Clin. Psychiatry*, **1**, 107–77.

Kuhl, D. E., Metter, E.J., Riege, W. H. and Hawkins, R. A. (1985) Patterns of cerebral glucose utilization in dementia. In: Greitz, T. (ed.) *The Metabolism of the Human Brain studied with Positron Emission Tomography*, pp. 419–31. New York: Raven Press.

Najlerahim, A. and Bowen, D. M. (1988) Regional weight loss of the cerebral cortex and some subcortical nuclei in senile dementia of the Alzheimer type. *Acta Neuropathol.*, **75**, 509–12.

Obrist, W. D. (1979) Electroencephalographic changes in normal aging and dementia. In: Hoffmeister, F. and Müller, C. (eds) *Brain Function in Old Age*, pp. 102–11. Berlin: Springer.

Pettergrew, J. W., Withers, G., Panchalingam, K. and Post, J. F. M. (1987) Nuclear magnetic resonance (NMR) spectroscopy of brain in aging and Alzheimer's disease. In: Wurtman, R. J., Corhin, S. and Growdon, J. H. (eds) *Topics in the Basic and Clinical Science of Dementia*, pp. 261–8. Vienna, New York: Springer.

Risberg, J. (1981) Non-invasive measurements of CBF during brain work in CCVD clinical applications to vasoactive drug studies. In: Scientific International Research (eds) *Drug and Methods in CVD*, pp. 197–201. Paris: Pergamon Press.

Saletu, B. (1981) Application of quantitative EEG in measuring encephalotropic and pharmacodynamic properties of antihypoxidotic/nootropic drugs. In: Scientific International Research (eds) *Drug and Methods in CVD*, pp. 79–115. Paris: Pergamon Press.

Saletu, B. (1987) The use of pharmaco-EEG in drug profiling. In: Hindmarch, I. and Stonier, P. D. (eds) *Human Psychopharmacology – Measures and Methods*, pp. 173–200. Chichester: John Wiley and Sons.

Saletu, B. (1989) Neurophysiological aspects of aging and gerontopsychopharmacology. *Mod. Probl. Pharmacopsychiatry*, **23**, 43–55.

Saletu, B. and Grünberger, J. (1985) Memory dysfunction and vigilance: neurophysiological and psychopharmacological aspects. *Ann. N. Y. Acad. Sci.*, **444**, 407–27.

Saletu, B., Linzmayer, L., Grünberger, J. and Mader, R. (1983) Spontaneous and drug-induced remission of alcoholic organic brain syndrome. *Psychiatry Res.*, **10**, 59–75.

Saletu, B., Saletu, M., Grünberger, J. and Pietschmann, H. (1985) Double-blind placebo-controlled, clinical, psychometric and neurophysiological investigations with oxiracetam in the organic brain syndrome of late life. *Neuropsychobiology*, **13**, 44–52.

Saletu, B., Anderer, P., Kinsperger, K. and Grünberger, J. (1987a) Topographic brain mapping of EEG in neuropsychopharmacology. Part II. Clinical applications (pharmaco-EEG imaging). *Methods Find. Exp. Clin. Pharmacol.*, **9**(6), 385–408.

Saletu, B., Grünberger, J. and Anderer, P.(1987b) Proof of antihypoxidotic properties of tenilsetam in man by EEG and psychometric analyses under an experimental hypoxic hypoxidosis. *Drug Dev.*, **10**, 135–55.

Saletu, B., Hochmayer, K., Grünberger, J., Böhmer, F., Paroubek, J., Wicke, L. and Neuhold, A. (1987c) Therapy of multi-infarct dementia with nicergoline: double-blind, clinical, psychometric and EEG-imaging investigation with two different drug administration schedules. *Wien. Med. Wochenschr.*, **137**(22), 513–24.

Saletu, B., Anderer, P., Paulus, E., Grünberger, J., Wicke, L., Neuhold, A., Fischhof, P. K., Litschauer, G., Wagner, G., Hatzinger, R. and Dittrich, R. (1988) EEG brain mapping in SDAT and MID patients before and during placebo and xanthinol-nicotinate therapy: reference considerations. In: Samson-Dollfuss, D., Guieu, J. D., Gotman, J. and Etevenon, P. (eds) *Statistics and Topography in Quantitative EEG*, pp. 251–75. Paris: Elsevier.

Saletu, B., Anderer, P. and Grünberger, J. (1989a) EEG brain mapping in gerontopsychopharmacology: on protective properties of pyritinol against hypoxic hypoxidosis. *Psychiatry Res.*, **29**(3), 387–90.

Saletu, B., Semlitsch, H. V., Anderer, P., Resch, R., Presslich, O. and Schuster, P. (1989b) Psychophysiological research in psychiatry and neuropsychopharmacology. II. The investigation of antihypoxidotic/nootropic drugs (tenilsetam and co-dergocrine-mesylate) in elderlies with the Viennese Psychophysiological test-system (VPTS). *Methods Find. Exp. Clin. Pharmacol.*, **11**, 43–55.

Saletu, B., Anderer, P. and Grünberger, J. (1990) Topographic brain mapping of EEG after acute application of ergotalkaloids in the elderly. *Arch. Gerontol. Geriatr.*, **11**, 1–22.

Semlitsch, H. V., Anderer, P., Saletu, B., Resch, F., Presslich, O. and Schuster, P. (1989) Psychophysiological research in psychiatry and neuropsychopharmacology: Part I: Methodological aspects of the Viennese Psychophysiological test-system (VPTS). *Methods Find. Exp. Clin. Pharmacol.*, **11**, 25–41.

Semlitsch, H. V., Anderer, P., Saletu, B. and Hochmayer, I. (1991) Topographic brain mapping of cognitive event related potentials in a double-blind, placebo-controlled study with a hemoderivative Actovegin in age-associated memory impairment. *Neuropsychobiology*, in press.

Tamininga, C. A., Foster, N. L., Fedio, P., Bird, E. D. and Chase, T. N. (1987) Alzheimer's disease: low cerebral somatostatin levels correlated with impaired cognitive function and cortical metabolism. *Neurology*, **37**, 161–5.

Van der Drift, J. H. A., Kok, M. K. D., Niedermayer, E., Maguet, R. and Viourous, R. Y. (1972) The EEG in relation to pathology in simple cerebral ischemia. In: Remond, A. (ed.) *Handbook of Electroencephalography and Clinical Neurophysiology*, p. 14a. Amsterdam: Elsevier/North-Holland.

13

Age-related Memory Impairment: A Longitudinal and Cross-sectional Comparison

S. G. Kilminster

Interphase UK, Billingshurst, UK

One of the difficulties in the area of research into the dementias is that of diagnostic criteria and terminology. Generally, the dementias appear to be largely defined in terms of exclusion of various signs and symptoms. Against this background is another confusing issue of whether the intellectual and information processing abilities of humans worsens with advancing age and, if so, by how much. In addition, it is not clear whether phenomena such as benign senescent forgetfulness (BSF) or age-associated memory impairment (AAMI) are the precursors of the dementias, in particular senile dementia of the Alzheimer type (SDAT).

It is imperative to be able to monitor any cognitive impairment with age, so that one can follow-up longitudinally any predicted relationship between AAMI and SDAT. Furthermore, the identification of variables that regress with age would be an obvious method of choosing dependent variables for examining the efficacy of any drug in terms of (a) slowing down the rate of impairment, (b) halting the dementing process, or (c) reversing the dementing process.

It would appear reasonable to be able to identify subjects who may later develop SDAT or a more serious form of AAMI as early as possible, the notion being that trying to preserve the functioning of the central nervous system (CNS) may be more effective than trying to regain lost or damaged brain tissue. The analogy may be that the horse has already bolted. At present, with a myriad of pharmaceutical agents and paradigms, there appears to be no evidence of any reversal or halting of SDAT. It may be that all we can hope for is a good attempt at slowing down any mental deterioration. Of

Dementia: Molecules, Methods and Measures. Edited by I. Hindmarch, H. Hippius and G. K. Wilcock
© 1991 John Wiley & Sons Ltd

course, one still has to develop the psychometric procedures to be able to specify on an individual basis that an impairment later in life is highly likely. We need to 'catch' the disease early enough and psychometric procedures are badly needed here.

The term BSF has been around for some time (Kral, 1962). The more specific term AAMI has been applied more recently by Crook *et al.* (1986). However, despite the increasing usage of this latter term and an almost passive acceptance of the phenomenon, we are still a long way from showing AAMI to be a definite condition.

Reviews in this area (Fozard, 1985; Poon, 1985) indicate that evidence is largely based upon cross-sectional studies. Such studies show older subjects with worsened sensory, short-term and long-term memory functioning when compared with younger subjects. Additionally, older subjects are slower to respond (Birren *et al.*, 1980). This latter effect has been suggested as a mechanism for worsened performance on many tests, including those of memory. Horn (1982) has argued that this effect may be a consequence rather than a cause of decreased intellectual functioning. Elderly subjects are not only thought to be mentally slower, probably reflecting an obvious physical slowing with age, but also respond to test situations more cautiously. Analysis of response bias by signal detection theory (SDT) has not substantiated any increased caution in the elderly compared with younger subjects (Fozard, 1985).

Another cognitive explanation for worsened performance of memory and reaction time is that it is due to increased anxiety levels in the elderly. The general finding of heightened levels of anxiety is associated with worsened performance on a wide variety of tests (Eysenck, 1983; Kilminster *et al.*, 1988). However, elderly subjects have generally lower not higher levels of state anxiety (Spielberger, 1983). There is as yet no evidence of elderly subjects being more cautious or anxious in test situations, although there is a paucity of studies in this area. Additionally, much of the difference in memory performance between young and elderly subjects can be ameliorated by cognitive training techniques including, among other things, mnemonic devices (Yesavage, 1985).

It has been said that the evidence for AAMI rests upon cross-sectional data. There are three broad criticisms that can be levelled at these data:

1. *No matching of appropriate controls.* Older subjects are not matched for socio-economic group, education, public health measures, dietary factors, etc. It may well be that elderly subjects, as a group, started off in youth with a lower level of cognitive performance than their present-day youthful counterparts. The regression of performance with age would then be an artefact.
2. *Set effects correlated with age.* How often has one been away on holiday for 2 weeks and returned to work to find a certain 'difficulty' in getting back into the swing of things. One is slower to respond and perhaps one makes a few little mistakes and excuses oneself since it is one's first day back. The point is that mental agility can be thought of, like physical agility, in terms of keeping fit. It can be argued that elderly subjects may have no need to study for exams, spend hours in computer parlours or at home with computer games (with major reaction time components). The life-style of the retired is probably very different from the youth at play or the life of a young executive. Perhaps the ways that the youth interact with their environment facilitates them in mental test situations, whereas the opposite is the case for the elderly.
3. *Confounding effects of increased morbidity in the elderly.* As age increases there is an increasing frequency of diseases and usage of drug therapy. Many elderly

subjects complain of sleep disturbance and receive hypnotic therapy. A large number of cross-sectional studies have not excluded subjects with physical or psychological disorders. Even diseases such as essential hypertension, accounting for some 10% of the adult population, is known to be associated with minor decrements in cognitive functioning (Francheschi *et al.*, 1982). These biases would increase the chance of an artefactual negative correlation between cognitive performance and age.

The above points led us to adopt an approach not reliant upon cross-sectional data using longitudinal studies where subjects act as their own controls. Subjects are trained to a performance plateau on all tests, even on those tests that have no learning effect over time. In addition, subjects must be fully screened for physical and psychiatric disturbances and for all CNS active drugs.

We have set up a database from our phase I unit where we regularly screen healthy subjects. At present we have data from about 300 subjects which we are updating on a longitudinal basis. This data includes all demographic, medical, psychiatric and psychometric variables. Below we outline a small subset of data for 51 healthy elderly subjects which we have analysed both by longitudinal and cross-sectional methods. The data covers a three and a half year period and so it is very much in its infancy. Subjects were tested at various periods, approximately at 6-month intervals. The data are therefore presented more as a pilot study, since we will probably need a 10-year period of measurement for reliable results.

The Sample

Males and females aged from 59 to 77 years were included. All subjects were healthy and screened on the following parameters: full electrocardiography, haematology, renal and liver function tests, electrolytes and lipids, haemodynamics, drug screen, medical and psychiatric history and psychometric training.

Methods

The dependent variables included the following: critical flicker fusion, choice reaction time, tracking reaction time, tracking accuracy, and the Sternberg Paradigm for Memory.

The independent variables included sex, age and time. The latter was the longitudinal variable of age and was assessed at seven levels. The analysis was by multiple linear regression with the use of forward and backward stepwise selection procedures. The psychological variables were regressed upon age, time, sex and first-order interaction terms.

By comparing equations with age and time factors we could approximate cross-sectional and longitudinal data sets.

Results

Longitudinal Data

These are presented graphically in Figures 1–5.

There were no significant regression effects with time with critical flicker fusion, total (choice) reaction times, tracking reaction times, tracking accuracy, and overall Sternberg memory variables.

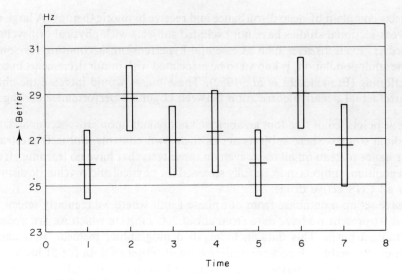

Figure 1. Critical flicker fusion

Cross-sectional Data

There were significant regression effects with age with critical flicker fusion, total reaction time, tracking reaction time, tracking accuracy and the Sternberg memory test (Table 1).

Summary

Overall there was a clear distinction between longitudinal and cross-sectional data. The former showed no deterioration of cognitive performance with advancing years but

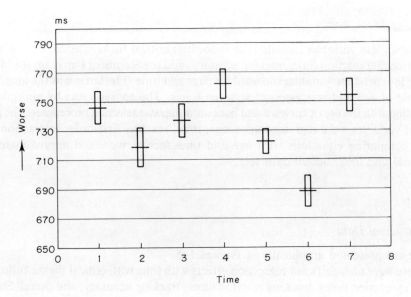

Figure 2. Total reaction time

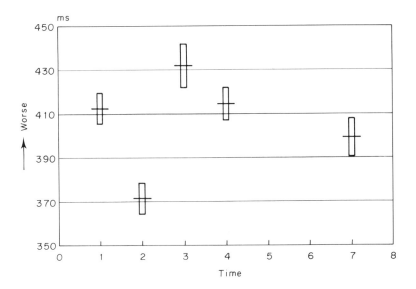

Figure 3. Tracking reaction time

the latter did. Examining the sign of the standard regression coefficients in the cross-sectional data revealed a worsening of cognitive performance with age. With tracking accuracy, both time and age×time terms were significant, revealing an improvement over the seven time points, but with the interaction term showing a decremental effect working against the former effect. In short, these data are easily interpreted. Longitudinal data does not support a worsening of cognitive performance with age, but cross-sectional analysis on the same data supports the opposite contention. The present longitudinal study can be criticized as being prone to floor effects (and hence type II errors) since

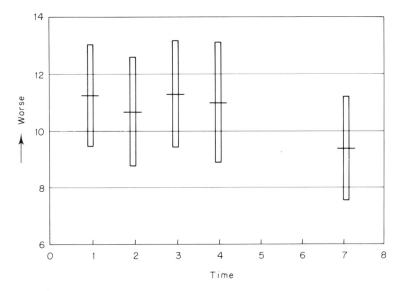

Figure 4. Tracking accuracy

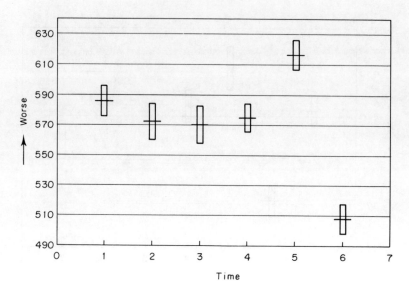

Figure 5. Overall memory

Table 1. Cross-sectional data

Variable	Coefficient	Standard coefficient	T	P(2-tail)
Critical flicker fusion				
Constant	36.718	0.000	9.366	0.000
Age	−0.106	−0.175	−1.946	0.054
Sex	−1.521	−0.274	−3.056	0.003
Total reaction time				
Constant	−20.317	0.000	−0.131	0.896
Age	11.006	0.414	4.894	0.000
Tracking reaction time				
Constant	120.773	0.000	1.013	0.314
Subject	−3.065	−0.617	−2.592	0.011
Age	3.779	0.242	2.334	0.022
Sex	71.665	0.484	2.026	0.046
Tracker accuracy				
Constant	6.567	0.000	5.209	0.000
Time	−2.924	−1.924	−2.338	0.022
Age × Time	0.038	1.724	2.097	0.039
Sex	3.562	0.484	4.909	0.000
Sternberg memory scanning				
Constant	−246.968	0.000	−1.613	0.110
Age × time	−0.151	−0.146	−1.633	0.106
Age	12.408	0.493	5.508	0.000

the sample size was modest and the study extended over a relatively short time period. In addition, the equations may well be better fitted by a non-linear, e.g. quadratic, function. This has not been tested with the present data set. However, as we have previously argued, cross-sectional data can give rise to artefacts favouring a type I error.

It has been previously stated that the evidence for the impairment of cognitive function with advancing age rests upon cross-sectional data and criticisms of this have been given. The present data set reveals a discrepancy between cross-sectional and longitudinally analysed data. Some longitudinal animal data exists, but the phylogenetic distance from rodents and even primates negates some of the usefulness of these animal paradigms in buttressing the conclusions of human cross-sectional studies (Bowden and Williams, 1984; Bartus *et al.*, 1983; Dean *et al.*, 1981; Bartus and Dean, 1985).

In conclusion we have presented a methodological critique and a comparison of longitudinal and cross-sectional data, and we recommend that the notion of AAMI and similar terms refer to a phenomenon which should be interpreted with caution. Until the appropriate psychometric data is available from well-controlled longitudinal studies, we prefer to remain open-minded as to whether human ageing is necessarily associated with impairments in cognitive functioning. If we can show that human ageing is often associated with impaired cognitive functioning, then we may additionally have discovered early predictions for later disease if AAMI does predispose to dementia. Furthermore, it may well be the case that AAMI (if it exists) does not predispose to dementia but may be of sufficient order to warrant some elderly individuals requiring treatment with cognitive activators. Either way, the field is wide open to discover new psychometric procedures or indeed combinations of tests that will allow not only the efficacy of any drug treatment to be assessed but also to predict early enough when treatment should be given.

References

Bartus, R. T. and Dean, R. L. (1985) Developing and using animal models in the search for an effective treatment for age-related memory disturbances. In Gottfries, C. G. (ed.) *Normal Aging, Alzheimer's Disease, and Senile Dementia: Aspects on Etiology, Pathogenesis, Diagnosis and Treatment*, pp. 231–67. Brussels: Editions de l'Université de Bruxelles.

Bartus, R. T., Dean, R. L., Beer, B. and Lippa, A. S. (1982) The cholinergic hypothesis of geriatric memory. *Science*, **217**, 408–17.

Bartus, R. T., Flicker, C. and Dean, R. L. (1983) Logical principles for the development of animal models of age related memory impairments. In: Crook, T., Ferris, S. S. and Bartus, R. T. (eds) *Assessment in Geriatric Psychopharmacology*, pp. 263–99. New Canaan, Connecticut: Mark Powley Associates.

Birren, J. E., Woods, A. M. and Williams, M. V. (1980) Behavioural slowing with age. Causes, organisation and consequences. In: Poon, L. W. (ed.) *Aging in the 1980s: Psychological Issues*, pp. 293–308. Washington, D.C.: American Psychological Association.

Bowden, D. M. and Williams, D. D. (1984) Aging. *Adv. Vet. Sci. Comp. Med.*, **28**, 305–41.

Crook, T., Bartus, R. T., Ferris, S. H., Whitehouse, P., Cohen, G. D. and Gershon, S. (1986) Age associated memory impairment: proposed diagnostic criteria and measures of clinical change. *Dev. Neuropsychol.*, **2**(4), 261–76.

Dean, R. L., Scozzafava, J., Goas, J. A., Regan, B., Beer, B. and Bartus, R. T. (1981) Age related differences in behaviour across the life span of the C57BL/6J mouse. *Exp. Aging Res.*, **7**(4), 417–51.

Eysenck, M. (1983) *Attention and Arousal*, Ch. 6, pp. 95–120. Berlin, Heidelberg, New York: Springer Verlag.

Fozard, J. L. (1985) Psychology of aging: normal and pathological age differences in memory. In: Brocklehurst, J. (ed.) *Textbook of Geriatric Medicine and Gerontology*, pp. 122–45. Edinburgh: Churchill Livingstone.

Francheschi, M., Tancredi, O., Smirne, S., Mercinelli, A. and Canal, N. (1982) Cognitive processes in hypertension. *Hypertension*, **4**, 226–9.

Horn, J. L. (1982) The theory of fluid and crystallised intelligence in relation to cognitive psychology and aging in adulthood. In: Craik, F. M. and Trehub, S. (eds) *Aging and Cognitive Processes*, Vol. 8, pp. 237–8. New York: Plenum.

Kilminster, S. G., Lewis, M. J. and Jones, D. M. (1988) Anxiolytic effects of acebutolol and atenolol in subjects with induced anxiety. *Psychopharmacology*, **95**, 245–9.

Kral, V. A. (1962) Senescent forgetfulness: benign and malignant. *J. Can. Med. Assn.*, **86**, 257–60.

Poon, L. W. (1985) Differences in human memory with aging: nature, causes and clinical implications. In: Birren, J. and Schaie, K. (eds) *Handbook of Psychology of Aging*, pp. 427–62. New York: Van Nostrand Reinhold.

Spielberger, C. D. (1983) *The Manual of the STAI*. Palo Alto: Consulting Psychologists Press.

Yesavage, J. A. (1985) Nonpharmacologic treatment for memory losses with normal aging. *Am. J. Psychiatry*, **142**(5), 600–5.

14

Critical Flicker Fusion in Gerontological Research: Clinical Implications for Alzheimer's Disease

Stephen Curran

Department of Psychology, The University, Leeds, UK

Introduction

The number of scientific papers on Alzheimer's disease appears to be growing 'exponentially' but the basic cause or causes of this syndrome remain unknown (Curran and Wattis, 1989). As the search for a therapeutic agent continues, it will be necessary for psychopharmacologists to be ready with reliable and valid measures to profile new compounds in both volunteer and patient samples.

Methodological Considerations

When assessing elderly subjects it is essential to be aware of the particular problems associated with this population who are different from normal young volunteer subjects in a number of important ways. In particular, their overall performance on a number of psychological tests is lower, e.g. visual information processing (Walsh, 1976), short-term memory (Craik, 1979), motor reaction time (Botwinik and Storandt, 1974), learning ability (Botwinik, 1973), attention/concentration (McGhie *et al.*, 1965), global cognitive function (Busse, 1978; Woods, 1982) and critical flicker fusion threshold (CFFT) (Curran *et al.*, 1990). A good rapport also needs to be established between elderly subjects and the investigator, and the level of arousal/motivation, emotional state and sensory function, especially the integrity of the visual and auditory systems, all need careful consideration (Vingoe, 1981). Hindmarch and Wattis (1988) have noted that 'the limiting factor of all psychopharmacological research in the elderly population is the

Dementia: Molecules, Methods and Measures. Edited by I. Hindmarch, H. Hippius and G. K. Wilcock
© 1991 John Wiley & Sons Ltd

appropriateness of the assessment measures used to determine the drug effect'. These concerns are even more important when dealing with patients with Alzheimer's disease. The use of pre-experimental screening, the control of confounding variables and the use of placebo and/or verum treatments will all improve the chances of identifying a drug effect.

There is currently no agreed test battery available for clearly differentiating between patients with Alzheimer's disease and normals or for the evaluation of anti-dementia agents in the clinical trial setting. Although a great many psychometric tests are available, it is unclear how many of these have been shown to be valid, reliable and pharmaco-sensitive in patients with Alzheimer's disease.

Many clinical rating scales are unsuitable for repeated measures designs because of the risk of learning effects, e.g. the Mini-Mental State Examination (Folstein *et al.*, 1975) and the Hodkinson scale (Hodkinson, 1972). In addition, the majority of clinical instruments are various types of rating scales. In general, rating scales are prone to many methodological problems. Broadly speaking, they can be subdivided into observer-rating (skilled, semi-skilled and unskilled) and self-rating scales. The general points of criticism include the subjective nature of the assessment and that a skilled and experienced interviewer is needed, especially when the interviewer has to elicit information which is not accessible to the subject, such as the presence of delusions and hallucinations. In addition, it is necessary to ensure that the individual items are independently scored, and it is important that constant errors are avoided, including the error of leniency, the halo effect, the error of proximity and the logical error. The personality of the rater (central or extreme tendency type) is also a factor that has to be taken into consideration. Other problems with rating scales include which items should be included in a particular scale, how individual items are to be weighted and how grades of severity are to be defined. Statistical problems are also present in that the assignment of numbers to grades of severity implies that the interval between one grade and the next are exactly equal. However, such a scale is ordinal in nature (Guilford and Fruchter, 1978), and to apply parametric statistics to such scales is statistically incorrect (Brown and Hollander, 1977). It is also strictly not correct to add scores from individual items together. Scores should be ranked to indicate the order in which the scores lie. Finally, a given total on a scale may be made up of different items in different patients or on different occasions in the same patient (Hamilton, 1987). For all these reasons, it would be preferable to use tests for repeated measures designs which have proven reliability, validity and pharmacosensitivity, in addition to being free from learning effects and providing an objective measure of performance (Table 1).

Table 1. The 'ideal' psychometric test

Reliable
Valid
Pharmacosensitive
Easy to use
No 'ceiling' effect
No 'floor' effect
Objective
Quantitative
No educational bias
No cultural bias
Minimal emphasis on verbal and numerical skills
Age sensitive

A Psychopharmacological Perspective

Psychopharmacologists are interested in measuring the effects of psychoactive drug-induced changes in cognitive and/or psychological behaviour. A great variety of measures have been described and used, and many of these have been automated (Cull and Trimble, 1987). However, it is often unclear what a particular test is supposed to reflect in terms of psychological function. In addition, many tests which have claimed to measure central nervous system (CNS) activity appear to have been developed in an entirely arbitrary fashion.

Hindmarch and Wattis (1988) have proposed a model of information processing. Input from the sense organs reaches the CNS and is processed before producing overt motor behaviour. This central processing can be influenced by a number of variables, including personality, motivation and memory. This model illustrates that a battery of psychometric measures is probably the most appropriate way to measure the effects of psychoactive drugs on CNS function.

It is preferable to use a small number of psychologically relevant measures as this will increase the chances of identifying a drug-induced change as relevant to a particular psychological function. In addition, as the number of tests increases, subjects, especially those with Alzheimer's disease, will find it increasingly difficult to cope with the test battery. One also runs the risk of identifying significant results by chance. Such results are clinically irrelevant (Kendall, 1987).

Despite the great number of tests available to psychopharmacologists (Hindmarch and Stonier, 1987, 1989), few attempts have been made to isolate those tests which are able to identify drug-induced changes in cognitive and/or psychological functions in the elderly, although such studies have been described in young volunteers (Hindmarch and Wattis, 1988). In normal volunteers some of the most pharmacosensitive measures include auditory vigilance and the digit-symbol substitution test (sensory), balance performance and hand tremor (motor), and mental arithmetic, digit span, verbal learning and CFFT (overall CNS activity) (Ott and Kranda, 1982; Hindmarch *et al.*, 1988; Hindmarch and Wattis, 1988). Although a small number of tests have been identified as being able to differentiate the effects of different anti-depressants in elderly depressed subjects (Siegfried *et al.*, 1984; Siegfried, 1985), a reliable, valid and pharmacosensitive test battery for the evaluation of anti-dementia drugs is still awaited.

Most of the available tests have been developed in healthy young volunteers. Before a psychometric test can be used with confidence in research into Alzheimer's disease, it is first essential to establish its face validity. This can then be followed by an examination of its age sensitivity, reliability, validity and pharmacosensitivity, the latter three in patient populations.

The Role of Elderly Subjects in Test Development

There is much debate about the relationship between normal ageing and Alzheimer's disease. Copeland (1987) has suggested that the two are separate processes. Giaquinto (1988) has presented detailed evidence both for and against this hypothesis, but a number of authors have argued that Alzheimer's disease is an exaggeration of the normal ageing process (U'Ren, 1987; Brayne and Calloway, 1988; Deary and Whalley, 1988).

It may therefore be useful initially to examine a new test in an elderly population for a number of different reasons. If the test is age and disease sensitive, it is possible that the measure may be of value for the identification of early cases of Alzheimer's disease when assessed longitudinally; the rate of fall in performance would be greater in the patient sample. In addition, if the test is age sensitive, it is probable that the measure would be able to detect small changes in performance induced by the administration of psychoactive drugs (either positive or negative). Patients with 'pure' clinical Alzheimer's disease are difficult to find and full assessment is time-consuming and expensive. The normal elderly may provide a useful screening population for test identification prior to use in patients with Alzheimer's disease.

CFFT

CFFT measurement has repeatedly been shown to be a valid and reliable technique (Curran, 1990), in addition to being one of the most successful pharmacosensitive measures in psychopharmacology (Turner, 1968; Smith and Misiak, 1976; Hindmarch, 1982). However, the majority of studies have concentrated on young healthy volunteers. It is not known if CFFT is also a reliable, valid and pharmacosensitive technique in patients with Alzheimer's disease.

Face validity refers to what a test is 'supposed to measure' (Anastasi, 1988). Unfortunately, there is little published work regarding guidelines for the establishment of face validity (Nevo, 1985; Nevo and Sfez, 1985). This does not obviate the need for objective validity, but is an initial first step before proceeding more formally with test evaluation.

Although there is debate regarding the neurobiological basis of the CFFT, there is considerable evidence that it reflects the central and/or cortical integrative function of the CNS (Curran *et al.*, 1990).

Cortical activity can be altered by exposure to flickering light and the change is maximal in the occipital cortex. In addition, the electroencephalographic activity recorded over the occipital cortex has been found to be synchronous with the frequency of the flicker. Other evidence includes differences between monocular and binocular vision and the fact that cortical lesions have been shown to be associated with reductions in the CFFT (see Curran *et al.*, 1990 for review). Soininen (1983) has found that slowing of the occipital rhythm in patients with Alzheimer's disease was the best electroencephalographic parameter for distinguishing between patients with Alzheimer's disease and normal controls. Marterer *et al.* (1990) using a positron emission tomography (PET) scan technique have demonstrated a specific left temporo-parieto-occipital metabolic dysfunction, and Pavlovic (1990) has reported neuropsychological dysfunction in a similar region. Neuropsychological testing revealed dysfunction that was most severe in the left and right parieto-occipital regions followed by the left frontal, right temporal and right frontal areas. These results are consistent with the notion that the posterior associative zones are particularly sensitive to the lesions characteristic of Alzheimer's disease. Although macro- and microscopic lesions may be relatively lacking in these regions (Esiri, 1989), this is consistent with the widely held view of a general lack of correlation between functional and anatomical parameters.

The CFFT is undoubtedly a complex phenomenon. It appears to reflect CNS function rather than being related to a specific anatomical structure or structures and may be the 'final outcome' or response of many interconnected regions within the CNS. The CFFT appears to reflect, at least in part, occipital lobe function. Since this has been demonstrated to be one of the areas to be functionally affected in patients with Alzheimer's disease, it is reasonable to examine this measure more closely in this patient population.

Measurement of CFFT

Subthreshold intermittent light is perceived as flicker. If the frequency is gradually increased the flicker becomes gradually less distinct until it is no longer perceived. This point of fusion is known as the fusion threshold (ascending method). Alternatively, if the flickering is suprathreshold and is gradually decreased, the point at which flicker is perceived is known as the frequency threshold (descending method). These are variations of the continuous method of limits (Woodworth and Schlosberg, 1958). The mean of the ascending and descending thresholds is the CFFT (Curran, 1990).

CFFT in Normal Elderly Subjects

A number of studies have demonstrated a decline in CFFT with increasing age in normal elderly subjects, e.g. Schmidtke (1951) and McFarland *et al.* (1958). Curran *et al.* (1990) examined for the first time different aspects of CFFT in normal elderly subjects. The sample consisted of 644 normal elderly, community-based, general practice patients (age range 60–91 years, mean 71.29 ± 6.97 years). Although CFFT and the descending and ascending scores were not found to be significantly correlated with age, the CFFT and descending scores did decrease as a trend, confirming a recent report by Coleston and Hindmarch (1989). This lack of a significant relationship is probably due to the narrow age range investigated. If the age range had been wider, it is likely that the trend would have become a significant relationship, as demonstrated by a number of different studies, e.g. McFarland *et al.* (1958). However, the difference (ascending – descending scores) was found to be significantly and negatively correlated with age. Most of this change can be explained by a fall in the descending scores with increasing age, as there was no change in the ascending scores with increasing age.

It was also demonstrated in this study that the descending scores were significantly greater than the ascending scores. This is in agreement with a number of other studies reviewed by Curran (1990).

Patients with DSM-III-R (APA, 1987) criteria for primary degenerative dementia of the Alzheimer's type [PDDAT] were then investigated (Curran *et al.*, 1991). Patients were all classified as mild-moderate (DSM-III-R) and were matched with volunteers of equal age, sex and occupational class (age range 67–89 years, mean 81.7 ± 6.05 years). Both the CFFT and the descending scores were able to distinguish between normals and patients with PDDAT at a high level of statistical significance. Sixty five per cent of patients had CFFT scores below 1.96 SD of the volunteer CFFT mean, and 85% of patients had descending scores below 1.96 SD of the volunteer descending mean. Ascending scores were unable to differentiate between the two groups. In addition, the descending scores in the patient group were significantly lower than the ascending scores. This represents a reversal of the situation in normal elderly subjects. Since the ascending scores are not significantly different in the two groups, it appears that one of the features of patients with PDDAT is a large reduction in the sensitivity of the CNS to suprathreshold flicker. This observation is unlikely to be due to a shift in response criterion or to the effects of increased reaction time, as one would expect the effect on both the ascending and descending thresholds to be equal rather than specific for the descending scores.

The CFFT and the descending scores have been demonstrated to possess a high diagnostic utility. These two measures may be candidates for the longitudinal assessment of normal elderly subjects and particularly those with borderline Alzheimer's disease. It is suggested that patients developing the condition would have a much greater and more rapid fall in the CFFT and especially the descending score. The identification of early cases of Alzheimer's disease is one of the major challenges in the field. The use of simple measures such as those described may provide a cheap and easily administered test for patient assessment. However, before undertaking such a project it would be necessary to establish, as a minimum, the reliability and validity of the technique. These areas are currently being evaluated by the author.

Implications for Alzheimer's Disease Research

Drug development in the field of dementia is time consuming and expensive, especially at the clinical trial stage. The use of animals during early drug development is not without its problems (Leonard, 1989). In addition, there is growing concern about ethical issues and the validity of animal models of human disease. Volunteer studies suffer from the disadvantage that a therapeutic compound is examined in a normal subject. Failure to demonstrate an efficacious effect may be due to inappropriate or insensitive tests, a lack of drug effect or because the individual is already functioning maximally. Administration of a therapeutic compound might fail to improve what is already 'normal'.

One solution to this problem is the use of volunteer models with artificially induced deficits in psychological function. Two models which have been examined include techniques to disrupt memory function. This has been achieved using either a benzodiazepine, e.g. flunitrazepam (Bhatti and Hindmarch, 1987), or scopolamine (e.g. Brazell *et al.*, 1989). Although memory impairment is one aspect of Alzheimer's disease, it is by no means the only problem seen in this complex syndrome.

Fagan and Deary (1989) examined the effects of 40% nitrous oxide on CFFT in normal young volunteers. A selective reduction in the descending scores was demonstrated, but no effect on the ascending scores was found. Since it has been demonstrated that one of the features of Alzheimer's disease (PDDAT) is a specific reduction in the descending threshold, it may be worth exploring the possible role of nitrous oxide as an additional model of Alzheimer's disease in volunteer studies. More extensive use of volunteer models would probably increase the possibility of identifying a suitable therapeutic agent and at an earlier stage.

Conclusion

Patient samples need to be clearly defined and the choice of test should be relevant to the psychological function under consideration. Large numbers of tests should be avoided to reduce the risk of identifying significant results by chance.

It is necessary for psychopharmacologists to develop reliable, valid and pharmaco-sensitive tests for the evaluation of anti-dementia agents. Psychometric tests developed in young healthy volunteers will need to be reexamined before they can be used with confidence in patients with Alzheimer's disease.

The CFFT is probably one of the most suitable measures available for this purpose. It has been demonstrated to be age sensitive and to have a high diagnostic utility in patients with Alzheimer's disease. It may also have a useful role in monitoring the cognitive progress of borderline cases of Alzheimer's disease and thus contribute to our understanding of the natural history of this syndrome.

References

Anastasi, I. (1988) *Psychological Testing*, 6th edn. New York: Macmillan Publishing Company.

APA (1987) *Diagnostic and Statistical Manual of Mental Disorders*, third edition (revised). Washington, D.C.: American Psychiatric Association.

Bhatti, J. Z. and Hindmarch, I. (1987) Vinpocetine effects on cognitive impairments produced by flunitrazepam. *Int. Clin. Psychopharmacol.*, 2(4), 325–31.

Botwinik, J. (1973) *Cognitive Processes in Maturity and Old Age*. New York: Springer.

Botwinik, J. and Storandt, M. (1974) Cardiovascular status, depressive affect and other factors in reaction time. *J. Gerontol.*, **29**, 343–8.

Brazell, C., Preston, G. C., Ward, C., Lines, C. R. and Traub, M. (1989) The scopolamine model of dementia: chronic transdermal administration. *J. Psychopharmacol.*, 3, 76–82.

Brayne, C. and Calloway, P. (1988) Normal ageing, impaired cognitive function and senile dementia of the Alzheimer's type: a continuum? *Lancet*, **ii**, 1265–6.

Brown, B. W. and Hollander, M. (1977) *Statistics: A Biomedical Introduction*. New York: John Wiley and Sons.

Busse, E. W. (1978) Duke longitudinal study I: senescence and senility. In: Katzman, R., Terry, R. D. and Bick, K. L. (eds) *Alzheimer's Disease: Senile Dementia and Related Disorders*, pp. 59–68. New York: Raven Press.

Coleston, D. M. and Hindmarch, I. (1989) Critical flicker fusion threshold (CFFT) and choice reaction time (CRT) in psychopharmacological research of aging. *J. Psychopharmacol.*, 3(4), 55p.

Copeland, J. R. M. (1987) The diagnosis of dementia in old age. In: Pitt, B. (ed.) *Dementia*, pp. 52–68. Edinburgh: Churchill Livingstone.

Craik, F. I. M. (1979) Human memory. *Annu. Rev. Psychol.*, **30**, 63–102.

Cull, C. A. and Trimble, M. R. (1987) Automated testing in psychopharmacology. In: Hindmarch, I. and Stonier, P. D. (eds) *Human Psychopharmacology: Measures and Methods*, Vol. 2, pp. 113–53. Chichester: John Wiley and Sons.

Curran, S. (1990) Critical flicker fusion techniques in psychopharmacology. In: Hindmarch, I. and Stonier, P. D. (eds) *Human Psychopharmacology: Measures and Methods*, Vol. 3, pp. 21–38. Chichester: John Wiley and Sons.

Curran, S. and Wattis, J. P. (1989) Round-up: searching for the cause of Alzheimer's disease. *Geriatr. Med.*, **19**(3), 13–14.

Curran, S., Wattis, J. P., Shillingford, C. and Hindmarch, I. (1990) Critical flicker fusion in normal elderly subjects; a cross-sectional community study. *Curr. Psychol. Res. Rev.*, **9**, 25–34.

Curran, S., Wattis, J. P., Shillingford, C. and Hindmarch, I. (1991) Critical flicker fusion in primary degenerative dementia of the Alzheimer's type: Clinical implications. *Curr. Psychol. Res. Rev.*, in press.

Deary, I. J. and Whalley, L. J. (1988) Recent research on the causes of Alzheimer's disease. *BMJ*, **297**, 807–10.

Esiri, M. M. (1989) Patterns of cortical and subcortical pathology in Alzheimer's disease. In: Davies, D. C. (ed.) *Alzheimer's Disease: Towards an Understanding of the Aetiology and Pathogenesis*, pp. 33–41. London: John Libbey.

Fagan, D. and Deary, I. (1989) A study of the influence of artificial pupils in the use of the critical flicker fusion test to detect CNS depression due to nitrous oxide. *J. Psychopharmacol.*, 3, 99p.

Folstein, M. F., Folstein, S. E. and McHugh, P. R. (1975) 'Mini-Mental State'. A practical method for grading the cognitive state of patients for the clinician. *J. Psychiatr. Res.*, **12**, 189–98.

Giaquinto, S. (1988) *Ageing and the Nervous System*, pp. 207–17. Chichester: John Wiley and Sons.

Guilford, J. P. and Fruchter, B. (1978) *Fundamental Statistics in Psychology and Education*, 6th edn. Tokyo: McGraw Hill.

Hamilton, M. (1987) Assessment of psychopathology. In: Hindmarch, I. and Stonier, P. D. (eds) *Human Psychopharmacology: Measures and Methods*, Vol. 1, pp. 1–17. Chichester: John Wiley and Sons.

Hindmarch, I. (1982) Critical flicker fusion frequency (CFFF): the effects of psychotropic compounds. *Pharmacopsychiatria*, **15**(1, suppl.) 44–8.

Hindmarch, I. and Stonier, P. D. (eds) (1987) *Human Psychopharmacology: Measures and methods*, Vol. 1. Chichester: John Wiley and Sons.

Hindmarch, I. and Stonier, P. D. (1989) *Human Psychopharmacology: Measures and Methods*, Vol. 2. Chichester: John Wiley and Sons.

Hindmarch, I. and Wattis, J. P. (1988) Measuring effects of psychotropic drugs. In: Wattis, J. P. and Hindmarch, I. (eds) *Psychological Assessment of the Elderly*, pp. 180–97. Edinburgh: Churchill Livingstone.

Hindmarch, I., Aufdembrinke, B. and Ott, H. (1988) *Psychopharmacology and Reaction Time*. Chichester: John Wiley and Sons.

Hodkinson, H. M. (1972) Evaluation of a mental test score for assessment of mental impairment in the elderly. *Age Ageing*, **1**, 233–8.

Kendall, M. (1987) Drugs for dementia. In: Pitt, B. (ed.) *Dementia*, pp. 265–80. Edinburgh: Churchill Livingstone.

Leonard, B. E. (1989) From animals to man: advantages, problems and pitfalls of animal models in psychopharmacology. In: Hindmarch, I. and Stonier, P. D. (eds) *Human Psychopharmacology: Measures and Methods*, Vol. 2, pp. 23–66. Chichester: John Wiley and Sons.

Marterer, A., Fischer, P. and Danielczyk, W. (1990) Gerstmann's syndrome in dementia of Alzheimer's type and multi-infarct dementia. *Proceedings of the III International Brain Workshop: Neurodevelopment, Aging and Cognition*, Dubrovnik, Yugoslavia, p. 22.

McFarland, R. A., Warren, A. B. and Karis, C. (1958) Alterations in critical flicker fusion as a function of age. *J. Exp. Psychol.*, **56**, 26–32.

McGhie, A., Chapman, J. and Lawson, J. S. (1965) Changes in immediate memory with age. *Br. J. Psychol.*, **56**, 69–75.

Nevo, B. (1985) Face validity revisited. *J. Educ. Measurement*, **22**, 287–93.

Nevo, B. and Sfez, J. (1985) Examinees' feedback questionnaires. *Assess. Eval. Higher Educ.*, **10**, 236–49.

Ott, H. and Kranda, K. (1982) *Flicker Techniques in Psychopharmacology*. Weinheim, Basel: Beltz Verlag.

Pavlovic, D. (1990) Visual perception in dementia of Alzheimer type. *Proceedings of III International Brain Workshop: Neurodevelopment, Aging and Cognition*, Dubrovnik, Yugoslavia, p. 23.

Schmidtke, H. (1951) Uber die Messung der psychischen ermudung mit Hilfe des Flimmertest. *Psychol. Forsch.*, **23**, 409–63.

Siegfried, K. (1985) Cognitive symptoms in late-life depression and their treatment. *J. Affective Disord.*, **1** (suppl.), 33–40.

Siegfried, K., Jansen, W. and Pahnke, K. (1984) Cognitive dysfunction in depression. *Drug Dev. Res.*, **4**, 533–53.

Smith, J. M. and Misiak, H. (1976) Critical flicker fusion (CFF) and psychotropic drugs in normal human subjects – a review. *Psychopharmacology*, **47**, 175–82.

Soininen, H. (1983) Electroencephalographic signs of senile dementia. *Geriatr. Med. Today*, **2**(10), 39–47.

Turner, P. (1968) Critical flicker frequency and centrally acting drugs. *Br. J. Ophthalmol.*, **52**, 245–50.

U'Ren, R. C. (1987) History of the concept of dementia. In: Pitt, B. (ed.) *Dementia*, pp. 1–18. Edinburgh: Churchill Livingstone.

Vingoe, F. J. (1981) *Clinical Psychology and Medicine: An Interdisciplinary Approach*. Oxford: Oxford University Press.

Walsh, D. A. (1976) Age differences in central perceptual processing: a dichoptic backward masking investigation. *J. Gerontol.*, **31**, 178–85.

Woods, R. (1982) The psychology of ageing: assessment of deficits and their management. In: Levy, R. and Post, F. (eds) *The Psychiatry of Late Life*, pp. 68–113. Oxford: Blackwell Scientific Publications.

Woodworth, R. S. and Schlosberg, H. (1958) *Experimental Psychology*. London: Methuen.

15

The Assessment of Quality of Life in Nootropic Drug Research: Some Questions

*Walter Deberdt and †Anne Brems

*UCB-Pharmaceutical Sector, Braine L'Alleud, Belgium and
†Pasteelsblokweg 3, Kessel-Lo, Belgium

Introduction

Since the World Health Organization defined health as 'a state of complete physical, mental and social well-being and not as the absence of disease and disability' (WHO, 1948) and as 'a level of the individual's satisfactory functioning on each of the basic dimensions of health: physical, mental, social and economical activities of daily living' (WHO, 1984), a lot of research has been done. Numerous measures have been used, and a variety of studies have been done on the multidimensional impacts of disease on the sick (Greenwald, 1987). In the case of quality of life in the elderly population, there are some questions concerning the concept of health, the approaches to investigating health and the problems of assessment in clinical and epidemiological practice (Kozarevic and Israël, 1987) which need to be answered.

In psychogeriatrics, and more particularly in the assessment of nootropics, there are two specific reasons why we should look beyond the effect on symptoms and disease:

1. Dementia and cerebral ageing lead essentially to pathological or problematic behaviour, and many aspects of this behaviour are affected in a very complex way. A therapeutic effect on a symptom does not indicate how much 'daily life' functioning has improved, neither does it indicate whether the improvement is satisfactory for the patient himself.

Dementia: Molecules, Methods and Measures. Edited by I. Hindmarch, H. Hippius and G. K. Wilcock
© 1991 John Wiley & Sons Ltd

2. The socioeconomic benefit of a medical treatment must be known. Again, functional capacities of the patient determine the physical and mental burden for his social environment and so they determine also the cost-benefit ratio for the society.

In this chapter we will discuss the concept of quality of life in its individual and intra-individual meanings and try to evaluate some corresponding efforts to assess quality of life. We will then consider some of the questions and solutions concerning the assessment of quality of life in the clinical research on nootropics.

The Inter- and Intra-individual Dimensions of Quality of Life

Looking at the concept of quality of life in its most extensive meaning, we can distinguish four aspects. Even if one could consider quality of life as a purely subjective matter, the actual functional capacities would be critical in the discussion. Speaking about quality of life, it is necessary to consider:

1. The individual dimension, or the level of coping abilities of the patient.
2. The inter-individual dimension, or the level of autonomy or dependency.

Furthermore, both dimensions contain subjective and objective parameters.

Table 1 shows some examples of instruments testing the four extreme aspects of the quality of life of the patient and his surroundings. It must be mentioned that, even if this description of quality of life seems rather extensive, the notion is distinct from concepts like 'life satisfaction' or 'adjustment'. Satisfaction as a purely subjective feeling has been interpreted and elaborated in the form of questionnaires, evaluating happiness, life satisfaction and morale (Neugarten *et al.*, 1961; Wood *et al.*, 1969; Wiendieck, 1969; Löhr and Walter, 1974). The fact that in these instruments present happiness, satisfaction with the past and future-orientated morale are mixed, makes them useless for clinical research. Moreover, the authors discarded from their questionnnaires any allusion to a practical life situation or a functional capacity.

'Adjustment' is another frequently used notion in this context (Barrabee *et al.*, 1955; Katz *et al.*, 1963; Linn, 1967). With the exception of the scale of Linn, which measures personal satisfaction and self-fulfilment, the notion of adjustment also points to a social normative concept. This mixture of individual and subjective parameters with social and objective parameters should be avoided in clinical research, otherwise the specificity

Table 1. Common assessment of the four aspects of quality of life

	Subjective aspect	Objective aspect
Individual aspect (coping)	Life Satisfaction Index (Neugarten *et al.*, 1961)	Performance Test of ADL (Kuriansky and Gurland, 1976)
Inter-individual aspect (autonomy/dependency)	Zarit Burden Scale (Zarit *et al.* 1980)	Health Care Costs (Coughlin and Liu, 1989)
	Caregiving Hassles Scale (Kinney and Parris Stephens, 1989)	

and sensitivity of the individual point of view would be lost and there could be a lack of hard facts to calculate the social burden the mental deterioration is causing.

Cognitive measures such as the Mini-Mental State Examination (MMSE) (Folstein *et al.*, 1975) can be considered to be an example of objective individual coping capacities. Another example is the activities of daily living (ADL) test of Kuriansky and Gurland (1976), which is also a real performance test, not a rating scale like the well-known instrumental ADL (IADL)-PSMS (Physical Self-Maintenance Scale) scales of Lawton and Brody (1969). ADL scales would be situated more to the subjective side of the diagram in Table 1, as there are always some subjective appreciations that slip into the scoring of a scale.

The other aspect of quality of life, the inter-individual one, can be described as the level of autonomy or dependency of the patient with regard to his environment. Zarit *et al.* (1980, 1986) used the Zarit Burden Scale to study the changes over time for caregivers of dementia patients cared for at home. Subsequent nursing home placement was more strongly associated with subjective factors (caregivers perceived burden) than with the objective cognitive and functional capacities of the patients.

Finally, we come to the assessment of the objective inter-individual or social parameters. An example of this is a recent study by Coughlin and Liu (1989) assessing the health care costs of older patients with cognitive impairments.

One could question in this overview of Quality of Life assessment the position and role of the multitude of observation rating scales, such as the GRS (Geriatric Rating Scale) (Plutchick *et al.*, 1970), the Sandoz Clinical Assessment-Geriatric (SCAG) (Shader *et al.*, 1974), the GBS (Gottfries-Bräne-Steen Scale) (Gottfries *et al.*, 1982), etc. These kinds of scales assess more or less globally or specifically the dementia syndrome, and not the suffering of the patient or the social burden. Although most of the items are relevant to the measurement of the well-being of the patient and his surroundings, these instruments do not aim to and do not assess quality of life.

In most instances researchers are interested in the global level of the quality of life: social and cognitive functioning, IADL, mood, physical status and complaints, and financial possibilities and worries. However, it can be worthwhile to study the consequences of an intervention in a specific and more detailed aspect of human functioning. Brendemühl *et al.* (1988) found a significant difference in the results of the orientation task for elderly drivers after a 6-week piracetam treatment compared with placebo. That such a difference has consequences for daily life, more specifically for car accidents involving elderly drivers, is obvious.

Assessment of the Quality of Life in Clinical Research

A lot of parameters and corresponding assessment instruments may give a global or specific idea of quality of life. The problem of assessment in clinical research comes, however, from the multitude of independent variables interfering with the drug effect. Some particular aspects of the clinical research on nootropics make it especially difficult:

1. At the behavioural level, the development of the deterioration is slow and chronic. For instance, in a double-blind study on 39 elderly outpatients with a mean MMSE score of 22 we observed over a period of 12 weeks not the slightest change on the IADL-PSMS scale of Lawton and Brody (1969) in neither the treated group nor the

placebo group. In this kind of population, still living in the community, it is necessary to do a long-term follow-up. However, there is then a high risk of other independent variables, such as other concomitant diseases, other drug treatments, and changes in the social, emotional or physical surrounding of the patient, interfering with the drug effect.

2. In elderly patients there is an important heterogeneity of pathology and deterioration rate. About 30% of the clinical diagnoses in severely demented patients are contradicted by the autopsy (Chan-Palay, 1990, personal communication; Wilcock, 1990, Chapter 5). Cerebrovascular dementia may appear to be Alzheimer's disease or mixed, and vice versa. So it is an illusion to believe we could know, when selecting mildly deteriorated patients, which pathology has been treated and, *a fortiori*, what will be the spontaneous deterioration rate of an individual patient. Yesavage *et al.* (1988) found significant changes over a period of 1 year using the Alzheimer Disease Assessment Scale (ADAS) (Rosen *et al.*, 1984), the MMSE and the Brief Cognitive Rating Scale and Global Deterioration Scale (BCRS-GDS) (Reisberg *et al.*, 1983) in 30 Alzheimer patients with a mean MMSE score of 16.5. However, the inter-individual variation in these changes (SD) was at least as high as the mean change itself.

3. Actual problems in the daily life functioning of people with mild deterioration may vary a lot from one person to another, depending on social class, individual interests, sex and sex-linked expectations, premorbid intelligence and functioning, social microenvironment, availability of formal and informal home-care, concomitant chronic disease, etc.

From the nature of the problems and from the difficulties of assessment, it is clear that solutions should not be sought solely in other, better or newer assessment instruments.

First, it must be clear what the researcher wants to obtain. Quality of life could mean everything, but it is impossible to study and assess everything. If the goal of a study is to convince the authorities of the refund of a product, it is logical to focus on the costs of care and on the benefits brought by the treatment. In this context, we developed the Home Care Registration, that gives a good indication of the patient's need of help and of the kind and quantity of help the patient actually gets from his environment, volunteer and professional caregivers (Figure 1). The scale provides the objective number of hours of help, using a conversion chart for that kind of help that is more difficult to quantify.

Second, totally different from this objective, social point of view, is the question of whether the treatment is worthwhile for the patient, whether the improvement in attention, memory or psychomotor functioning is perceived and appreciated by the patient in daily life functioning. This question is pertinent in mildly deteriorated patients or patients with age-related memory impairment. Even if the used test battery has high face validity, for example the computerized testing of Larrabee and Crook (1988), the question of the problem of content validity remains. As indicated before, the researcher is confronted with a multitude of what could be important problems for the individual patient.

One solution to this problem of heterogeneity could be the use of a battery of rating scales, covering more or less all dimensions of life quality. However, a change in a few items, important for that particular patient, will get completely lost in the variability generated by the multitude of other items. A structured interview during which all

HOME—CARE REGISTRATION

PATIENT:name:.................................nr:...............

Rated by:.................................Date:..........

	NEED OF HELP	HELP: kind,hours a week				OTHER AIDS COMMENTS
		professional kind	hours	volunteer kind	hours	
1.bathing	0 1 2 3					
2.washing face and hands	0 1 2 3					
3.hairdressing and shaving	0 1 2 3					
4.getting dressed,undressed	0 1 2 3					
5.toileting	0 1 2 3					
6.taking medication	0 1 2 3					
7.daily care	0 1 2 3					
8.walking (inside)	0 1 2 3					
9.mobility (outside)	0 1 2 3					
10.exercises	0 1 2 3					
11.shopping	0 1 2 3					
12.food preparation	0 1 2 3					
13.eating	0 1 2 3					
14.daily housekeeping	0 1 2 3					
15.cleaning	0 1 2 3					
16.laundry	0 1 2 3					
17.jobs in/around the house	0 1 2 3					
18.financial administration	0 1 2 3					
19.social activities	0 1 2 3					
TOTAL NEED OF HELP		TOTAL HOURS PROF.HELP		TOTAL HOURS VOL.HELP		

0:no help ; 1:supporting help ; 2:partial help ; 3:complete help
registration of hours: total hours per week.

Figure 1. Home-care registration

dimensions are discussed with the patient could be a better solution. For each item the patient would be asked whether it is a relevant problem and how much distress it is causing. In each section the interviewer should have the possibility to add a specific problem of the patient that was not mentioned in the checklist. The restriction of such an instrument is that the individual's subjective opinion can only be asked of mildly deteriorated patients.

However, all these reliable and valid instruments cannot prevent the necessity of following the patient for a long time, at least 6 months, to see the effect of the treatment on parameters such as institutionalization rate. A solution could be to enhance learning and adaptation processes by providing not only a cognition enhancer but also a stimulating environment, for example memory training groups. A double-blind placebo-controlled trial with a 12-week piracetam treatment performed in this way appeared to be successful (Israël, 1990).

Concerning the heterogeneity of the pathology and the deterioration rate, a few possibilities could be considered. Even when objective, internationally accepted selection criteria are used, when patients with a certain well-defined deterioration level are selected and when the study population is stratified according to premorbid intelligence, social situation, etc., the variability remains high. The variability caused by the placebo effect and the effect of the care-taking could be diminished by a wash-out period of 3–4 weeks before starting active treatment. But the problem of some patients being quite stable and others showing a rapid decline still remains. The number of patients should be reasonably high, but it is very difficult to set up a trial of more than 200 outpatients, and even a study with 100 patients is a big undertaking. Perhaps the opposite study design, a kind of single case orientated design, could provide a solution.

Patients could be followed for cognitive decline with sensitive psychometric measures for 3 to 6 months. They then receive active treatment for another 6 months, and at the end the results on whatever parameter could be analysed in view of the individual rate of decline measured during the first period. The spontaneous deterioration rate during the second period could differ from the first period, but it is necessary to at least know whether the patient was really declining or not. Otherwise, a clear therapeutic effect on a few rapidly deteriorating patients could be masked by a majority of patients that would never change just because of their chronic, nearly normal, progression of age-related problems.

Finally, the problem with the assessment of the quality of life in nootropic drug research is not to find the appropriate tool of measuring, but to detect, neutralize or avoid a multitude of factors interfering with quality of life. As one cannot stop life going on, and as quality of life assessment is supposed to pick up all that noise of daily living, it seems that there is no clear solution; a lot of preparatory research must be done and conclusions and generalizations must be handled with the most precaution.

References

Barrabee, R., Barrabee, E. L. and Finesinger, J. F. (1955) A normative social adjustment scale. *Am. J. Psychiatry*, **112**, 252–9.
Brendemühl, D., Schmidt, U. and Schenk, N. (1988) Driving behaviour of elderly motorists in standardized test runs road traffic conditions. In: Rothengatter, J. A. and de Bruin, R. A. (eds) *Road User Behaviour: Theory and Research*, pp. 310–8. Maastricht: Van Gorcum.
Coughlin, T. A. and Liu, K. (1989) Health care costs of older persons with cognitive impairments. *Gerontologist*, **29**(2), 173–82.
Folstein, M. F., Folstein, S. E. and McHugh, P. R. (1975) 'Mini-Mental state': A practical method for grading cognitive state of patients for the clinician. *J. Psychiatr. Res.*, **12**, 189–98.
Gottfries, C. G., Bräne, G. and Steen, G. (1982) A new rating scale for dementia syndromes. *Gerontology*, **28**(2), 20–30.

Greenwald, H. P. (1987) The specificity of quality-of-life measures among the seriously ill. *Med. Care*, **25**, 642–51.

Israël, L. (1990) Communication at the symposium on piracetam. *Hellenic Association of Neurology and The Foundation Ciencia y Medicina*, Athens, 29th April.

Katz, S., Ford, A. B., Moskowitz, R. W., Jackson, B. and Jaffe, M. (1963) Studies of illness in the aged – The index of ADL. *JAMA*, **185**, 94–9.

Kinney, J. M. and Parris Stephens, M. A. (1989) Caregiving Hassles Scale: Assessing the daily hassles of caring for a family member with dementia. *Gerontologist*, **29**, 328–32.

Kozarevic, D. J. and Israël, L. (1987) Disabilities and the level of affected activities of daily living. *Rev. Epidemiol. Sante Publique*, **35**, 248–56.

Kuriansky, J. and Gurland, B. (1976) The performance test of activities of daily living. *Int. J. Aging Hum. Dev.*, **7**, 343–52.

Larrabee, G. J. and Crook, T. (1988) A computerised everyday memory battery for assessing treatment effects. *Psychopharmacol. Bull.*, **24**(4), 695–7.

Lawton, M. P. and Brody, E. M. (1969) Assessment of older people: self maintaining and instrumental activities of daily living. *Gerontologist*, **9**, 179–86.

Linn, M. W. (1967) A rapid disability rating scale. *J. Am. Geriatr. Soc.*, **15**(2), 211–4.

Löhr, G. and Walter, A. (1974) Die LZ-Skala. Zur Erfassung der subjektiven Lebenszufriedenheit im Alter. *Diagnostica*, **20**(2), 83–91.

Neugarten, B. L., Havighurst, R. J. and Tobin, S. S. (1961) The measurement of life satisfaction. *J. Gerontol.*, **16**, 134–43.

Plutchik, R., Lieberman, M., Bakur, M., Grossman, J. and Lehrman, N. (1970) Reliability and validity of a scale for assessing the functioning of geriatric patients. *J. Am. Geriatr. Soc.*, **18**(6), 491–500.

Reisberg, B., Schneck, M. K., Ferris, S. H., Schwartz, G. E. and deLeon, M. J. (1983) The brief cognitive rating scale (BCRS): findings in primary degenerative dementia (PDD). *Psychopharmacol. Bull.*, **19**, 47.

Rosen, F. L., Mohs, R. C. and Davis, K. L. (1984) A new rating scale for Alzheimer's disease. *Am. J. Psychiatry*, **141**, 11.

Shader, R. I., Harmatz, J. S. and Salzman, C. (1974) A new scale for clinical assessment in geriatric populations: Sandoz Clinical Assessment-Geriatric (SCAG). *J. Am. Geriatr. Soc.*, **22**(3), 107–13.

WHO (1948) *Constitution of the World Health Organization. Basic Documents*, 15th edn. Geneva: World Health Organization.

WHO (1984) Scientific Group on the Epidemiology of Aging: The uses of epidemiology in the study of the elderly. *Technical Report Series*, No. 706.

Wiendieck, G. (1969) Entwicklung einer Skala zur Messung der Lebenszufriedenheit im höheren Lebensalter. *Z. Gerontol.*, **3**(3), 215–24.

Wood, V., Wyllie, M. L. and Schaefor, B. (1969) An analysis of a short self-report measure of life satisfaction. *J. Gerontol.*, **4**, 465–9.

Yesavage, J. A., Poulsen, S. L., Sheikh, J. and Tanke, E. (1988) Rates of change of common measures of impairment in senile dementia of the Alzheimer's type. *Psychopharmacol. Bull.*, **24**, 531–4.

Zarit, S. H., Reever, K. E. and Bach-Peterson, J. (1980) Relatives of the impaired elderly: correlates of feelings of burden. *Gerontologist*, **20**, 649–55.

Zarit, S. H., Todd, P. A. and Zarit, M. J. (1986) Subjective burden of husbands and wives as caregivers: a longitudinal study. *Gerontologist*, **26**, 260–6.

16

Intrusion Errors in Dementia:
A New Look at an Old Measure

Thomas Lorscheid and Sharon Thompson

*Clinical Research Department, F. Hoffmann-La Roche AG,
Basel, Switzerland*

In 1974 Drachman and Leavitt published their influential study on the cognitive impairment observed in normal volunteers treated with the anti-muscarinic agent scopolamine. One of the tasks administered to assess the detrimental effects of scopolamine required the subjects to generate words within a given category (e.g. birds). The authors reported that over half the subjects intruded words that did not belong to the given category. This was the first study that documented the occurrence of intrusion errors in subjects who were cognitively impaired as a result of a cholinergic deficit. In the following decade research in dementia began to look for the occurrence of intrusion errors, and morphological data confirmed that there was a strong relationship between senile plaque counts (i.e. the severity of the dementia) and the frequency of intrusions. In the past several years, however, research has nearly forgotten this very important sign of dementia.

In this chapter we will discuss the cholinergic hypothesis of memory functioning and its relationship to intrusion errors. Behavioural data from demented patients and scopolamine-impaired normal subjects, and morphological data from patients with Alzheimer's disease (AD), support the claim that there is a link between the incidence of intrusion errors in demented patients and the dysfunction of the cholinergic system. We will then discuss the hypothesis that the dysphasia observed in demented patients is the result of a loss of semantic distinctions causing related items to become interchangeable. This hypothesis was tested in patients with a major depressive episode (DSM-III; APA, 1980) and varying degrees of cognitive impairment using a new task that systematically measures intrusion errors. The frequency of intrusion errors was compared in patients classified as primarily demented or primarily depressed. The chapter closes with a discussion of the results of this study, and of the practical and theoretical relevance of such a task.

The Link to the Cholinergic Hypothesis

In 1973 behavioural data suggested that the cholinergic system may be critically involved in human memory functioning (Crow and Grove-White, 1973). This cholinergic hypothesis has since received wide support from both behavioural and neuropathological data. In particular, AD, known for its prominent clinical symptom of widespread memory loss, has been linked to a deficit of the cholinergic system in a multitude of publications (see Brinkman and Gershon, 1983 for review).

Crow and Grove-White (1973) studied the effect of the cholinergic blocker scopolamine on memory processes. They found that scopolamine produces a specific impairment of memory processes that cannot be accounted for by attentional disorders. The impairment observed in normal individuals under the effects of a cholinergic blocker has since been described as similar to the impairment in elderly patients with signs of memory loss (Drachman and Leavitt, 1974). The majority of the research into the effects of scopolamine in healthy young adults has supported the conclusion that the drug produces a memory deficit that is specifically related to its anti-cholinergic properties, because these effects on memory cannot be reversed by subsequent amphetamine administration (Drachman, 1977).

Other evidence for a connection between the cholinergic system and memory processes comes from studies with drugs that enhance cholinergic functioning. Agents such as physostigmine (an anti-cholinesterase drug that inhibits the breakdown of acetylcholine) and arecoline (a cholinomimetic drug that acts directly on the cholinergic receptors) have been found to have variable enhancement effects on human memory (Davis *et al.*, 1982). This enhancement appears to be a specific effect on the ability to store new information in the long-term memory (LTM), but not on the ability to retrieve information from the LTM or on the short-term memory. This is critical because a sign of AD is a deficit in the encoding of new information into the LTM (Miller, 1975).

A study by Rusted and Warburton (1989) found that scopolamine may disrupt the organization of verbal material at input so that, even though items may be durably stored, they are not accessible during free recall. Some of the results that led to this conclusion came from a recognition task. There was not a significant change in the number of correct responses after scopolamine administration, suggesting that because the items could be correctly identified during recognition, they had in fact been stored. In addition, scopolamine-treated subjects accepted more of the distractor items as target items. In other words, there was a significant increase in false alarms after treatment with scopolamine.

Is there, therefore, an encoding dysfunction linked to a cholinergic deficit that can be measured by intrusion errors? Behavioural data from three types of research suggest that this is indeed a plausible hypothesis. First, intrusion errors are one of the most reliable symptoms of AD patients (Gainotti *et al.*, 1989). In a study by Fuld (1983), word intrusions were observed in 88% of patients with a neurological diagnosis of AD. Fuld also reported that intrusions occurred even in patients without severe memory impairment or language problems, suggesting that intrusions are not a consequence of other functional impairments but of the AD-related changes. Second, intrusion errors and similar errors (i.e. false positive responses) are usually observed in animals following the administration of anti-cholinergic drugs (Gainotti *et al.*, 1989). This supports an older hypothesis that one of the main functions of the cholinergic system may be the inhibition of inappropriate responses and the reduction of interference effects (Miller, 1978). Third, a reduction in intrusion errors is a characteristic outcome of cholinergic drug administration in AD patients (Gainotti *et al.*, 1989). In a review of methods assessing memory in clinical trials, Brinkman and Gershon (1983) identify learning tasks that provide an index of intrusions as one of the most useful methods for detecting treatment effects. In several studies of cholinergic drug effects on memory dysfunction (e.g. Smith and Swash, 1979) the only significant treatment effect was in the reduction of intrusion errors.

According to Brinkman and Gershon (1983), 'the tendency of cholinomimetics to alter the number of intrusion errors is interesting, in view of the finding that intrusion errors may have been a relatively specific indicator of AD when diagnosis was verified at autopsy' (p. 143). Indeed, there are morphological data supporting the relationship of intrusion errors to the cholinergic system. In the study by Fuld (1983), intrusion errors were significantly associated with low choline acetyltransferase levels and high senile plaque counts when the diagnosis of AD was confirmed by autopsy findings. Fuld proposes that word intrusions may mirror the dysfunction of the cholinergic neurotransmitter system of the brain, because there is almost a one-to-one correlation between the amount of cholinesterase in the brain and the number of intrusions. Similarly, in a study of the effects of physostigmine and lecithin, the reduction in intrusion errors was highly correlated with a decrease in cholinesterase activity in the cerebrospinal fluid (Thal *et al.*, 1983). There is, therefore, both pharmacological and morphological evidence for a strong link between the functioning of the cholinergic system and the occurrence of intrusion errors.

This link provides a solid justification for examining intrusion errors in drug treatment studies. Most of the research in the field of dementia focuses on more direct assessments of memory (e.g. digit recall, face recall). The few studies that do consider intrusion errors have merely examined those that occurred during other tasks. For example, the most popular measure of intrusion errors comes from the category-retrieval task in which a subject is asked to name as many items as possible in a short time period from a specific category. An index of intrusions is determined by the number of inappropriate items (not belonging to the given category) that are named. While this method has been used with success in the past, given the importance of intrusion errors as explained above, there should be a more direct way to measure them. The measurement of intrusion errors has been unsystematic because there is not a task that is specifically designed to assess them. The Picture Recall and Recognition Task (PRRT) was designed with this in mind. Additionally, the previous method of assessing intrusion errors could require several hours of testing with a multitude of tasks. Fuld (1983) remarks that patients must be given sufficient opportunity to make intrusions, because the number of intrusions within each test was usually limited to only one or two. Rather than waiting for the spontaneous occurrence of intrusion errors, the PRRT attempts to provoke them in a time-economical manner. It was designed to systematically assess intrusion errors, thereby providing a sensitive and valid drug outcome measure.

The Dysphasia of Dementia

The language problems accompanying dementia are well known. Nominal aphasia is frequently reported in demented patients, and the degree of the naming difficulty may be a reliable indicator of the severity of the dementia (Skelton-Robinson and Jones, 1984). Originally naming errors were thought to be the result of a failure in recognition (Rochford, 1971), but more recent studies reporting that demented patients *can* in fact recognize objects they cannot name (Bayles, 1982) suggest that the problem is far more complex. Demented patients who are capable of describing the function of an object still tend to make dysphasic errors when trying to name it (Church and Wattis, 1988); for example, when asked for the name of the hands on a watch, a patient could identify the function (e.g. 'handles, showing the time') but make an error in naming the object (e.g. 'digitals') on a forced naming task (Church and Wattis, 1988, p. 158).

Two cases studies describing the language disorder in demented patients both arrive at the conclusion that there is a loss of semantic distinctions causing related items to merge into a single category. Schwartz *et al.* (1979) describe a patient who was not only unable to properly apply verbal labels to pictures in different categories (dogs, cats and birds), but was also unable to sort the pictures into their proper groups. Although the patient appeared to recognize the features that differentiated the categories, she did not utilize these features as criteria for the classification or identification of the items. The authors explained the dysfunction as a breakdown in the perceptual representation of knowledge, resulting in the loss of semantic distinctions. Similarly, Warrington (1975) reported that general aspects of meaning were preserved (e.g. superordinate class membership) in three demented patients, while more specific, distinguishing characteristics were not. For example, a patient could respond that a bee was an animal, but could not answer questions about its colour or size.

One explanation for the language deficit in dementia is that the demented patient has suffered a loss of semantic distinctions, leaving an incomplete set of features associated with a given label, which will therefore be applied indiscriminately to all items with a similar set of features. This parallels the pattern of errors that occurs during the acquisition of language in children. It has been suggested that in early stages of language development children overextend verbal labels because they do not yet know the relevance of the dimensions on which the two items differ (Clark, 1973). In other words, children have an incomplete set of semantic features associated with a verbal label. For example, a child has a set of features associated with the label 'daddy' that is incomplete, so when the child encounters another item, a different man, with the same features, the label 'daddy' is erroneously applied. This same pattern could be used to explain the naming deficit in dementing patients. If, in dementia, as Schwartz *et al.* (1979) hypothesize, a breakdown in the perceptual representation of knowledge occurs, one could predict that there would be a 'progressive loss of the semantic features which define reference terms; and that, moreover, this loss occurs systematically, with more specific, distinguishing features lost before more general ones' (Schwartz *et al.*, 1979, p. 285). Like the young child, the demented patient would then have an incomplete set of features associated with a label, and a name would therefore be applied indiscriminately to all items with a subset of features identical to this incomplete set. The indiscriminate labelling of items within a common category is the pattern reported in various studies of demented patients (Schwartz *et al.*, 1979).

If the language dysfunction seen in demented patients can be explained in terms of semantic distinctions, predictions can be made about the type of errors a demented patient would be most likely to make. If the information that distinguishes two semantically related items has been lost, these two items should be more readily interchanged. This leads to the hypothesis that on a recognition task a demented patient would more likely falsely accept a semantically related item than an unrelated item. It is this hypothesis that serves as the basis for the PRRT developed for the current study.

The PRRT

The PRRT yields five scores: measures of immediate recall, delayed recall and correct recognition, a measure of intrusion errors (i.e. false positive responses to semantically related distractors), and a measure of false alarms (i.e. false positive responses to semantically unrelated distractors). Hypotheses were made concerning each of these scores. It was predicted that demented patients would score significantly lower on the measures of working memory – delayed recall and correct recognition – than patients who were classified as depressed. This difference would be consistent with other reports of a deficit of the working memory in cognitively impaired subjects (see Rusted and Warburton, 1989 for review). Along these lines, no differences between patient groups were anticipated for immediate recall scores.

The main hypothesis of this study was that demented patients tend to make more false recognitions of semantically related distractor items than of unrelated items. Depressed patients should experience no loss of semantic distinctions, and, therefore, these patients should be no more likely to accept semantically related items than unrelated items. In other words, it was predicted that there would be a significant interaction between the condition of the patient (demented or depressed) and the type of error, with demented patients making a higher number of intrusion errors. These results would provide support for the theory that there is a loss of semantic distinctions in patients with cognitive decline that is related to the severity of the dementia. Because the majority of demented patients have AD (Brinkman and Gershon, 1983), this would also provide support for the link between the functioning of the cholinergic system and the occurrence of intrusion errors.

Methods

The subjects. In total, 207 patients were included in these analyses. All patients participated in an on-going, placebo-controlled, double-blind, multicentre trial of drug treatment effects on depression and cognitive symptoms with the monoamine oxidase A inhibitor moclobemide (Aurorix); only the baseline data from this study are considered here. Before entry into the study, all patients were required to meet general and psychiatric inclusion and exclusion criteria; males and females of all races between the ages of 60 and 90 years were eligible to participate either as in- or outpatients. All patients met the criteria for either major depressive episode, with additional cognitive deficits, or dementia, with depression (DSM-III; APA, 1980). This diagnosis was confirmed by a score of at least 6 on the Geriatric Depression Scale (Yesavage *et al.*, 1983), at least 15 on the first 17 items of the 24-item Hamilton Depression Scale (Hamilton, 1967), a score between 12 and 27 on the Mini-Mental State Examination (MMSE) (Folstein *et al.*, 1975), and a score above 8 for the first four items and above 40 for all 18 items of the Sandoz Clinical Assessment-Geriatric Scale (Shader *et al.*, 1974). Patients with specific physical impairments that could influence any of the assessments or with other psychiatric disorders were excluded from the study. Clinical details and outcomes of this study will be presented elsewhere (Baumhackl *et al.*, 1991; Hebenstreit *et al.*, 1991).

The average age of the subjects was 74 years, and the majority (81%) were female. According to DSM-III criteria, 97 patients were diagnosed by the treating physician as having dementia with depression and 107 were diagnosed as having a major depressive episode with cognitive deficits. (This data was missing for three patients.)

The materials. Three parallel forms of the PRRT were constructed to measure immediate recall, delayed recall and recognition. The pictures were taken from a set of standardized pictures (Snodgrass and Vanderwart, 1980) in a modified, colour version (Kessler *et al.*, 1987; drawings used with permission of the authors) and each form was matched on name agreement, image agreement, familiarity and visual complexity. They were designed in the following way: the recognition set of pictures contained the eight items presented during the learning period (target items), eight pictures which were identified as semantically related distractors and eight semantically unrelated pictures. For example, if a picture of a cigar was presented during the learning period, both this target item and a picture of a cigarette, the semantically related distractor, would be part of the recognition set.

The PRRT was designed to be an objective and sensitive measure of dementia that is easy to administer with only minimal training for the testing personnel and that is not too difficult to perform for even moderately demented patients.

The procedure. Before administering the picture recall and recognition test, the patient was informed that pictures would be shown to him which he should name and remember. The eight target items, each individually presented as a colour drawing on 21 cm × 15 cm white card, were shown to the patient one picture card after the other; the patient was asked to name each target item and the response was recorded. Immediately after all the cards were shown, the patient was asked to recall all the pictures he had seen (the maximum amount of time allowed was 30 s). For each picture it was noted whether it was recalled or not (the patient's designation was decisive for this). A finger-tapping task involving four 15 s trials was then performed. For the delayed recall task the patient was asked to name the objects that he could remember from the picture cards shown before (maximum amount of time allowed was 30 s). Again, the corresponding responses were recorded. A trail-making test then intervened. For the subsequently performed recognition task, the patient was told that a series of pictures would be shown to him of which some had been presented to him before. The patient was told to say for each picture whether he thought that he had already seen it before or not. Three scores were computed from the recognition task: the number of correct recognitions of the pictures that had been seen before, the number of intrusion errors and the number of false alarms.

Results

The patients were classified as either primarily demented or primarily depressed based on their score on the MMSE, divided around the median MMSE score of 20 (primarily

Table 1. Means [standard deviation] for PRRT scores of primarily demented and primarily depressed patients (*P* values indicate statistically significant differences between the groups)

Task	Primarily demented	Primarily depressed	$P \leq$
Immediate recall	4.2 [2.9]	4.8 [1.8]	n.s.
Delayed recall	1.9 [1.5]	3.8 [1.3]	0.001
Recognition	3.9 [2.9]	7.0 [1.7]	0.001
Intrusion errors	1.3 [1.6]	0.4 [0.8]	0.001
False alarms	0.6 [1.3]	0.2 [0.8]	n.s.

Note: n.s. = not significant.

demented ≤ 20, primarily depressed > 20). This classification had a high agreement with the physicians' diagnoses of dementia with depression or depression with cognitive deficits. The Kappa reliability statistic comparing the two methods of classification was highly significant ($K = 0.644$, $P \leq 0.0001$).

The data were analysed with one-way ANOVAs to detect differences in PRRT scores between those patients classified as primarily depressed and those classified as primarily demented. The means and standard deviations of the scores from each task for the primarily demented and primarily depressed patients are given in Table 1. There was no significant difference for immediate recall scores between the two patient groups [$F(1, 205) = 2.98$, n.s.], but the difference was highly significant for delayed recall scores [$F(1, 205) = 91.80$, $P \leq 0.001$] and for recognition scores [$F(1, 205) = 87.35$, $P \leq 0.001$]. These differences are illustrated in Figure 1. Additionally, the number of errors made were analysed with a repeated-measures two-way ANOVA to look for an interaction between the primary diagnosis of the patient (primarily depressed or primarily demented) and the repeated factor of type of error (intrusion error or false alarm). There was a significant main effect for both patient diagnosis, $F(1, 205) = 18.91$, $P \leq 0.001$, and type of error, $F(1, 205) = 19.44$, $P \leq 0.001$, and a significant interaction between diagnosis

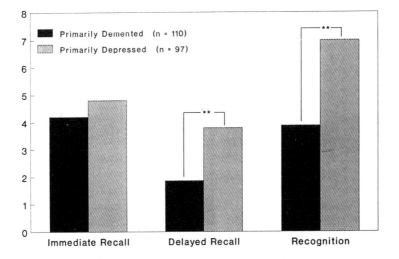

Figure 1. Average number of correct responses for immediate recall, delayed recall and recognition on the PRRT in primarily demented and primarily depressed patients (**indicates $P \leq 0.001$)

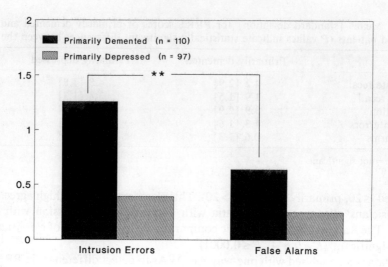

Figure 2. Average number of intrusion errors and false alarms on the PRRT in primarily demented and primarily depressed patients (**indicates $P \leq 0.001$)

and error type was also found $F(1, 205) = 7.61$, $P \leq 0.01$. Follow-up t-tests to determine the source of the interaction indicated a significant difference between the type of error for demented patients $(n = 110)(t = 4.21, P \leq 0.001)$ but not for depressed patients. This interaction is presented in Figure 2.

Discussion

As hypothesized, there were significant differences between the primarily demented and primarily depressed patients for delayed recall and correct recognition scores, but not for immediate recall scores. These results are in agreement with previous findings that the deficit in dementia is of the working memory (see Miller, 1975). The results also indicate that, generally, primarily depressed patients make fewer errors than primarily demented patients, irrespective of the type of distractor provoking the mistake. More prominent, however, is the difference between the two types of errors: more intrusion errors occur than false alarms. This pattern is much more pronounced in demented patients, as indicated by the significant interaction in the repeated-measures ANOVA. This lends support to the hypothesis that patients with more severe cognitive impairment have a tendency to make more intrusion errors than false alarms on the recognition task. This trend was observed in primarily demented but not in primarily depressed patients.

If patients with a cognitive impairment, probably induced by a cholinergic deficit, produce more intrusion errors (Fuld, 1983), and if cholinomimetic drugs such as arecoline and physostigmine reduce the occurrence of intrusion errors (Gainotti *et al.*, 1989; Smith and Swash, 1979), the measurement of intrusion errors might be a valuable tool not only for diagnostic purposes but also as an outcome measure in clinical trials with cognitively active compounds. The PRRT provides a direct and systematic method of assessing intrusion errors in cognitively impaired patients; additionally, the task is quick and easy to administer, is simple enough for patients with mildly or moderately severe dementia, and does not produce either floor or ceiling effects.

One criticism of the current form of the PRRT is the high amount of overlap between the error scores from the two patient groups. There was a mean difference of only one intrusion error between demented and depressed patients, and the range of scores for both patient groups was from zero to eight for both types of errors. Part of this overlap might be due to the patient population that was sampled. All of the patients, as part of the trial inclusion criteria, were required to show some signs of cognitive decline; therefore, all of the patients classified as primarily depressed were, to some degree, cognitively impaired. It would be natural to expect, therefore, that intrusion errors would be seen even in the primarily depressed group of patients. The significant differences that were obtained between the patient groups, considering the rough classification technique used, are a mark of the sensitivity of the task to different levels of cognitive impairment. However, the high overlap suggests that the PRRT might not be as useful as a diagnostic tool as it would be as a drug treatment outcome measure.

While the practical value of the PRRT may be limited to large clinical trials, the study has important theoretical relevance to the nature of linguistic functioning in normal and demented patients. The tendency for demented patients to falsely recognize items that are conceptually closer to target items and to make dysphasic errors can be considered in terms of Eleanor Rosch's prototype theory (Rosch, 1973): only prototypical representations, and not specific items, are encoded into memory. In AD patients the memory deficit is not a question of whether or not encoding occurs but to what level material is encoded. This means that a patient might not be able to retrieve a certain item but only the related semantic concept (e.g. not the actual representation of a boot is recalled but only the fact that a 'shoe' was presented). The closer a certain item is related to its prototype (i.e. the shorter the semantic distance from the prototype), the more likely the prototype would intrude on the recall of a specific item, and therefore increase the occurrence of intrusion errors. Figure 3 presents a visual representation of this notion of semantic distance. Various footwear can be thought of in terms of semantic distance to the prototypic picture one has of a 'shoe', and this is represented as concrete spatial distances in the figure. Items that are close to the prototype of 'shoe' are likely to share a host of common features, while more remote items will be fairly

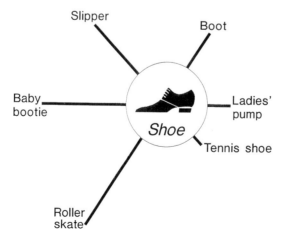

Figure 3. Visual model of the theory of semantic distance from a prototypic exemplar

different. In other words, this concept of a prototypic exemplar can be used to illustrate semantic relationships.

In the current study the results demonstrated that a primarily demented patient is more likely to falsely recognize an item that has some semantic relationship to a target item than an item that is unrelated. If this is taken one step further and considered in terms of the notion of semantic distances, one could hypothesize that, in demented patients, items that are very similar (differing only in specific details) to the prototype of a given category may more readily evoke intrusion errors. Future studies should try to answer the question of whether demented patients are more likely to falsely recognize items that are semantically closer (i.e. have more common features) to the target items than other related but more remote items. A test with several semantically related distractors for each target item, differing in semantic proximity to the target item, could be constructed for such a purpose. Studies such as this could yield significant information as to the nature and mechanisms of not only the demented, but the normal mind as well.

Summary

Pharmacological and morphological data exist to support the importance of intrusion errors in memory tasks to the study of dementia. There may be a loss of semantic distinctions linked to a deficit in the cholinergic system that manifests itself as a dysphasia in demented patients; this loss could be assessed using intrusion errors. The Picture Recall and Recognition Task (PRRT) developed for this study provides a measure of intrusion errors (i.e. false recognition of items semantically related to target items). The results taken from baseline data of a clinical trial with geriatric patients with major depressive episode and dementia indicate that intrusion errors occur more often than false alarms (i.e. false recognition of semantically unrelated items) in those patients with more severe cognitive decline. This indicates the usefulness of intrusion errors as a sensitive measure for the detection of changes in the severity of dementia.

References

APA (1980) *Diagnostic and Statistical Manual of Mental Disorders*, 3rd edn. Washington, D. C.: American Psychiatric Association.

Bayles, K. A. (1982) Language function and senile dementia. *Brain Lang.*, **16**, 265–80.

Baumhackl, U., Chan-Palay, V., Grüner, E., Hebenstreit, G. F., Kasas, A., Katschnig, H., Krebs, E., Kummer, J., Martucci, N., Radmayr, E., Rieder, L., Saletu, M., Schlegel, S. and Lorscheid, T. (1991) Improvement in cognitive symptoms after treatment with moclobemide in geriatric depressed patients with dementia. *Dementia*, in press.

Brinkman, S. D. and Gershon, S. (1983) Measurement of cholinergic drug effect on memory in Alzheimer's disease. *Neurobiol. Aging*, **4**, 139–45.

Church, M. and Wattis, J. P. (1988) Psychological approaches to the assessment and treatment of old people. In: Wattis, J. P. and Hindmarch, I. (eds) *Psychological Assessment of the Elderly*, pp. 151–79. New York: Churchill Livingstone.

Clark, E. V. (1973) What's in a word? On the child's acquisition of semantics in his first language. In: Moore, T. E. (ed.) *Cognitive Development and the Acquisition of Language*. New York: Academic Press.

Crow, T. J. and Grove-White, I. G. (1973) An analysis of the learning deficit following hyoscine administration to man. *Br. J. Pharmacol.*, **49**, 322–7.

Davis, K. L., Mohs, R. C., Davis, B. M., Levy, M. I., Horvath, T. B., Rosenberg, G. S., Ross, A., Rothpearl, A. and Rosen, W. (1982) Cholinergic treatment in Alzheimer's disease: implications for future research. In: Corkin, S. *et al.* (eds) *Alzheimer's Disease: A Report of Progress.* New York: Raven Press.

Drachman, D. A. (1977) Memory and cognitive function in man: does the cholinergic system have a specific role? *Neurology*, **27**, 383–90.

Drachman, D. A. and Leavitt, J. (1974) Human memory and the cholinergic system: a relationship to aging. *Arch. Neurol.*, **30**, 113–21.

Folstein, M. F., Folstein, S. E. and McHugh, P. R. (1975) 'Mini-Mental State': A practical method for grading the cognitive state of patients for the clinician. *J. Psychiatr. Res.*, **12**, 189–98.

Fuld, P. A. (1983) Word intrusions as a diagnostic sign in Alzheimer's disease. *Geriatr. Med. Today*, **2**, 33–41.

Gainotti, G., Nocentini, U. and Sena, E. (1989) Can the pattern of neuropsychological improvement obtained with cholinergic drugs be used to infer a cholinergic mechanism in other nootropic drugs? *Prog. Neuropsychopharmacol. Biol. Psychiatry*, **13**, 847–59.

Hebenstreit, G. F., Baumhackl, U., Chan-Palay, V., Grüner, E., Kasas, A., Katschnig, H., Krebs, E., Kummer, J., Martucci, N., Radmayr, E., Reider, L., Saletu, M., Schlegel, S. and Lorscheid, T. (1991) The treatment of depression in geriatric depressed and demented patients by moclobemide: results from the international multicenter double blind placebo controlled trial. *Dementia*, in press.

Hamilton, M. (1967) Development of a rating scale for primary depressive illness. *Br. J. Soc. Clin. Psychol.*, **6**, 278–96.

Kessler, J., Denzler, P. and Markowitsch, H. J. (1987) *Der Demenztest.* Weinheim: Beltz-Verlag.

Miller, E. (1975) Impaired recall and the memory disturbance in presenile dementia. *Br. J. Soc. Clin. Psychol.*, **14**, 73–9.

Miller, E. (1978) Retrieval from long-term memory in presenile dementia: two tests of an hypothesis. *Br. J. Soc. Clin. Psychol.*, **17**, 143–8.

Rochford, G. (1971) A study of naming errors in dysphasia and demented patients. *Neuropsychologia*, **9**, 437–43.

Rosch, E. (1973) On the internal structure of perceptual and semantic categories. In: Moore, T. E. (ed.) *Cognitive Development and the Acquisition of Language.* New York: Academic Press.

Rusted, J. M. and Warburton, D. M. (1989) Effects of scopolamine on verbal memory; a retrieval or acquisition deficit? *Neuropsychobiology*, **21**, 76–83.

Schwartz, M. F., Marin, O. S. M. and Saffran, E. M. (1979) Dissociations of language function in dementia: a case study. *Brain Lang.*, **7**, 277–306.

Shader, R. I., Harmatz, J. S. and Salzman, C. (1974) A new scale for assessment in geriatric populations: Sandoz Clinical Assessment-Geriatric (SCAG). *J. Am. Geriatr. Soc.*, **22**, 107–13.

Skelton-Robinson, M. and Jones, S. (1984) Nominal dysphasia and the severity of senile dementia. *Br. J. Psychiatry*, **145**, 168–71.

Smith, C. M. and Swash, M. (1979) Physostigmine in Alzheimer's disease. *Lancet*, **i**, 42.

Snodgrass, J. G. and Vanderwart, M. (1980) A standardized set of 260 pictures: norms for name agreement, image agreement, familiarity, and visual complexity. *J. Exp. Psychol.* [*Hum. Learn.*] **6**, 174–215.

Thal, L. J., Fuld, P. A., Masur, D. M. and Sharpless, N. S. (1983) Oral physostigmine and lecithin improve memory in Alzheimer's disease. *Ann. Neurol.*, **13**, 491–6.

Warrington, E. K. (1975) The selective impairment of semantic memory. *Q. J. Exp. Psychol.*, **27**, 635–57.

Yesavage, J., Brink, T., Rose, T., Lum, O., Huang, O., Adey, V. and Leirer, V. (1983) Development and validation of a geriatric screening scale: a preliminary report. *J. Psychiatr. Res.*, **17**, 37–49.

17

Molecules, Methods and Measures: Issues and Comments

Christine Shillingford

Clinical Research, Interphase House, Hindhead, UK

What follows is a résumé of the discussions, comments, critiques and suggestions made following the presentation of the various papers that are included in this volume. They are included here to give the reader some idea of the nature and flavour of the debate which followed the lectures for, as is almost always the case when a group of clinicians and scientists with a shared interest in dementia meet, the individual contributions prompted a wide-ranging and lively discussion.

Awareness of Dementia

The increasing socioeconomic impact of dementia, as the population of developed countries live longer, has heightened awareness of the disease and increased research activity accordingly. However, major breakthroughs in the aetiology and pathology of dementia have been elusive; differential diagnostic criteria are difficult to define as the heterogeneous nature of the symptoms of dementia makes any attempt at differentiation into discrete groups unreliable, even when post mortem data are available. To attempt to investigate behavioural effects of putative therapeutic agents in the light of these existing uncertainties is one of the most difficult challenges in pharmaceutical research and development today. While much attention and effort has focused on the quality of life and well-being of patients suffering from dementia, too little attention has been paid to the physical and psychological effect on carers attending to the needs and demands of relatives and friends with dementia. There is evidence that caring for dementia sufferers in the home and community increases the incidence of psychological and physical disorders in those carers involved on a day-to-day basis. Paying attention to the needs of the carers raises issues as regards the development of appropriate anti-dementia agents.

Dementia: Molecules, Methods and Measures. Edited by I. Hindmarch, H. Hippius and G. K. Wilcock
© 1991 John Wiley & Sons Ltd

It is not sufficient for the patient to be activated. This might improve a patient's reactivity, but at the same time it might make the patient more difficult to handle, more liable to wander, and even more irritable and aggressive.

'Age-associated Memory Impairment'

There have been attempts to discriminate between patients with dementia and a non-dementing population of older individuals who, while being psychologically and physically normal, complain of memory loss and have poor mnestic functions relative to the general population. This so called age-associated memory impairment (AAMI) does not result from a specific pathophysiological process and does not relate to any biological construct other than that of increasing age. There are severe methodological problems in comparing the performance of elderly individuals against norms derived from physically healthy, psychologically sound, intelligent people in their twenties. There does not seem to be proof from observations of elderly persons with memory deficits that there is a specific syndrome of memory loss equivalent to the AAMI criteria. The AAMI classification was specifically developed to provide a rationalization for entering otherwise 'normal' subjects in commercial studies of potential anti-dementia agents. Since no clinical underpinnings for AAMI exist, any pharmacological treatment which changes the AAMI ratings should not be regarded as an anti-dementia agent. Although some pharmaceutical manufacturers would see commercial reasons for so doing, AAMI concepts must be regarded as both inappropriate and counterproductive for those involved in dementia diagnosis and treatment. Furthermore, regulatory authorities warn researchers and manufacturers to avoid claims for medical conditions that are not generally accepted as entities in themselves. The 'nature versus nurture' debate continues and it is felt that much of the cognitive decline observed in cross-sectional studies is due to a confounding of the factors of date of birth, i.e. age, with environmental influences. Furthermore, unless study populations are adequately screened for physical pathologies, to which cognitive problems may be secondary, any results from cross-sectional studies can be misleading. Indeed, in studies where the subjects were rigorously screened for physical disease and where psychometric measures and continuous electro-encephalography (EEG) recordings were databased, the correlation between age and cognitive decline, at least over a 3-year period, was not clearly demonstrated.

Anti-dementia Drugs and Measures of Clinical Efficacy

At the moment it would appear there is no consensus as to the classification and nomenclature of the various classes of pharmaceutical agents used for the treatment of dementia. There are agents classified as 'promnestic', 'nootropic', 'anti-hypoxydotics', 'cognitive or cerebral metabolic enhancers', 'mentalerting drugs' and substances which are 'behavioural activators' which improve the 'quality of life' of the patient. Much of the problem in deciding the appropriate labelling of these compounds is a lack of knowledge and a continued uncertainty concerning the pathological and neuro-biochemical basis of the disease. It would appear that there is a confusing profusion of clinical measures for use in assessing demented patients and the efficacy of the substances that they have been given. However, it is noteworthy that the clinical global impression (CGI) remains the pivotal measure, both in Europe and the USA, for the assessment of the therapeutic activity of drugs used in the treatment of patients with dementia. The widespread acceptance of the CGI is disturbing as it is a subjective and non-specific assessment scale. Its importance has probably occurred by default due to an absence of objective measures of symptoms and the progress of the disease. It would seem that for the CGI to be useful, more attention must be paid to the factors that clinicians are using in their assessment of the patients and their response to treatment. The CGI has limited use as a research tool because of its lack of specificity, and its pre-eminence in the eyes of the drug regulatory authorities may therefore be limiting the acquisition of specific pharmacodynamic data from new putative anti-dementia agents. While the CGI is an assessment of the subjective impressions of a patient by the clinician, similar quality of life scales (QOLS) are often used for patient, carer and clinician QOLS have the same problems as the CGI – heterogeneous construct and subjectivity. However, the ratings of a patient by a carer, bearing in mind the more frequent contact, may be more accurate and may also be more relevant in socioeconomic terms than those derived from clinicians with a less-informed knowledge of the daily behaviour of the patient.

Models of Dementia

Most anti-dementia drugs are first researched in healthy volunteers. This is necessary as the action of drugs in the intact nervous system must be known. However, this knowledge should be limited to acquiring pharmacokinetic and pharmacodynamic information and should not be taken as evidence of clinical efficacy, even if AAMI volunteers are used or even if the drug has been tested in volunteers under some drug-induced amnesia. There are many models for dementia which have been suggested, but none is universally accepted as useful in preclinical studies for predicting the therapeutic efficacy of compounds in clinical use. Manipulation of the cholinergic and dopaminergic systems, as well as benzodiazepine-induced amnesia, have been used in volunteer populations, but extrapolations into patient populations are, at best, unreliable. It is also an oversimplification to suggest that the syndrome of dementia is attributable to a deficit in one single neurotransmitter system (e.g. cholinergic pathways). Indeed, the diversity of central nervous system transmitters involved in the range of clinically effective anti-depressants mitigates against the monotransmitter theory of psychological disturbance. It is not felt that dementia, in this respect, is any different from depression. Indeed, some of the partial inverse agonists of the 'benzodiazepine receptor' on the gamma-aminobutyric acid (GABA)-chloride ion receptor complex have been shown to have anti-dementia properties. While it is possible to suggest a mechanism which involves GABA in cholinergic transmission, it is also possible that other, non-cholinergic systems are involved.

Objective Measures

The potential of EEG brain mapping and other brain scanning systems has not yet been fully realized. The main concern centres on the relationship, if any, between topographical representations of electrical activity and underlying brain functions. Furthermore, there does not yet seem to be a clear indication of how electrophysiological changes reflect clinically relevant behaviours, although there is some evidence of correlations between

EEG variables and geriatric rating scales, particularly in multi-infarct dementia. The development of tests for quantifying the degree of dementia is time-consuming and laborious and there are few psychologically relevant and reliable assessments available (one exception being the Syndrom-Kurtz Test) to the researcher and clinician concerned with the development of new molecules and/or the management of the demented patient.

Future Prospects

It is clear from the pharmaceutical development programme of most major companies that there is a plethora of putative anti-dementia agents. That they are active in some way is not in doubt. The onus for the development of efficacious compounds now rests with the manufacturers and those clinical research organizations conducting studies and trials on the new molecules. It is only by using measures which have a proven validity and reliability that any advance in developing new treatment modalities will be made. However, measures without the appropriate methodological and theoretical framework are isolated and without any clinical relevance. Progress towards finding clinically efficacious agents for the management of patients with dementia has so far been slow. However, the essential ingredients for progress have now been identified, namely valid and reliable measures within an appropriate methodological framework. Thus proper experimentation and an appropriate clinical protocol will, in the future, allow for the development of agents with a generally accepted and proven efficacy in improving the well-being of patients and their carers.

Index

A4 protein, β-amyloid precursor protein, 65
Acetylcholine, precursors, 1
Acetylcholine-associated enzymes, loss, 12
Activities of daily living (ADL),
    face validity, 84–85
    instrumental (IADL)
        data, 130
        defined, 84
        raters, 133
    Katz index, 133
    NOSGER scale, features, 83, 84–85, 132
    performance test, 130
    problems of multifactorial measurement, 83,
        84–85
    quality of life assessment, 179
ADAS, *see* Alzheimer's Disease Assessment Scale
Adenosine, cellular reuptake, inhibition, 27
Age-associated memory impairment (AAMI),
    criteria, 198
    longitudinal and cross-sectional data,
        161–167
Alcohol,
    interaction with NCE, 124
    performance-enhancing effects, 121
Alkaloids, *see* Ergot alkaloids; Vinca alkaloids
Alkylxanthines,
    chemical structure, 23
    inhibition of cyclic nucleotide phospho-
        diesterase isoenzymes, 24–25
Alpha-2 agonists, volunteer studies, 71–72
Alzheimer's disease,
    heterogeneity
        age effect, 61–62
        consequences for drug design, 48–51
        indications, 48–49
        other evidence for, 62–63
    NINCDS-ADRDA criteria, 48, 80

PDDAT (primary degenerative dementia,
    Alzheimer type) CCF2 test, 173–174
scientific basis for therapeutic developments,
    61–66
senile dementia, Alzheimer-type (SDAT)
    criteria, 93
    DSM-III-R criteria, 114–115
    EEG mapping in dementia, 151–158
specific scales
    Dementia Rating Scale
        of Hughes, 129
        of Mattis, 97
    Global Deterioration Rating Scale (GDS),
        81, 129, 137
Alzheimer's Disease Assessment Scale (ADAS),
    attention deficit, changes over 1 year, 54
    content, 129
    data and characteristics, 132, 139
    DSM-III-R recognition, 97
    nootropic drug assessment, 84
    problems of multifactorial measurement, 83
    variability and standardization, 144
American Psychiatric Association,
    DSM-III-R criteria, 80, 97
        multi-infarct dementia, 114–115
        SDAT, 114–115
        test batteries, 118–119
    see also USA
AMP-A receptor stimulation, potentiation by
    aniracetam, 22
Amphetamine, performance-enhancing effect, 121
β-Amyloid precursor protein, 65
Anchor test (DSST), 111
Angiotensin converting-enzyme (ACE)
    inhibitors,
    anxiolytic properties, 34
    see also Captopril; Ceranapril

Animal tests,
    cognitive function, new anti-dementia
        molecules, 34–36
    Morris water maze, 35, 41
    primates, object discrimination reversal task,
        41
Aniracetam,
    chemical structure, 21
    potentiation of AMP-A receptor stimulation,
        22
Anoxia, survival time, drug enhancement, 26
Anti-cholinesterases, effect on M_2 receptors, 64
Anti-dementia drugs,
    classification, 198–199
    international development, 89–98
    methodology of clinical trials, 47–56
    see Drugs
    volunteer studies, predictive value, 66–76
Arecoline,
    memory effects, 186
    volunteer studies, 74
Attention,
    cholinergic drugs
        attentional switching, 11
        selective, 11
        sustained, 10–11
    Mackworth Clock task, 12
Attention deficit,
    changes over 1 year, 54
    clinical subtype of AD, 48
Attrition, clinical trials, 82

Behavioural Mood Disturbance and Stress
    Scale, 131
Benign senescent forgetfulness, as precursor to
    dementia, 161–167
Benzodiazepines,
    in AD research, 174
    no performance effects, 121
    receptor ligands, 122
β-amyloid precursor protein, A4 protein, 65
β-carbolines, 122–123
Bifemelane,
    effects on mossy fibre–CA_3 system of guinea
        pig hippocampus, 23
    pharmacology, 20
Bilan d'évaluation du Syndrome Démentiel, 136
Biological measures, nootropic drugs, 84
Biopterin, levels, 63
Blessed Dementia Rating Scale (BDRS), 130
    longitudinal studies, 142
Brain catecholamine levels, vinca alkaloids, 24
Brain mapping in dementia, *see* EEG mapping
Brief Cognitive Rating Scale (BCRS),
    data, 131, 139
    and Global Deterioration Scale (BCRS-GDS),
        180

longitudinal studies, 142
Bromvincamine, volunteer studies, 69–70
BSF *see* Benign senescent forgetfulness

Caffeine,
    performance-enhancing effects, 121
    structure, 23
Camdex,
    data, 132
    diagnostic criteria, 80
Captopril, anxiolytic properties, 34
β-Carbolines, 122–123
Ceranapril,
    animal tests, 36–44
    see also ACE inhibitors
Cerebral atrophy, PSD *vs* SD, 49
Cerebral blood flow, metabolically active com-
    pounds, 26
Cerebral metabolism, drug enhancement
    studies, 68–71
Check List Differentiating Pseudo-dementia
    from Dementia, 130
Chlorpromazine, effect on mossy fibre–CA_3
    system of guinea pig hippocampus, 23
Cholinergic drugs,
    attentional switching, 11
    benzodiazepine antagonist, 122–123
    information processing theory, 6–12
    long-term memory, 8–10
    selective attention, 11
    sustained attention, 10–11
    volunteer studies, 74
    working memory, 6–8
Cholinergic hypothesis,
    dysphasia in, dementia, 185–189
    intrusion errors, 185–194
Cholinergic system,
    GABA, 123
    marker enzymes, no diminution, 63
    role in information processing, 1–2
    strategies aimed at improvement, 63–64
Cholinesterase inhibitors,
    acetylcholine, amount, 2
    intrusion errors, 187
    see also Physostigmine; Tacrine hydro-
        chloride
Clifton Assessment Procedures for Elderly
    (CAPE), 131
Clinical Dementia Rating Scale (CDR),
    data, 131
    longitudinal studies, 142
Clinical Global Impression (CGI),
    pivotal measure, 198–199
    scales, 56
Clinical instruments, *see* Psychometric
    instruments

Clinical Rating Scale for Symptoms of Psychosis in Alzheimer's Disease (SPAD), 132
Clinical trials,
attrition, 82
comparability of studies, 81
comprehensive clinical rating scales, 55
cross-over studies, 50
degree of dementia, 81
dose range, 82
European approaches to design, 79–85
exclusion criteria, 81
global impression scales, 56
methodology, 47–56
multicentre trials, 82
multifactorial measurement, 83
new chemical entities (NCE)
anchor test, 111
EEG, 111
healthy volunteers, 109–124
Phase I trials, dose titration, 111
representativeness of studies, 81
sample size, 82
see also Drugs
Clonidine, volunteer studies, 71–72, 73
Co-dergocrine,
inhibition of cyclic nucleotide phosphodiesterase isoenzymes, 24–25
see also Ergot alkaloids
Co-dergocrine mesylate, *see* Hydergine
Cognitive Capacity Screening Examination, 137
Cognitive enhancers,
psychometric testing, 109–124
see Nootropics
Comparability of studies, clinical trials, 81
Comprehensive Psychiatric Rating Scale
(CPRS), 131
Confusion Assessment Schedule, 137
Cornell Scale for Depression in Dementia, 132
Critical flicker fusion test (CFFT), 169–175
advantages, 172
effect of nicotine, 13
effects of nitrous oxide, 174
implications for research, 174
measurement, 173
normal elderly subjects, 173–174
performance index, 122
regression with age, 164
Cross-over studies, clinical trials, 50
Cyclic nucleotide phosphodiesterase
isoenzymes,
drug inhibition, 24
five families, 24–25

D Test, Rating scales, 130
Data structures,
procedural *vs* declarative, 4
semantic *vs* episodic, 4

Dementia,
awareness, 197
critical issues, 91
definitions, 93
degree of dementia, clinical trials, 81
dysphasia in, cholinergic hypothesis, 185–189
EEG mapping in dementia, 151–158
mild *vs* severe, rating scales, 134
models, acceptability, 199
motivational issues, 91–92
severity
assessment through functional levels of
organisation, 140–141
praxis/gnosis, 140–141
Dementia Behaviour Scale, 131
Dementia Rating Scale,
of Blessed, 130, 142
of Mattis, 97
Denbufylline,
inhibition of cyclic nucleotide phosphodiesterase isoenzymes, 24–25
structure, 23
Dextroamphetamine, performance-enhancing
effect, 121
Differential diagnosis of dementia, *see* Clinical
instruments
Digit-symbol substitution test (DSST), floor
effects, 109
Dihydroergocritine, inhibition of cyclic
nucleotide phosphodiesterase, 24
Dopamine,
and nootropics, enhancement of release, 24
release, and nootropics, 22
Drugs,
development of new anti-dementia molecules
(NCE), 109–124
animal tests, 34–36
cognitive enhancing action
ACE inhibitors, 42–43
5-HTreceptor antagonists, 42–43
design and methodology, 95–96
diagnosis and severity of illness, 97
early decisions, 93–94
efficacy assessment, 97–98
general problems, 109–110
Phase II studies, 94–95
Phase III studies, 95
preclinical indicators of cognitive enhancing
potential, 36–42
trials, *see* Clinical trials
dose titration, 111
enhancement studies, cerebral metabolism,
68–71
see also Clinical trials; Nootropics
DSM-III-R criteria, *see* American Psychiatric
Association

Dysphasia,
    dementia, cholinergic hypothesis, 185–189
    semantic distinctions, 188–189

Edinburgh Psychogeriatric Dependency Rating
    Scale, 130
EEG mapping in dementia, 151–158
    pharmaco-EEG mapping, 155
    results, correlations
        EEG and CT, 154
        EEG and psychometric measures, 154
        EEG and psychopathology, 154
    results, summary and discussion, 157–158
    therapeutic monitoring of demented patients,
        155
Elaborative processes, 4–5
Elderly subjects, normal,
    CCFT, 172–174
    role in test development, 171–172
Encoding processes, 4–5
    dysfunction, intrusion errors, 186
Enrichment procedures, clinical trials, 50
Entiracetam, structure, 21
Ergot alkaloids,
    chemical structure, 22
    inhibition of cyclic nucleotide phospho-
        diesterase isoenzymes, 24–25
European approaches to design of clinical trials,
    79–85
European Consensus Conference,
    design of trials, 81–82
    diagnostic criteria and selection of patients,
        80–81
    ethical protection of patients, 85
    outcome measures, 82–85
    terminology of drugs, 80, 81
Exclusion criteria, clinical trials, 81
Extended Scale for Dementia, 136, 139
Extrapyramidal abnormalities, in AD, 62–63

Flumenazil, receptor ligands, 122
Flunitrazepam, in AD research, 174
Functional Assessment Staging Test (FAST),
    132
Functional Dementia Scale of Moore, 131

GABA, cholinergic system, 123
GBS Scale (Gottfries), 131
Generosity effect, defined, 56
Geriatric Evaluation by Relatives (GERRI), 131
Geriatric Mental State Schedule, 137
Germany, nootropics, 79
Global assessment,
    drug development, 97–98
    and rating scales, 128–137
Global clinical measures, 84

Global Deterioration Rating Scale (GDS), 81,
    129, 131
Glutamate, excessive release, NMDA receptors,
    27
Guanfacine, volunteer studies, 71–72

Halo effect, defined, 56
Haloperidol, effect on mossy fibre–CA$_3$
    system of guinea pig hippocampus, 23
Hippocampus, CA$_3$ system, long-term
    potentiation, 21
Hodkinson scale, learning effects, 170
Home Care Registration, quality of life
    measure, 180–183
Homovanillic acid, levels, 63
Hydergine, volunteer studies, 68–69
Hydroxyindoleacetic acid, levels, 63
5-Hydroxytryptamine receptor antagonists,
    effect on limbic-cortical circuitry, 33–34
    see also Ondansetron
Hypoxia, survival time, drug enhancement, 26

IADL, see Activities of daily living
Ideberione,
    effects on mossy fibre–CA$_3$ system of guinea
        pig hippocampus, 23
    pharmacology, 20
Imipramine, effect on mossy fibre–CA$_3$ system
    of guinea pig hippocampus, 23
Indeloxazine,
    effects on mossy fibre–CA$_3$ system of guinea
        pig hippocampus, 23
    pharmacology, 20
Information processing theory,
    cholinergic drugs, 6–12
    processing descriptions
        encoding processes, 4–5
        retrieval encoding processes, 5
    structural descriptions
        data structures, 4
        long-term memory storage, 3–4
        short-term memory storage, 3
International development, anti-dementia
    drugs, 89–98
Intrusion errors,
    assessment, Picture Recall and Recognition
        Test (PRRT), 187
    cholinergic hypothesis, 185–194
    cholinesterase activity, correlation, 187
    encoding dysfunction, 186
    senile plaques, 185
Investigators, homogeneity issues, 92
Ischaemia,
    Ischaemia Score, 130
    neuronal protection, 27
Italy, nootropics, 79

Japan, anti-dementia drugs, 79

Katz index of ADL, 133
Kendrick Battery for the Detection of Dementia in the Elderly, 136
Kunitz-type protease inhibitor, 65

Language,
   construction of psychometric instruments, 53
   problems in AD, clinical subtype, 48
Long-term memory,
   cholinergic blockade, 8–10
   storage, 3–4
Long-term potentiation, CA$_3$ system, hippocampus of guinea pig, 21–22

Mackworth Clock task, sustained attention, 12
MANOVA, EEG drug effects, 155–158
Mattis Dementia Rating Scale, 97, 129
Memory,
   overall, regression with age, 166
   selective deficit of memory subprocesses, 5–6
Memory impairment,
   clinical subtype of AD, 48
   see also Age-associated memory impairment (AAMI)
Memory Information Test, 97
Mental status questionnaires, 135–137
   Abbreviated Mental Test, 137
   Bilan d'évaluation du Syndrome Démentiel, 136
   Cognitive Capacity Screening Examination, 137
   Confusion Assessment Schedule, 137
   Dementia Screening Scale, 137
   Extended Scale for Dementia, 136, 139
   Geriatric Mental State Schedule, 137
   Kendrick Battery for the Detection of Dementia in the Elderly, 136
   Mental Test Score, 137
   Orientation Scale for Geriatric Patients, 137
   Philadelphia Geriatric Mental State Schedule, 137
   Short Portable Mental Status Questionnaire, 137
   Stimulus Recognition Test, 136
   Three Dimensional Praxis Test, 136
   Tooting Bec Questionnaire, modified, 137
   see also Mini-Mental State Examination
Metabolically active compounds,
   defined, 20
   effects on cerebral blood flow and metabolism, 26
   enhancement of cognition, 24
   neuronal protection, 27
   summary, 27–28

Methamphetamine, effect on mossy fibre–CA$_3$ system of guinea pig hippocampus, 23
MID, *see* Multi-infarct dementia
Midazolam, effect on mossy fibre–CA$_3$ system of guinea pig hippocampus, 23
Mini-Mental State Examination,
   applications and data, 136
   attention deficit, changes over 1 year, 54
   degree of demtnia, shortcomings, 81
   DSM-III-R recognition, 97
   learning effects, 170
   longitudinal studies, 142, 143
   quality of life assessment, 179
Mitochondrial respiratory rate, drug enhancement, 26
Motivational issues, dementia, 91–92
Multi-infarct dementia,
   DSM-III-R criteria, 114–115
   EEG mapping, 151–158
Multicentre clinical trials, 82
Multifactorial measurement, clinical trials, 83
Multiple reaction time test, 120
Munich, conference, *see* European Consensus Conference
Muscarinic agonists,
   cholinergic system, 2
   volunteer studies, 72–74
Muscarinic receptors (M$_2$ receptors),
   presynaptic autoreceptor function, 2
   in SDAT, 2
   selective change in density, 64
Myoclonus in AD, 62

Nerve growth factor (NGF),
   clinical trials, 65
   Meynert's nucleus, 64
Neuropsychological Test Battery, CERAD, 139
Neuropsychological tests, 138–143
   application, 142
   clinical relevance and use as outcome criteria, 145
   conditions required, 138
   differentiation from psychometric instruments, 138
   longitudinal studies, 142
   Neuropsychological Test Battery, CERAD, 139
   relevance and use as outcome criteria, 145
   selection, 144
   selection of instruments, 144
   test batteries
      computer-supported psychoexperimental, 117–120
      reliability, 120
      DSM-III-R criteria, 118–119
   variability, 143–144
   see also Psychometric instruments

Neurotrophic factors, clinical trials, 64–65
New chemical entities (NCE), *see* Drugs
New Hierarchic Dementia Scale, 132
Nicergoline, *see* Ergot alkaloids
Nicotine,
    effects on SDAT, 13–14
    performance-enhancing effects, 121
    therapy, 64
    see also Smoking
Nicotinic receptors, role in cholinergic system,
    12–14
NINCDS-ADRDA criteria for Alzheimer's
    disease, 48, 80
Nitrous oxide, effects on CCFT, 174
NMDA receptors, excessive glutamate release
    in cerebral ischaemia, 27
Nootropics,
    defined, 20
    effects on cerebral blood flow and
        metabolism, 25
    effects on cognition, 20–25
    enhancement of cerebral metabolic activity,
        26
    European Consensus Conference (1989), final
        report, 68
    pharmaco-EEG mapping, 155–158
    research, quality of life, 178
    structure of piracetam and derivatives, 21
    see also Drugs
NOSGER *see* Nurse's Observation Scale for
    Geriatric patients
Nucleus basalis,
    ascending pathway, deterioration in SDAT,
        12
    magnocellularis, lesion, impairment of
        habituation patterns, 36–39
    Meynert, no diminution of neurons in AD, 63
Nurse's Observation Scale for Geriatric patients
    (NOSGER), 83, 84–85, 132

Ondansetron,
    animal tests, 36–44
    see also 5-Hydroxytryptamine receptor
        antagonists
Orientation Scale for Geriatric Patients, 137
Oxiracetam, structure, 21

Pauli memory performance test, 120, 121
PDDAT (primary degenerative dementia,
    Alzheimer type) CCF2 test, 173–174
Pegboard test, 120, 121
Pentoxifylline, structure, 23
Performance Test of Activities of Daily Living,
    130
Philadelphia Geriatric Mental State Schedule,
    137

Phosphodiesterase inhibitors,
    effects, 25
    see also Rolipram
Physostigmine,
    memory effects, 186
    volunteer studies, 74
Picture Recall and Recognition Test (PRRT),
    assessment of intrusion errors, 187
    materials, 190
    methods, 189
    procedure, 190
    results, 191–192
    subjects, 189
    summary and discussion, 192–194
Pilocarpine, volunteer studies, 74
Piracetam,
    effects on adenylate kinase, 26
    effects on ischaemic tissue, 26
    orientation task, 179
    structure, 21
    volunteer studies, 70–71
    see also Nootropics; Nootropics, structure
Positron emission tomography (PET), left or
    rightsided hypometabolism, 63
Pramiracetam, structure, 21
Praxis Test, 136
Primates, object discrimination reversal task, 41
Propentofylline,
    action, 27
    structure, 23
Psychometric instruments,
    assessment uses, 51
    construction, 52–55
        language functions, 55
        recent memory, 53
        working memory, 53–54
    content, 129
    differentiation from neuropsychological tests,
        135
    global assessment and rating scales, 128–134
    ideal, 170
    neuropsychological tests, 138–143
    scaling, 129
    sensitivity, 83
    validity, 171
    see also Mental status questionnaires;
        Neuropsychological tests; Rating Scales
Psychostimulants, *see* Nootropics
Pyritinol,
    effects on mossy fibre–CA_3 system of guinea
        pig hippocampus, 23
    pharmaco-EEG mapping, 155–158
    pharmacology, 20

Quality of life,
    assessment
        ADL test, 179

MMSE test, 179
  subjective *vs* objective, 178
  inter/intra-individual dimensions, 178–179
  measurement, Home Care Registration, 180–183
  nootropics research, 177
Questionnaires, *see* Mental status questionnaires

Rapid Disability Rating Scale, 131
Rating scales,
  changes in dementia, 134
  classification
    according to use, 135
    and review, 133–137
  learning effects, 170
  main objectives and rationale, 134
  severity of dementia, 134
  specificity, 135
Rating Scales, *see also* Clinical instruments
Rating scales, titles,
  Alzheimer's Disease Assessment Scale (ADAS), 132, 139
  Behavioural Mood Disturbance and Stress Scale, 131
  Brief Cognitive Rating Scale (BCRS), 131, 139
  Camdex, 132
  Check List Differentiating Pseudo-dementia from Dementia, 130
  Clifton Assessment Procedures for Elderly (CAPE), 131
  Clinical Dementia Rating Scale (CDR), 131
  Clinical Rating Scale for Symptoms of Psychosis in Alzheimer's Disease (SPAD), 132
  Comprehensive Psychiatric Rating Scale (CPRS), 131
  Cornell Scale for Depression in Dementia, 138
  D Test, 130
  Dementia Behaviour Scale, 131
  Dementia Rating Scale, 129
  Dementia Scale, 130
  Edinburgh Psychogeriatric Dependency Rating Scale, 130
  Functional Assessment Staging test (FAST), 132
  Functional Dementia Scale, 137
  GBS Scale, 131
  Geriatric Evaluation by Relatives (GERRI), 131
  Global Deterioration Rating Scale (GDS), 137
  Instrumental Activities of Daily Living Scale, 130
  Ischaemia Score, 130
  Neuropsychological Test Battery, CERAD, 139
  New Hierarchic Dementia Scale, 132

  Nurse's Observation Scale for Geriatric patients (NOSGER), 132
  Performance Test of Activities of Daily Living, 130
  Rapid Disability Rating Scale, 131
  Rating Scale for Diagnosis of Alzheimer's and Pick's Disease, 131
  Sandoz Clinical Assessment—Geriatric (SCAG), 130
  Stockton Geriatric Rating Scales, 130
Recent memory, construction of psychometric instruments, 53
Representativeness of studies, clinical trials, 81
Retrieval processes, 5
Rockville FDA symposium, USA, 80, 81, 84
Rolziracetam, structure, 21
RS 86, volunteer studies, 72–74

Sample size, clinical trials, 82
Sandoz Clinical Assessment—Geriatric (SCAG) study, 81, 130, 142, 143
Scopolamine,
  in AD research, 174
  cholinergic blockade, 8–9, 186
  disruption of verbal organization import, 186
  effect on mossy fibre–CA_3 system of guinea pig hippocampus, 23
  impairment of cognitive performance, animal tests, 34–37
  model of age-deficit paradigm, 123
  recognition task, 186
Semantic distance, theory, visual model, 193
Semantic distinctions, dysphasia, 188–189
Senile dementia, Alzheimer-type (SDAT),
  criteria, 93
  DSM-III-R criteria, 114–115
  EEG mapping in dementia, 151–158
Senile plaques, intrusion errors, 185
Short-term memory,
  model, articulatory loop and visuaspatial scratch-pad, 3
  scopolamine
    articulatory suppression task, 8
    spatial tapping task, 8
  smoking, 13–14
  storage, 3
SIDAM, diagnostic criteria, 80
Signal detection theory (SDT), 162
SKT, *see* Syndrom–Kurtz Test
Sleep, polygraphic sleep parameters, volunteer drug studies, 66–76
Smoking,
  short-term memory, 13–14
  see also Nicotine
Stimulus Recognition Test, 136
Stockton Geriatric Rating Scales, 130

Syndrom–Kurtz Test,
    applications in clinical practise, 103–104
    construction, 102–103
    development, 101–108
    material and test procedure, 105–108

Tacrine hydrochloride, cholinesterase pathways,
    63
Tapping test, 120, 121
Tenilsetam, structure, 21
Term test, 128
THA, *see* Tacrine hydrochloride
Theophylline, structure, 23
Three Dimensional Praxis Test, 136
Tooting Bec Questionnaire, modified, 137
Total reaction time, regression with age, 165
Tracking accuracy, regression with age, 165
Tracking reaction time, regression with age, 165
Trophic factors, clinical trials, 64–65

USA,
    anti-dementia drugs, 79
    FDA, anti-dementia drugs, assessment, 80, 81
    see also American Psychiatric Association

Vasodilator therapy contraindications, 26
Video tracking test, 120, 121
Vinca alkaloids,
    brain catecholamine levels, 24

chemical structure, 22
effect on mossy fibre–CA_3 system of guinea
    pig hippocampus, 23
inhibition of cyclic nucleotide phospho-
    diesterase isoenzymes, 24–25
neuronal protection, 27
vincamine derivatives, volunteer studies,
    69–70
Visual analogue scales, 120, 121
Visuospatial ability, deficit, clinical subtype of
    AD, 48
Volunteer studies,
    anti-dementia drugs, predictive value, 66–76
    healthy volunteers
        cognitive enhances, psychometric testing,
            109–124
        predictive value of studies, 66–76

Wisconsin Test Apparatus, animal tests, 35, 41
Working memory, 3, 6
    cholinergic blockade, 6–8
    construction of psychometric instruments,
        53–54
    see also Short-term memory

Xanthinol, clinical changes in SOAT and MID
    patients, 156

ZK 93426, performance enhancement, 123

Index compiled by June Morrison